In the Psychiatrist's Chair II

Anthony Clare is Medical Director of St Patrick's Hospital
and Clinical Professor of Psychiatry at Trinity College, Dublin.

Also by Anthony Clare
and available in Mandarin

In the Psychiatrist's Chair

ANTHONY CLARE

In the Psychiatrist's Chair

II

Mandarin

A Mandarin Paperback
IN THE PSYCHIATRIST'S CHAIR II

First published in Great Britain 1995
by William Heinemann Ltd
This edition published 1996
by Mandarin Paperbacks
an imprint of Reed International Books Ltd
Michelin House, 81 Fulham Road, London SW3 6RB
and Auckland, Melbourne, Singapore and Toronto

A CIP catalogue record for this title
is available from the British Library
ISBN 0 7493 1904 6

Printed and bound in Great Britain
by Cox & Wyman Ltd, Reading, Berks.

To Jane who has been my constant source
of support, encouragement and love.

Acknowledgements

I gratefully record my thanks to Carmel O'Kelly who helped with the preparation of the text, Kate Goodhart, an excellent desk editor, Helen Fraser for her steady confidence in the enterprise, Michael Ember whose skills as a producer are legendary and Liz Ember whose role in ensuring that these interviews took place and were appropriately recorded has been immeasurable. I am also grateful to the following for permission to reproduce extracts from copyright material: Penguin Books for Elias Canetti, *Crowds and Power* 1975; Grove Press for Frantz Fanon, *Black Skin, White Masks*.

Contents

Colin Blakemore

Looking back at over ten years of *In the Psychiatrist's Chair*, I am struck by the fact that amongst the many people interviewed, a handful of medical doctors apart, there is not a single scientist. Why such an omission? Is it that scientists are an extraordinarily dull and balanced lot in contrast to artists, writers, actors, media stars, film-makers, even politicians? Is it that scientists are less reflective and less intuitive, more likely to be practical and pragmatic, logical and bland? Or is it merely a reflection of the fact that the artist in our society is much fêted, admired and highly visible while the scientist goes about his or her business unnoticed and, to an extent at any rate, undervalued.

To remedy the lack, Colin Blakemore is certainly the obvious candidate. Firstly, there is the fact that he is one of a handful of top-class scientists in Britain not only able but willing to argue the role and value of science in the public marketplace of ideas. In a hard-hitting article in the *Daily Telegraph* in 1990, he argued that 'writing for ordinary people about what scientists do is an important part of the new contract between science and the country'. In the same article he quoted a Gallup poll which earlier that year revealed that the public don't trust scientists to tell the truth – doctors, priests and solicitors were way ahead on the public scale of trust.

Then there is the fact that he is a scientist whose area of interest is the brain. It was this interest and expertise which qualified him to present *The Mind Machine* for BBC2. Brain research, he argued in a *Radio Times* supporting piece, is vital because it confronts 'the greatest problems faced by society: depression, madness, ageing, violence'. His research field is the physiology of vision but his wider interest in psychiatric illness is reflected in the fact he is a key and influential scientific adviser to the pressure group, SANE (Schizophrenia: a National Emergency), and has been enormously supportive of SANE's successful efforts to raise over six million pounds to initiate a chair for research into schizophrenia at Blakemore's own university, Oxford. And then there is the fact that Blakemore is not a scientist in the twilight of his years and therefore relatively immune to the criticisms and backbiting that can happen to scientists prepared to involve themselves with the media. He is at the peak of his work, is internationally renowned and is a fellow of the prestigious Royal Society.

Is it true that scientists as a group are less likely to suffer from psychiatric illness? Yes, according to a recent study undertaken by British psychiatrist, Felix Post. He selected world-famous people with outstanding and original achievement who have been alive during the past 150 years and for whom expertly researched biographies written after their death are available. He extracted the 'factual' information from the biographies, firmly eschewing the biographers' speculations and interpretations concerning their subjects' psychological make-up. He compared innovative and and world-famous novelists and dramatists with famous scientists. Of note, incidentally, is Post's comment to the effect that it was relatively easy to select his fifty-five writers but much more difficult to find scientists who had attracted biographies of high quality. Indeed to bring his number of scientists up to a reasonably acceptable level, he had to bring in applied scientists and doctors. Even then out of some sixty scientists only thirty-five had biographies written of sufficient depth to permit Post to include them in his study.

Post analysed his data in terms of 1) life-long characteristics (personality disorder) and 2) episodic impairment of mental heath (psychiatric illness). 30% of the writers but only 12% of the scientists had a history of having suffered episodes of mild psychiatric symptoms, while 33% of the scientists and 54% of the writers were classed as having had at some stage an episode of definite phychiatric illness. 30% of the writers had severe psychiatric ill-health and nearly one in six had engaged in serious suicidal behaviour. In contrast, only 15% of the scientists had ever been seriously psychiatrically ill and only two had attempted suicide. Whereas 15% of the writers had regularly taken drugs and alcohol, only two scientists had done so. Marital difficulties also figured more prominently among the writers – 52% had broken marriages against only 12% of the scientists!

Such findings, and they are not without qualification, lend support to the conventional picture of the scientist as controlled, detached, and impassive. Initially at any rate, Professor Blakemore is inclined to agree, emphasising the value of detachment while at the same time at pains to insist that the day-to-day business of being a scientist is not all that different from being an engineer or a bank manager. He was not all that comfortable during the interview but this only adds to the impression he gave me of a man thinking carefully about the questions I was asking. He is honest about this – 'I don't like sitting down and working through my problems,' he declares at one point, 'I'd rather keep them below the surface and concentrate on control and presentation and just dealing with the world as it is.'

Throughout the interview there is a perceptible conflict between the scientist he would like to be and the man he is. For he is actually drawn to the notion of the scientist as someone who has a 'detachment from one's emotional investment' and he promptly contrasts such a figure with the scientist 'who waves his hands around a lot, or the scientist who is just a bit too emotionally committed to his or her ideas'. Blakemore has always been inclined to be controlled and self-reliant, characteristics often to be found in bright only children who grow up to be exceptionally bright adults. He dislikes showing his feelings. Even though or perhaps because he is quite sensitive, he can be impatient and from time to time feels intensely and passionately about things. Revealingly, he compares the process of research to the process of personal control. Scientific work, he remarks, is often 'amazingly random and haphazard and disorganised' but the publication that results from it is 'terribly controlled and absolutely disciplined'. That is how he thinks people work as well – or perhaps, more accurately, that is how he functions – 'a kind of hot-house of ideas and emotions down below and a level of control and presentation in which they're displayed to the rest of the world'. So those scientists that Post studied may well have been as emotionally churned-up as their artistic counterparts but they had learned to keep those feelings well submerged and confined!

The observation which stirred up more listener response than almost anything said by anyone else during the series is when Colin Blakemore declares he no longer has religious faith. He goes further and declares that no scientist, 'who seriously goes into the laboratory to try and study how the brain works', can entertain the hypothesis that man has a soul, that there is, so to speak, a ghost in the machine. Peter McKay in the *Evening Standard* was particularly cross and in a piece entitled 'The meaning of life, perhaps' mocked brain research for contributing so little to 'our understanding or our control' of the things that matter about human nature. Others wrote despairingly about Blakemore's reductionism and his unequivocal materialism. But others again welcomed as profoundly refreshing his insistence that, speaking personally, he can face the notion that what we have inside our heads is 'a machine that has remarkable capacities . . . to generate feelings, to generate consciousness, to generate emotions, to create an internal world for translating behaviour into a language, an internal language of explanation'. The brain struggling to understand the brain is, as he put it elsewhere, society trying to understand itself.

Yet if Freud is right and much religious belief stems from a desire to make unpalatable truths about life, disease and death more palatable, then Colin Blakemore has good reason to be a religious believer. His own father died of Alzheimer's disease and he, as a scientist, is well placed to know that having a close family member suffer from the disorder increases the risk for oneself. His own wife periodically suffers from depressive illness. For this reason I put to him the question of human suffering. Given his rigorous insistence that the material, physical world is all we have, what does he say to those who face in their daily lives the death of a child from a tumour of the eye or of a parent from dementia, whose young husband is left permanently brain damaged through a road accident caused by somebody else's wilful behaviour or whose wife's daily life is regularly disturbed by severe dips in mood? Professor Blakemore does not flinch from the question nor does he answer evasively but quite bluntly draws the inexorable conclusion given his own flatly stated philosophy. Life deep down has no purpose and accordingly suffering has no purpose either. We are here in this world and we have to deal with both – with life *and* with suffering. And he himself deals with it by asking questions, understanding experiments, testing results and by never standing still, never stopping, never not working, never, or hardly ever, pausing long enough to acknowledge that self-same nagging, insistent question posed in so many of the letters his interview provoked – what is the point of it all then?

There will be those of a more analytical persuasion than I who may be tempted to make a connection between the rupture between Blakemore and his father and between him and the deity in which he himself once believed. Blakemore is one of those people, and in the post-Butler era there are many, who were moved by the educational opportunities facilitated by the hard work of their parents and the provisions of State education away from the lives and experiences of the rest of their families. Education meant that any possibility of true communication between Colin and his father was made remote. His regret concerning the drift away from his father is a familiar elegy – lost opportunities to express feelings, lost moments for simple communication – but there is, too, an honest and moving recognition that whatever the gap in education and knowledge they may well have shared more than divided them. The less educated father, vicissitudes of whose own life robbed him of so much opportunity, is nonetheless portrayed in a final musing passage as a man better able, perhaps, to show his true feelings than the gifted, renowned and cerebral fellow of the Royal Society.

CLARE: Professor Colin Blakemore is one of the most eminent research scientists in this country with an academic career peppered with prestigious lectureships and fellowships in European, American, Japanese and Chinese universities as well as Oxford and Cambridge. He was born in Coventry on June 1st, 1944. He comes from a working-class family and was educated at King Henry VIII school in Coventry and won a state scholarship to Cambridge where he read medicine. After three years he was, as he puts it, seduced by the excitement of academic research, which he has been pursuing ever since, into the workings of the brain. He was the BBC's youngest Reith Lecturer in 1976 and three years later at the age of thirty-five became the country's youngest professor of physiology and fellow of Magdalen College, Oxford and was named Man of the Year by the Royal Association for Disability and Rehabilitation. In 1989 he was given the Michael Faraday Award by the Royal Society for services rendered to the cause of science. Like most high profile scientists, he is not without his detractors; some describe him as ruthless, ambitious and combative, adding somewhat grudgingly that he may just possibly be a genius. In the popular press he is occasionally represented as a modern Frankenstein and has been on the hit-list of animal rights extremists and suffered, with his wife and three daughters, kidnap and death threats, fake bombs, poisoned pen letters and insulting telephone calls. Last year he was elected to be a fellow of the Royal Society.

Colin Blakemore, are you yourself curious about the way your own mind works?

BLAKEMORE: I don't think I'm a very self-analytical person, no. I don't spend much time thinking about my motives or what drives me.

CLARE: So when you're researching into the brain, when you're actually looking at this extraordinary organ, you don't reflect back from that to think, what I am looking at I am thinking with, what I'm uncovering is indeed how I work.

BLAKEMORE: Almost the opposite. I think one needs a certain detachment from one's own mental experiences and one's own conscious state in order to try to approach the scientific problem of understanding how the brain, as a machine, a very complex machine, works. I mean, no doubt one day we have to have on the agenda explaining how we perceive things, how we intend things and choose things and feel things. I feel that's rather a long way down the road and if one becomes too obsessed with the immense difficulty of accounting for personal experience, it makes the much more straightforward, though difficult, challenge of understanding the brain as a piece of biological machinery that much more difficult.

CLARE: Well, now, you used the word 'detachment'. People are curious about scientists in this society particularly, I think it's true to say. They are intrigued to know if there is a way of thinking that is scientific? I think one of the key features in this stereotype of a scientist is the notion of 'detached'. Now, do you think first of all that's true, that there is a quality that distinguishes scientists as a general group from other people?

BLAKEMORE: No, I don't think so any more than anyone who's professionally qualified is distinguished from the population by those qualifications. Science is a way of thinking about the world but the day to day business of being a scientist is not actually that different from being an engineer or producing something on the shop floor or, for that matter, managing a bank. It's a job with a certain set of routines and rules, much of the work is very mundane. Detachment is important because often the challenges that nature presents to the scientist don't have self-evident explanations and, in fact, intuition very often leads to wrong starting points for research, to wrong background or hypotheses. I think it's generally recognised that there are two ways that scientists work – the idealistic way where they simply observe the universe, gather data, and then try at the end to put it all together into a hypothesis, to try to understand it, fit it together; the other way, which is actually slightly less reputable in the philosophy of science is to have an idea first and then pursue it to try to find evidence for it, the hypothetical deductive method. It's very difficult for scientists to detach themselves from prejudice and from prior expectation. People become very committed to their ideas long before their ideas are generally accepted or before they have the evidence to prove them, so one needs a curious mixture of detachment and the ability to know when an idea is wrong, to accept the evidence of nature, but also the sort of resolute commitment initially to a particular way of thinking that can drive you on through, frankly, the boredom of doing research in the hope of finding out how things really do work.

CLARE: How far back do you go in your own life to identify your interest in science, your interest in that process of either proposing hypotheses, imaginative ideas about how things work or indeed, the more painstaking way of accumulating large amounts of information? When you go back to the young Blakemore, can you find evidence of those traits that have subsequently served you well?

BLAKEMORE: Not many, at very early stages.

CLARE: What would your earliest memory be of yourself?

BLAKEMORE: I don't have a terribly good early memory. I remember a few events of the first few years. I remember very clearly the first television set that my father brought home because he worked in the television trade and that was when I was four. I have a very clear and vivid memory of dragging a teacher home from nursery school to have a look at this wondrous monster in the corner of the room. Not that we could pick anything up because we lived in Coventry and there wasn't a transmitter nearby. Even the flickering light was a sort of technological miracle. I can remember the first tricycle that I owned, I suppose I must have been two or three or something like that, and being very proud of riding on it and actually being quite interested in how it worked. I liked to take things apart, did not succeed always in putting them back together again but I'm not sure that scientists are terrible good at those kind of mechanical things anyway, but I did have an interest in how things worked. Not that that, I think, is a prerequisite for a scientist. I mean it could be. An artist could be equally interested in simply how things work and how they're created. I didn't go to university with any intention of being a scientist. I didn't know what a scientist was. I'd never met a scientist. I didn't know much about how science worked. I went to university intending to be a doctor because that was the only profession really that I'd had any contact with from my, my background so it was a natural thing to aspire to when I had the chance to go to university.

CLARE: How had you contact with that from your background? Your father worked in what capacity?

BLAKEMORE: He worked in the television trade. He was in the airforce for the whole of the war. He joined up at the age of seventeen, came out of the airforce with no sort of professional training, with some experience in radio transmission, and went into the only job that seemed to be available. He went into a local television and radio shop. Soon left and delivered batteries in a big blue van, which actually I remember very well. I must have been three then. I remember riding in the van to nursery school. And then he became a sales representative, a commercial traveller really for television companies, one or two of them, through much of his working life. So that was the contact with the television industry.

CLARE: What sort of man was he?

BLAKEMORE: A complicated man. I think to sum him up in a word, he was a very restless man. And because of that I didn't see that much of him and he found it difficult to stay in one place, and that included the home. He didn't stay at home very much either because he was travelling, working, or because he had his own life and he was often out in the evenings and I didn't see very much of him. This is not to say he was an uncaring father, actually he was very caring.

CLARE: Affectionate, then?

BLAKEMORE: I'm not sure that he was a man who could easily show his affections.

CLARE: For example, do you feel he knew you?

BLAKEMORE: No. And I'm not sure that I knew him, not at least until maybe the last few years before his death, paradoxically, because he died from Alzheimer's disease and therefore was actually a very different person, but for the first time really in my life I felt that I became closer to him during those last few years than I had been when I was young. We were very different people. I mean obviously different in academic inclination – that's not to say that he wasn't able but he'd been deprived by history from having any chance to exercise whatever intelligence he had. I was very different in the world into which I wanted to move and had aspirations to move. He didn't understand that. He was very supportive but really couldn't give me any advice or support that was relevant to what I wanted to do.

CLARE: And your mother, what was she like – she's still alive?

BLAKEMORE: My mother's still alive, yes. My mother was immensely practically supportive. She was and still is a very organised lady. I think she projected on to me a lot of the ambition that I had when I was young. She's a bright person and I think had great hopes for me. I'm an only child and that, I think, makes parents project all of their hopes and desires on to that one product of a marriage and I felt that quite strongly. My mother was there. She wasn't pushy, she wasn't terribly forceful but I knew that she was proud of what I could do and wanted me to do well.

CLARE: And did she give you the feeling that you would do well? Was she the sort of mother who drove you to achieve more and more to satisfy or was she the sort of mother who took great relaxed satisfaction in the things you were doing?

BLAKEMORE: Yes, I think the latter. I think she had confidence in what I could do and she certainly didn't push me beyond my limits. I think she was pleased at what I achieved and had immense confidence, misplaced confidence in what I could do, and simply sat back and did what she could to provide an environment that would make it happen.

CLARE: Did you ever feel that she invested you with too much? It sounds from what you say that your father wasn't there a great deal and so you must have been very important to this woman. You were the only other person in the house?

BLAKEMORE: Yes, I was aware, very aware of that and aware of the dilemma that that created. I mean the responsibilities that fell on my shoulders and the demands, emotional and supportive demands, that fell on my shoulders, yes.

CLARE: Did your mother work outside the house or was she full time with you?

BLAKEMORE: Not after the age of three or four. When I got to that age she decided to give up work and essentially devote herself to the family home.

CLARE: Which meant you really?

BLAKEMORE: Yes.

CLARE: Yes. And how early did you realise that you were bright?

BLAKEMORE: I draw a distinction between feeling bright and feeling capable. I realised from quite early that I could do things and get them done. I could pass the hurdles and get on and pass the tests. I did well in examinations. I started by going to primary school in the working-class area where we lived and obviously did well there and moved ahead in the school to the point where the school suggested that my parents should try, somehow, to find the wherewithal to send me to the local grammar school, the primary section of the local grammar school, which they did, to my immense gratitude. I certainly wouldn't be where I am now without that tremendous financial sacrifice that they made when I was seven. And I passed the eleven plus exam and I passed other exams and I got on. I never had the feeling of being terribly intelligent. I think the first time that I had that feeling that maybe I was brighter than the people around me was when I got to Cambridge because I had absolutely no expectation of doing well in Cambridge. I imagined that I had just somehow clawed my way into this position of distinction and that I would have a middling career in university and I did reasonably well. I got a first and found that I was able to compete with people around me from much more powerful schools and family back-grounds than mine. For the first time I thought, God, maybe I am brighter than I thought.

CLARE: Do you remember any particular moment or event at Cambridge that you felt, 'Good God, I'm as good as anyone here?'

BLAKEMORE: I remember very, very well talking to my tutor at the end of my first year when, really, to my immense surprise I got a first in my first year examinations and although tutors were not, and still are not, by the way, really permitted to reveal scores or marks, there were informal ways in which one could get an indication. I wanted to know really which subject because I thought it must only be one that I'd done best in so I could think about how to concentrate on that in the rest of my time at Cambridge and I remember so well my tutor saying, 'Well you got a first in physiology and you got a first in biochemistry,' and then saying, 'well, you got a second in anatomy.' I was amazed that I could have got a first-class result in two subjects and what happened was I concentrated an awful lot in anatomy in my second year and got a first in that as well!

CLARE: You mentioned that your decision to do medicine was related to the fact that that was one activity, one area, that you actually had some knowledge of. How did that come about?

BLAKEMORE: Well, the local doctor was one of the few professional people that I came in contact with but the reason I came in contact with the family doctor quite frequently was that I had a fairly prolonged illness through my teenage years, probably starting, I think, around the age of eleven, which was eventually, and with some disbelief, diagnosed as a duodenal ulcer. I had an ulcer and had a lot of episodes of pain whenever I was stressed around examination times and that kind of thing and also two or three rather serious haemorrhages. I was in hospital for a while and so on, so I had quite a lot of contact with the medical profession at the receiving end.

CLARE: We've talked about your mother's ambition for you. In a sense, of course, what's really interesting in people such as you who do achieve a great deal is the extent to which from very early on the person in a sense drives himself or herself. It may, of course, come from an interaction with expectations outside but sometimes what's really propelled such a person forward is that wherever they are, even on a desert island, they drive themselves. Would you describe yourself like that? Would you say that actually you set yourself these targets, you put yourself under stress from fairly early on?

BLAKEMORE: Absolutely. I'm very aware of that, and more and more aware of it as time goes by because if you keep demanding more and more of yourself as you get older, the day gets fuller and fuller and fuller and the stress becomes greater and greater. I'm a workaholic. I know a lot of scientists who are. They're driven by all sorts of things. I mean obviously to some extent personal ambition to get on, to fulfill their careers, but also driven by the nature of things that they do, desperately anxious to solve the problem – this immense curiosity that a scientist has got to have to overcome the boredom of much of what they do. It creates an enormous ambition just to know. Scientists, I mean many scientists that I know, who are successful, work the most ridiculous hours with no proportionate rewards. I mean there's no piece rate for being a scientist. If you're slaving away till two or three in the morning every day it's you that's driving yourself and has to be.

CLARE: You used the term 'workaholic'. Do you actually, yourself, experience withdrawal symptoms when you, for one reason or another, are not working?

BLAKEMORE: I'm almost never not working.

CLARE: Really?

BLAKEMORE: Yes. I find it very difficult to stop work.

CLARE: For instance, do you take holidays?

BLAKEMORE: Well, they pass for holidays but I think if you ask my family they would say they were just a different sort of work.

CLARE: What would they say? What sort of holidays would they say that you have?

BLAKEMORE: Well, I would take my computer with me and sit in front of it from the start of the day and work whenever I could and probably rather grudgingly do the things that one ought to do on holidays, like taking trips to see the sights or sitting on the beach. I hate sitting on the beach. Pretty soon I retreat to a book or a computer.

CLARE: What about seeing the sights?

BLAKEMORE: Yes, I quite like doing that and, and have developed great skills in seeing sights quickly! Going to conferences and so on which is part of the business of being an academic, often conferences are held in attractive places for obvious reasons, to try to encourage people to come to them, and the way things usually turn out, I often accept an invitation to go to a meeting because of the marvellous place that it's in with every intention of staying and looking at the sights for a few days. As it gets nearer, the time available compresses so I jump on an aeroplane and go into a lecture theatre from the aeroplane, give my talk and race back to the airport. So one becomes very skilled at seeing the sights on the way to the airport!

CLARE: Let's just consider the extent to which being an only child provides you with a number of things. Particularly if you're bright, there is the sense in which there are expectations and in the case of the dynamics of your family, with your father not being terribly present and your mother clearly aware that she had a bright son on her hands, there's that additional influence. But you also have described the extent to which you developed a sense of pushing yourself and testing yourself, perhaps to the point of even, from time to time, over-stressing yourself. There's the extent to which an only child, and this can be seen as an advantage or a disadvantage, an only child is really thrown in on himself, or herself, himself in your case. Was that so? How much of a circle of friends would you have had? How early, in other words, is the Colin Blakemore that you've just described, very involved with computers and work, not outward looking to that extent, or gregarious? How much was that a feature of your childhood? Do you remember it as a time when you spent a lot of time inside your own head?

BLAKEMORE: Friendship is not a dominant feature of my memory of childhood. I can reconstruct the range of friends that I had and some of those friendships were very strong. Some of them still survive. Not least the friendship with my wife who I met when I was really quite young. But, if I pick up the sense of what you said, I learnt to be self sufficient and to depend more on myself than on people around me. I learnt when I was young, for instance, to appreciate being alone and actually enjoyed being alone. Not in a sort of egoistic sense of enjoying my own company but almost liking the challenge of having to cope. When I was seventeen I went to the United States and sort of bummed my way around the States for four or five months between school and university.

CLARE: On your own?

BLAKEMORE: On my own and I think I must have been alone almost not speaking to anyone for periods of weeks on end. I was hitching my way round. I suppose I must have spoken to the people in the car as a form of conversation but no close conversational contact with anybody over long periods of time, and I don't remember it being a stressful or a difficult time. I quite enjoyed it, dealing with the challenge of being alone.

CLARE: And that's something that you still would count as one of your characteristics?

BLAKEMORE: No, interestingly, and I try and analyse this for myself. I dislike being alone now. I still spend quite a lot of time alone but I don't like it and I need to bounce ideas and feelings off other people very much more than in the past and I think that that's something which is increasing rather than decreasing with age.

CLARE: Do you know why?

BLAKEMORE: Well, if the logic is that I don't feel that I needed company when I was young because I was self sufficient, the inverse of that would mean that I feel I need people more now because I'm not so self confident, and I think that's true.

CLARE: And you're not so self confident because?

BLAKEMORE: Because life now is not at the stage of discovering what you can achieve, of having new challenges and moving through them. For me, life is very much more a matter of coming to terms with what I have achieved and trying to do the scope of things that I have to do as well as possible. So it isn't that the environment presents challenges in quite the same way. I need a different sort of feedback, if you like, about myself and my own capacities than just achieving new things, which was what was happening when I was younger.

CLARE: You mention that you met your wife when you were quite young, and indeed, you married quite young, twenty-one I think?

BLAKEMORE: Yes.

CLARE: Would she have been your first serious girlfriend?

BLAKEMORE: Yes.

CLARE: The adolescence that you passed through, would it have been marked by this self sufficiency?

BLAKEMORE: In what respect? In dealing with the opposite sex?

CLARE: Yes, that's right.

BLAKEMORE: No, I was enormously inept with dealing with girls. I just didn't have any contact with girls, really.

CLARE: When would you have had your first contact with girls? When you went to Cambridge?

BLAKEMORE: No, no, no, no.

CLARE: No?

BLAKEMORE: Oh, no. I had cousins who lived next door, but the first time I went to a party with boys and girls, I suppose I must have been thirteen, twelve, thirteen, fourteen, that sort of age, but didn't become involved with any girl really before I met my wife.

CLARE: And you met her where?

BLAKEMORE: Well, she's from Coventry as well. She was the sister of someone who went to the same school that I did. I went to a concert, bumped into him and was introduced to his younger sister.

CLARE: And did you marry shortly after you met or was . . . ?

BLAKEMORE: Oh, no. We met I suppose when I was sixteen, she was fifteen. We married when I was twenty-one, so we'd known each other for several years.

CLARE: Now what does she make of this self sufficiency?

BLAKEMORE: She, I hope, has come to terms with it. She's had rather a long time to come to terms with it.

CLARE: But in those days, when you started out, because that's when it would have been at its most marked?

BLAKEMORE: I don't know very much about her motives in those days. I guess I projected assumptions on to her. I suppose the same kind of assumptions that I have about my mother. That she was happy to see me do the things I was doing and trying to get on with my career.

CLARE: And was that dynamic similar? Were you out of the house a lot?

BLAKEMORE: Yes.

CLARE: She got on rearing your three daughters?

BLAKEMORE: Three daughters now. Our first child was born after we'd been married for, I think, nine years so there was a long period of time when my wife pursued her career and worked.

CLARE: But nonetheless, the example you gave me of working every hour God or whoever it is gave you, fits those early years.

BLAKEMORE: Very much so. You see, we married just after I finished at Cambridge, went off immediately to the United States where I had a fellowship to be a research student, to work for the doctorate and that was very hard work. I did a PhD in the University of California in two and a half years 'cos I didn't have any more time to do it than that and that involved a tremendous amount of very hard work.

CLARE: And while you were doing that, what was she doing?

BLAKEMORE: She was working at the *San Francisco Chronicle* as an editorial assistant.

CLARE: And when you started out and got married, did you intend to have children? Was there any assumption that you would have a family? Because nine years is a long time.

BLAKEMORE: I can't remember the issue ever arising except, you know, some discussion about contraception which must imply that we didn't intend to have children, but it wasn't a serious issue that occupied our thoughts or worried us. It was, I'm glad to say, in retrospect, a very natural thing to do that we had to put off having children until we'd reached a more stable state and I'm absolutely sure that was the right thing to have done. Right for us and certainly right for our kids.

CLARE: Now you say those early years you're not absolutely clear how it evolved. What about in later years when the children began to arrive, because this is, of course, where one of the great dilemmas of our time, the balancing of public and private life becomes very apparent and you do very frankly describe yourself as someone with an enormous pull into public, professional life, your research and your work as a professor and so on. What about the tension that that creates from someone who's looking for something else, who's placing, in a sense, a demand on you? One of the first people I suppose would have been your wife to place a real demand on you other than your work and your career and your academic advancement. Did that lead to conflict? What's it like, in other words, to be married to a workaholic?

BLAKEMORE: Well, I don't know because I'm not married to one.

CLARE: You're not married to one. What does she say?

BLAKEMORE: My wife has a much more balanced view of the relationship between work and play than I do. She, as I said, must have come to terms with it. Here we are, still married after twenty-seven years or however long it is.

CLARE: Would she work on you to put limits to your own work?

BLAKEMORE: She did at the early stages of our marriage, to some extent, although she always, I think, yielded to arguments about what I felt was necessary for my career and wanted to be supportive and was immensely supportive. Now I think she's just come to terms peacefully with the kind of problems that being married to me must create in her life. I mean she just accepts that I do work very hard, that I'm unpredictable in my movements, that I get home very late, that I can bring home the problems of my work to her and to the home and ask her to help me deal with them, as anyone does in a marriage. She's a very tolerant person.

CLARE: You described your father as restless. Would you say you are?

BLAKEMORE: I think I'm intellectually restless. I certainly don't have the kind of geographical restlessness that he just had to be somewhere else, had to move on all the time. I hope I have that at an intellectual level. I want to move on to new challenges in my mind. I'm well aware I don't do that in the same way that I used to when I was young. But, there's a restlessness there. Yes. I know a feeling that I want to get, and I think my father had it too, want to get as much done in the time that's available as possible, to squeeze in as much as can be done in the time that one's given.

CLARE: Where does that come from, do you think? What feeds that desire to put as much in as possible?

BLAKEMORE: I think in my own case it partly come from the sort of intimations of mortality that I had after this prolonged illness when I was young. Since then I always had the feeling that I'm not going to live for very long. Hence the desire to get done what I could within my allotted time. Sometimes I'm surprised that I'm still alive now.

CLARE: Really?

BLAKEMORE: Yes.

CLARE: During that time you were ill as a child, you say you had a number of haemorrhages. On any one of those occasions did you feel you were going to die?

BLAKEMORE: I can remember one occasion very vividly. I was

working on the post, delivering the post at Christmas and had to get up very early to get to the sorting office and got up before my parents did, made some breakfast in the kitchen, jumped on my bicycle, rode down the road and blacked out and fell off my bicycle, picked myself up feeling rather strange and came back home and was taken into hospital and so on where I was for quite a long time and I was worried then. I was extremely worried, partly because I didn't know what was going on and wasn't actually sure that the doctors were terribly confident about what was going on at the time. I lost a great deal of blood, actually, in that episode. Yes, I was afraid.

CLARE: So there's a sense of living on borrowed time? That this is time you hadn't expected. You pack it full. In fact that particular problem has eased, has it, the ulcer and the bleeding?

BLAKEMORE: I had an operation when I was, I think, twenty, a gastrectomy which, thank goodness, doesn't have to be done these days because of drugs that are available and treat ulcers very, very effectively. But I had a gastrectomy, major surgery. Fortunately, I mean fortunately because I discovered afterwards what the probability of complete success in that operation is and it's not high, I'm one of the positive statistics, yeah, and I've recovered reasonably well.

CLARE: Yes. Your desire to do medicine was related to that, it clearly and understandably made quite an impression on you. What happened to that career? Did you qualify as a doctor?

BLAKEMORE: No, I didn't. I did medicine in Cambridge, pre-clinical medicine, the sort of scientific part of medicine, three years, and got a scholarship to go to St Thomas' Hospital. I was very keen to do that but I'd got the bug of the United States by this trip to America that I'd taken before I went to university, hitch-hiking around, and I wanted to go back and I applied for and got something called a Harkness Fellowship which would have paid for eighteen months or something of working in the United States between pre-clinical and clinical work. I went to work in Berkeley and started in research and just became more and more committed to it and it actually went very well.

I was very fortunate at the stage that I started in the project that I did. Things went very well.

CLARE: What sort of research would that have been? Can you remember?

BLAKEMORE: I was working, oh, yes, I remember it very distinctly. At this stage in the 1960s, it was 1965 when I went, there was a sudden blossoming of activity, of understanding of how the visual parts of the brain work, and really that's been the centre of my interest ever since and I got in at a very early stage in that area of research which involves recording from single nerve cells in the visual part of the brain in an anaesthetised animal, trying to find out what those cells do, what they're telling the rest of the brain about the things that are in front of an animal's eyes. And I got interested in depth perception, how we judge the distances of objects and was working on the mechanisms in the brain that might be responsible for that. And it was just such a fascinating problem. The thing about science is that if it goes well, then you can't ever stop. Every finding leads to a new question and every question is as interesting as the last and you can't ever stop. Science doesn't stop. There are no boundaries to it so it pulls you along whether you want it or not, if things go well. Now things don't always go well for everybody and I've seen people drop out of science very disappointed, looking around them and saying, 'Why do other people get this buzz out of this crazy business of slaving away with very few rewards, this boring stuff in the lab?' It just depends whether things go right or not. You are fortunate if they go right at the beginning, but for me they did. There was, for a while, the conflict then between what I should do in my career. Should I go back to medicine, or carry on with science. A turning point was a visit to Berkeley in California where I was working as lecturer from Cambridge, for a man from the department that I'd studied in as an undergraduate a few months before I got my doctorate. He talked to me and he was one of this breed of physiologist, himself medically qualified who does everything in his power to persuade people not to qualify in medicine. He would love to see people go into science. So he did. He said, why not come and work in Cambridge and get a teaching job? Remember this was the 1960s, 1968, when I have to say that it was ridiculously simple to find an academic teaching post. The universities were expanding. The money was there. It was just crazily easy. I got a job at Cambridge, which essentially, was a permanent job on the basis of a curriculum vitae that I'd typed on one of these fold up airmail letters. There was plenty of room on the airmail letter because my curriculum vitae consisted of about four lines and one publication. Nowadays, people who've been working for ten years right at the forefront of their field with fifty, sixty world-quality publications can't get a job in the universities. So, it was made very easy for me.

CLARE: And, because some listeners won't understand this, those first three years you would have had no contact with patients at all. It was laboratory-based or basically anatomy and whatever. So you never experienced the patient contact which drew you to medicine in the first place. You were a patient at the receiving end of a number of doctors' interventions.

BLAKEMORE: Yes. I mean I'm not saying that I never regretted not carrying on with medicine. For a long time I did and actually still toyed with the possibility of going back to finish those two and a half years, or whatever it would have been, to have qualified, but with time I realised first of all it would have been increasingly difficult to do so, to go back to being a student, particularly a medical student and all the discipline involved in that and secondly the realisation that I didn't really need it. That ambition had gone out of my life and something else had been substituted for it and something that I knew gave me pleasure and intense satisfaction and I wasn't at all sure that medicine would have done that. So gradually the feeling that I ought to go and finish my clinical work receded. Much of my research is concerned with clinical problems and twenty years ago it would have been extremely difficult for someone in my position, that is working in a medical school, in medical research, without a medical degree, to be able to pursue questions of clinical interest. It's very different now and there's very good collaboration and interaction between the clinical and the pre-clinical departments and I have worked directly with clinical patients with the cooperation of my clinical collegues.

CLARE: Do you often wonder what kind of doctor you would have made?

BLAKEMORE: Yes, I do. I had, of course, a very idealistic image of myself as a doctor when I was young, I think that's very important in being a medical student, that there is a kind of vocational image of what it's like to be a doctor, something that I have to say is sadly lacking in some medical students these days because very often, because of the difficulty of getting into medical school, they are simply the intellectual cream of their schools. They're told they're good enough to be able to do medicine and they haven't really thought through the vocational challenges and why they're doing it. No, I had a very clear view of wanting to be a good doctor. I wanted to be a neurologist. I hoped I would be a compassionate and successful doctor, curing people and helping people. Ridiculously naïve, with no contact with medical education at that stage.

CLARE: No, but you'd experienced it directly as a patient. Just as a matter of interest, did they interview you to go to medical school in those days? You and I will remember that some people said, 'Don't say that kind of thing if you're asked' because somehow it was not the right thing to say to experienced doctors screening medical students, and yet many of us did feel that that's why we were going in. Were you actually interviewed?

BLAKEMORE: Yes, of course. I was interviewed both at Cambridge and then afterwards by St Thomas' for the clinical place that I never took up. I went to Cambridge with every intention of doing medicine so I was interviewed with that career in mind. I then later, myself, became a medical tutor at Cambridge and saw this from the other side and, frankly, I tried to be sympathetic to kids who had this burning vocational desire to do medicine who perhaps weren't at the same kind of intellectual level that medical schools then were able to demand. I wouldn't have got in, I wouldn't get into medical school now with the grades at A-level that I got at school. I got into Cambridge and got a state scholarship. I wouldn't get in now. I think that's wrong. It's a pity that because medicine is a relatively secure profession, though not quite as secure as it was in those days, people turn to it as a safe haven and the criterion for those who are able to turn to it becomes academic performance. That's sad.

CLARE: What about this sense of detachment and the buzz in solving problems? Do you think that would have been useful had you gone on to be a doctor? Do you think that in a sense you are better suited to be the full-time researcher?

BLAKEMORE: Yes, I think so. I think temperamentally I'm better suited to that. I think that medicine, at least at the forefront of technological medicine, if one can call it that, the growing areas of medicine, applications of the most modern techniques in biochemistry and pharmacology and now genetic manipulation and so on, medicine is just as large an intellectual challenge as science, is just as difficult a tussle to find solutions to extremely complicated problems and I'm sure there can be the same kind of rewards in that, but I'm not sure that I'm actually very well suited to the day-to-day slog, important though it is, of diagnosis, of seeing the routine array of everyday medical problems and dealing with the counselling aspect of medicine that are so important, certainly for a general practitioner. I'm not sure that I would have been very well cut out for that, frankly. I would like to have thought that I would, but I don't think I would.

CLARE: Are you a patient man in interpersonal situations? I don't mean now as a researcher, you may well be exceedingly patient, but I mean in dealing with other people.

BLAKEMORE: I try to be controlled. I think I'm reasonably well controlled so there's a difference between the external persona and, sometimes, what's going on inside. I don't think I'm a terribly patient person. I get restless and unhappy with problems that aren't solved quickly and easily but I try very hard and I think I'm reasonably successful at it. I try to conceal those kinds of worries and frustrations and even aggressions. I think I do a pretty good job of controlling myself.

CLARE: You mention control. Is that because inside you're quite passionate? You feel things quite deeply?

BLAKEMORE: Yes, I think so.

CLARE: Would people know that?

BLAKEMORE: Occasionally. I suppose they see the outbursts every now and then and I'm aware occasionally that I say things out of turn that I regret afterwards and have said on impulse and I try and control that to the extent that I can.

CLARE: Would people see you as cold, calculating?

BLAKEMORE: Yes, I think people see me as distant, as hard to penetrate. I don't think many people would claim to know me very well.

CLARE: And why is that?

BLAKEMORE: Well, I think probably because I don't reveal myself very easily. I don't enjoy revealing. I don't enjoy analysing myself. I'm not particularly enjoying this experience, actually, but it's an interesting exercise, but not something that I'm very familiar with. I don't sit down working through my problems and other people's problems with them. I'd rather keep them below the surface and concentrate on control and presentation and just dealing with the world as it is.

CLARE: That brings me to an area that interests me. One of the reasons I wanted to interview you concerned the area of feelings. You did a BBC television series, *The Mind Machine*, which was very remarkable. I took you to task because you used the word 'machine'. You defend it in the book and point out very resonably that the brain is the most astonishing machine that we know and unravelling how it works is a lifetime's endeavour. The reason I was interested and a bit irritated and now I have you I can raise it with you because it's crucially related to what we're just talking about, is this issue of feelings. In every way except that, it seems to me, the brain and machine analogy is reasonable. The problem is this question of feelings. They provide a lot of problems for even the most sophisticated of machine analogies. They're not predictable and they do involve things like intuition and they're messy and they demand control.

BLAKEMORE: Well, I suppose I could slip out of this question you're asking simply by saying that you underestimate the nature of the machine that we have inside our heads. Clearly it is the kind of machine that can have feelings and emotions. It is the kind of machine that can have regrets and doubts and fears, the kind of machine that can fall in love and all of those things that we experience. I think you have to recognise that we live our lives at two levels. We live our lives at the level of believing that we, that is the internal eye, the agent that propels us through the world, this thing inside us that sees the world, that has feelings, that has desires, that has hatreds, that has ambitions, we feel ourselves to be that way. And yet, if we look at another person and ask ourselves really, what do we know of this person, all we know of is their behaviour and then there is always an equation between the way people behave and the way they feel. The job of a scientist therefore, since the nature of feelings is such that they can never be directly observed, they are private experiences that can't be measured with a meter or probed with an electrode, the only legitimate way that a scientist can approach the question of feelings is to examine behaviour.

CLARE: Now, you prefaced all that by saying you could slip away. What is the other way of responding to this issue of the faulty analogy with machine because of this messy area of feelings?

BLAKEMORE: Well, of course it could be that I, and I have to say the vast majority of brain researchers, are wrong in our assumption that the spiritual world of self-awareness is really just a product of the machinery of the brain. It might be that there's something very distinctly different that is separate from the physical world, call it a soul or whatever you will, that we'll never understand in scientific terms. I don't believe that and actually I don't believe that anybody who seriously goes into the laboratory to try and study how the brain works can actually entertain that hypothesis, at least while they are doing experiments, because if you really believed there was a soul, a ghost in the machine, then how could you study such a machine with tools, with methods, that can only look at machines, not ghosts?

CLARE: You said that when you look at someone else, in the final analysis, you can only really observe their behaviour, but isn't this where intuition has a role? That is to say, that as a result of analysing your own feelings and their relationship with the way you behave, that you interpret another person's behaviour? Of course it's a hazardous exercise. You can get it wrong. But you have an insight into what someone else is feeling, whatever they're behaving, because you have an insight into your own feelings and indeed the issue of feelings in general. That's the great artistic achievement, to be somehow able to enter into how another person feels.

BLAKEMORE: Well, indeed, and this is the essence of the hypothesis of a good friend of mine, Nicholas Humphrey, about the nature and the biological value of consciousness, that it gives us a kind of internal meter for judging the significance of the behaviours and the actions of other people. We can for instance, if we see another person turning red in the face and their eyes bulging and their fists raising, we could say, 'My God, if I was behaving like that I know I would feel angry, I would be feeling anger. That is what this other person must be feeling.' It's a way of translating from the behavioural world into the world of feelings. I think it's an interesting idea and it in no way negates the mechanistic hypothesis about how the brain works. As I said, this machine we have in our heads is a machine that has remarkable capacities. It has the capacity to generate feelings, to generate consciousness, to generate emotions, to create an internal world for translating behaviour into a language, an internal language of explanations. The problem is that this spiritual world that we feel that we have gives us an account of how we actually work. It tells us that we're rational. It tells us that we sit and think through problems. It tells us that we have choice, that we can think which decision we will take on the basis of either factual evidence or moral inclinations or just chance, whatever we want to do. It gives us sensations like being in love or being in pain. It gives us a complete description of how we work. In a sense, it is an alternative to a science of the brain and we have it already in our heads. What one has to say is: 'Where has this internal self-reflective science of the brain come from?' It's come from us. It's come from our evolution. There's absolutely no reason to believe that it should be accurate. I know perfectly well from my knowledge and others' of the visual part of the brain that my apparent awareness of the world, my internal privy experiences of seeing the world are a totally inaccurate description of how my brain is giving me those impressions. I have no sense of the computational machinery behind it and the complexity of the processing that's going on. So, if my visual experiences don't tell me about the visual processes that I know are going on in my brain, why should my experiences of hate or pleasure or love or choice or moral values really tell me how my brain is working.

CLARE: So, given what you've said, the objection is often put to that view, that it is reductionist, that it leaves us prey to a feeling that in one sense, nothing very much matters, that it is the scientific justification of doing your own thing, since a moral system is largely the creation of what you've just described, the final stage of processes we haven't the faintest idea how they work, then why pay too much attention to them, particularly when there are times when it's so much more satisfying to breach them?

BLAKEMORE: Well, I think there will always be two ways of seeing the world. The way that evolution has given us to see the world and the way that science tells us the world really is. I put it to you that just because you know that the sun doesn't go round the earth, it hasn't altered your way of seeing a magnificent sunrise or glorying in the beauty of a sunset. I mean, those are internal experiences which knowledge can never erode.

CLARE: Well, indeed, I was going to ask you just that. Does your knowledge affect your perception? You've answered in a sense. You say the two worlds – does that mean they don't actually come together?

BLAKEMORE: Well, as I said, we may one day, and we should certainly hope that we can, we may one day be able to give a description of how it is that our brains produce this inner world of personal experience, but when we know that the world of experience won't disappear. It actually works very well. We've probably had it as human animals for half a million years at least. It's a beautifully refined system for enabling people to understand the world and most of all to understand each other at a certain level of description. It is, it is a kind of naturally evolved theory of the brain.

CLARE: Let me ask you something. Colin Blakemore the scientist and those views that you have, studying the brain, looking at these two worlds, how does this affect you in your family? Are there times when your daughters or your wife would say, 'This is Colin Blakemore the scientist?' Do you take from one world inappropriately into another? Would they reprimand you that you're applying, if you like, principles or processes from one world in their own interpersonal world?

BLAKEMORE: Yes, that does happen. I think probably the reaction would be, 'Oh God, here's dad being boring again.' You know. We spend quite a lot of time talking about genetics, as I think anybody who knows anything about genetics should do with their children because the natural inclination of children to reject, or not to reject but to move away from, to detach themselves, to become different from their parents, which is a very strong and perfectly natural tendency, upsets parents, of course, enormously. Well it's useful to be able to say, 'Just a minute, do you know, you're half me, just think about that problem.' Or 'You know, you are one eighth of your cousin', or whatever. It gives a different perspective on relationships between children and parents. Of course, they know that, my children know I'm interested in the brain. I'm glad to say that my eldest daughter is herself now becoming interested in the brain. She's going to be studying psychology at Oxford. We spend a lot of time at home talking about the brain and they know I'm interested in it. They are interested in it. It actually is a fascinating area of science which can be of interest to anyone. It could be very hard if I was a particle physicist or a cosmologist to be able to convey the excitement of what I'm interested in to my family, as I do.

CLARE: You've mentioned genetics and your interest in the brain. There's something quite poignant about the fact that your father died in his mid sixties and that he died of Alzheimer's disease, of dementia.

BLAKEMORE: Yes.

CLARE: This is where, in a sense, knowledge doesn't necessarily free. I would anticipate that you actually would be very well aware of the possible risks that you yourself might be at in terms of dementia. Is that right?

BLAKEMORE: Well, of course, yes. I mean, every time I can't remember an address or a telephone number, I ask myself, 'Is this the beginning?' I suppose the first symptoms that my mother and then I began to see in my father was when he was in his mid-fifties. I'm forty-eight, so I'm very aware of that possibility.

CLARE: And the first symptoms were? What did you notice?

BLAKEMORE: Oh, forgetfulness, disorganisation in his life, just not being able to plan his life with the same efficiency.

CLARE: And is that another of the factors that contributes to your packing things in, living life to the full?

BLAKEMORE: I think that tendency was there long before I knew my father was ill, certainly long before I knew he had dementia, but it's kind of upped the stakes a little bit, yes.

CLARE: How do you deal with setback? Your career is, and you and I know that careers can be painted in this way, is logical progression of progress, promotion, achievement, recognition, appointment, but I assume there are setbacks there. Self reliant people I suppose, are at their most exposed when they really are tested. What do you think looking back, has been your most testing time? Or perhaps you think it's yet to come.

BLAKEMORE: I can imagine, tests, just to broach the second possibility that you raise, I can certainly imagine tests in the future, not least the test of what I do now. I'm forty-eight and I have a good job at Oxford as an academic. It's very hard to know where I could go from here, yet I have twenty years of working life left and that does worry me, particularly for someone who is intellectually restless, sees a need to move on. I don't deal terribly well with challenges and setbacks. I'm perhaps very much more easily hurt than people realise and it's part of the control that I try to exercise not to show my feelings. But at several times in my life I've been very deeply upset for long periods of time about disappointments in work, not achieving something I've wanted to achieve or being hurt by something that someone else has done, or even through all those normal human emotions of jealousy or passions of various sorts.

CLARE: Have you ever been depressed?

BLAKEMORE: I think I'm a pretty sanguine character. I'm actually very strongly optimistic. I'm able in the end to bounce back and just carry on. And I'm certainly not depressive in the way that you and I would use that word. I don't have a clinical condition that makes me depressed by any means. Pretty stable emotional character I think. But yes, I've had a couple of periods in my life when I've had what I've recognised as being the clinical symptoms of depression for a few weeks or months at a time.

CLARE: And during those periods, what do you think pulled you through, or certainly prevented it from becoming more like the serious clinical depressions that people like myself see?

BLAKEMORE: I think the recognition that there was no alternative but to pick oneself up. That the only alternative was to stay in this hell-hole of depression, which is the most awful state to be in, so the determination to get out of it. That's fine if the depression is reactive, if it is caused by events in the world because you can stand up and fight them, but to be in that position gave me, I think, an insight to the horrendous problems that people face who are by inclination depressive, whose depression is not caused by their world, not caused by what people do to them, not caused by their environment. It's caused by them, just as much as a duodenal ulcer is caused by them, or arthritis is caused by their body, by their chemical make-up and there's no way out of that, just by fighting against the problem, because the problems are inside.

CLARE: What are you like with illness in others, say with illness in your family?

BLAKEMORE: My wife has had several periods of illness. She is depressive and has endogenous depression, unipolar depression, so she has this dreadful experience from time to time of having a depression which is not caused by her environment and having to deal with it. I try to be sympathetic; don't we all when faced with illness in others? I'm sure I'm not as good at it as many people are. I'm sure I'm not as bad as some.

CLARE: You and I are very familiar with this idea of depression as a biological condition as well as a reactive one. That's to say, as you say, depression identified as springing from some change or changes which we do not fully understand or only partially understand within the brain and regulating mood and drives, zest, appetite, sleep, sexual drive and so on. You and I also know that there are people who are very critical of that model. They feel that it lets people off the hook in the sense that it means that we can say, if I personalise for a minute, the fact that Colin Blakemore is a twenty-two-hour-a-day working man, he's obsessed with cracking the brain, advancing scientific research, has nothing to do with his wife being depressed. If I didn't ask you this question they'd say, 'God, there were the two of them colluding in this narrow biological model of disease, two men, what's more, and here is this poor woman who periodically gets depressed.' So, I put that question to you. That's a challenge often put to me, the notion that a biological model of a disorder such as depression is often a sort of medical way out so that we don't have to look at social and psychological factors such as workaholic husbands who find, if you like, illness a bit difficult if it can't be pretty promptly treated.

BLAKEMORE: Well, to give the obvious excuse, my wife's father is also unipolar depressive. I don't think that my workaholic tendencies have caused his difficulties. But of course you know, and I think from my limited knowledge I know, that the tendency to be depressive is a real, deep biological problem. And, by the way, my wife would be the first to support the view that this is something which is just beyond the control of the world. If you are going to become depressed when you have this condition, there is nothing that can stop it. But equally there is an interaction. Events in life can trigger depressive episodes even in someone who has that biological disposition. I should hate to think that things that I've done might have triggered that in my wife's case. I don't think so. Perhaps I'm wrong.

CLARE: The extent to which you've become depressed has been nothing like as severe as that and you've always come out of them. As you've said, temperament is very important and you've a sanguine enough temperament. But several times in this interview you've mentioned spontaneously the issue of controlling your feelings and I wonder where did that come from. Why was it so important? You do place a lot of emphasis on control. I think of you as someone who keeps your feelings under control. I suspect that that's why people feel they don't know you because, reflecting an earlier element in our discussion, we think we know people when they behave in certain ways that suggest certain feelings. Someone who keeps his feelings under control; there's less of this penetration of the soul. We have less to go on. The behaviour is itself less varied and variable. So if you accept all of that, where do you think it comes from? Why do you place such a premium on keeping control of your emotions?

BLAKEMORE: Well, maybe I don't trust my emotions to be appropriate. I know the times that occasionally feelings do burst through. I can get angry or passsionate about a situation or extremely happy or temporarily even manic about some exciting occasion. I often regret that afterwards and feel that it wasn't quite appropriate. That people will think less of me for being too easily emotionally reactive.

CLARE: But isn't that very English? Why would they think it? Why wouldn't they see you as an enormously enthusiastic, spontaneous, effervescent man who's just brimming over with ideas?

BLAKEMORE: Maybe, you're absolutely right. I think I am very, very English in that respect. Maybe this is why the English have done disproportionately well in science because one needs that kind of detachment from one's emotional investment in something to be a good scientist. I suspect that the scientist who waves his or her hands around a lot, the scientist who is just a bit too emotionally committed to his or her ideas, the scientist who aggressively attacks an alternative view at a personal level is a less respected scientist and actually a less good scientist than one who tries to be dispassionate. As I've said earlier in this interview, we all have our commitments to ideas, to our inclinations and our intuitions in science. I think intuition is terribly important in science and good scientists are the ones who have that amazing knack to come up a priori with the right idea time after time and are proved right. But they mustn't show that they have a personal commitment to it or their science suffers. It's something like the relationship between doing scientific work, which is often amazingly random and haphazard and disorganised and blind alleys and wrong hunches and things, and then the publication, which eventually results from it which is terribly controlled and absolutely disciplined. This was done because of that and there were, you know, eighteen experiments, one after the other as if that's the way it was actually planned. It's a very odd relationship between the control or presentation of science and the way in which it's actually done and I think that's how people work as well. There is a kind of hot-house of ideas and emotions down below and a level of control and presentation in which they're displayed to the rest of the world. Maybe the British err a little bit too much on the side of the veneer of presentation.

CLARE: Because how much is operating here? How much are we confronting a sort of peer expectation, a peer pressure? That's to say, from what you're saying, I could suggest that Colin Blakemore actually under the surface is full of bubbling emotions and so on but in view of what you've said yourself, that were that to be manifested, it's not that you Colin Blakemore would be any less the scientist but you would be seen to be less the scientist. So we've a sort of interesting echo of what we were talking about earlier. We've got a situation where a certain kind of behaviour is taken to reflect a certain kind of internal life but you and I are now discovering that it doesn't actually. That the cool exterior of Colin Blakemore, which is what we expect of scientists because that's really the kind of detachment we want, is in fact very carefully constructed by Colin Blakemore because in truth, inside, he's passionate about his ideas. He probably is very identified in his own mind with certain ways of proceeding, but what he's learned is not that that's a bad thing – but that if you show it, it will seem to be a bad thing. That's not the way scientists are seen to be. Because, you see, I had this problem at the beginning when I said to you, 'Is there something about scientists that's particularly scientific?' and I actually used the word 'detachment' and you were very scathing about it. You didn't think there was really. Now we've come round full circle. You think, 'Well maybe there is.' I sense that you are controlled because there's something to control. You're not controlled because there's nothing to control. So where does that leave us? It leaves us, does it not, with the fact that you were right when you said detachment isn't the crucial feature of being a scientist. It's a crucial feature of being an English scientist.

BLAKEMORE: I know lots of detached people who are not scientists. They're often people who have the capacity to be in their projected image, a number of different personas. And I'm aware of that in myself. If one reveals completely openly the depths of one's feelings, then one is only one person. I suppose you might say the true person. If what you project is a translation of those inner thoughts which you believe to be appropriate for the situation that you're in, it gives you the capacity to be many people. And I'm aware of that in myself. I am different people on different occasions. I can control my inner feelings to produce a different image and I think that actually I'm not admitting this as a kind of crime or sin. I think it's a very useful capacity to have and I'm well aware of being able to turn on in different situations a different person, a different personhood, a different personality.

CLARE: And there might be situations where this sense of needing to control isn't so sharply developed, isn't so sharply present, that you can be more spontaneous?

BLAKEMORE: Well, I hope so. I mean in my own home, in my family, I hope that's true.

CLARE: Talking about the brain, you came down very squarely on the side of there being no ghost in the machine and you felt that the majority of brain researchers probably feel similarly and that's your theoretical position and you've argued it very powerfully in a number of places. In terms of your own individual life, where does that leave you? Do you ever have a desire, ever experience the desire to believe something different for the purposes of your own life's satisfaction? To feel that it doesn't all end with your dissolution? That there – which is one of the powerful impulses behind much religious beliefs, the sense that not just there's another dimension but that it would mean the lives we lead would be lived afterwards in another way, in another form – do you ever sense that yourself? Is there any religious sense in you that matches that kind of feeling?

BLAKEMORE: None at all. I lost my faith, because I did actually have religious faith for a while when I was young.

CLARE: Was your family religious?

BLAKEMORE: My mother was at least nominally religious. I'm not sure whether she retains a strong faith now. Certainly the great aunt of mine who brought my mother up after her mother died, was very deeply religious and so I had quite an extensive experience of going to church and all those things. I was confirmed in the Church of England when I think I was fifteen or sixteen but pretty soon afterwards lost my faith. It sounds very arrogant, but I don't have any doubts or worries or problems with that at all and I think this is somewhere where science helps and particularly a knowledge of biology helps, because modern biology, that is inevitably based on the Darwinian concept, the idea that we are evolved creatures, that we are the product of an amazingly protracted, complex process of chance, provides an alternative which I find much more deeply intellectually satisfying than the notion of a curious detached deity or souls floating around. It's easy, of course, to ridicule those views but, you know, I wouldn't want my soul with all the complications and the personal experiences and the memories and all the quirks that any individual develops with age, floating around waiting to hover above some poor innocent child to implant itself again for the next generation, or whatever primitive view one has of souls.

And if it's a matter of waiting around in some celestial space for the end of the world, then I just say, 'Well, you know, what's going to be in this other world? I'd like to know more about it to know whether it's actually more attractive than just not being here at all.'

CLARE: Another powerful, driving impulse behind religious belief is the problem of suffering and some people listening would say, well that's fine for Colin Blakemore, the Darwinian, evolutionary theory of life satisfies him, and in general I think you'll agree your life has been a good one, a fulfilling one and long may it prosper. The problem is, that confronted by people whose lives seem miserable from the word go, for all sorts of disasters that you and I are very familiar with, if we just focus on disease for a moment, it's a cold reassurance in contrast say with the Christian message with its notion of a God sending a son down to suffer, to dignify suffering, to give it some kind of meaning. I think you will agree that there's an understandable drive behind religion that has sustained it in Western civilisation. So I'm asking you really, what do you say to someone who says, 'Professor Blakemore, I feel you are probably right about this but it leaves the question of the suffering of children with renal blastomas and cancers and the awful problem of dementia itself and terrible accidents, head injured people, stroke, the whole litany of human misery, it leaves it not only unanswered but curiously unsatisfactory. We become, if you like, the detritus of Darwinian evolution. We're just sad casualties of the remorseless progression to a better world, a better person, a better human being.'

BLAKEMORE: You paint a very cold picture of the alternatives to religious belief. Not to believe in a deity doesn't rule out compassion for instance. I would class myself as a humanist. I think we have an obligation. It's part of our make-up, our social make-up as extremely social animals, to have concern for our fellow creatures and that extends to the whole of the animal world but most particularly to our same species, to other human beings. So to give the impression that someone without religious view really is abandoning the sick or the disabled to their fate and simply just say, well, to be that way is part of the inevitable down side of a selective process, not at all.

CLARE: But I meant the issue of the meaning of that suffering?

BLAKEMORE: Well . . .

CLARE: What's its purpose?

BLAKEMORE: If life itself has no purpose and I do believe that life has no purpose in the deep sense of that word, then suffering has no purpose. It is something that unfortuntely some people have to deal with and are helped to deal with it by their friends, their colleagues, by their doctors. Of course, if it works, by their priests and by their own religious belief. But to paint a picture that somehow there's some noble meaning in being ill I think actually diminishes what it is to be ill.

CLARE: So If I were to ask you in a sense as a final question, what do you feel is the purpose of your life, the point of your life, what would you say?

BLAKEMORE: I don't feel that life has a purpose in the sense that you could ask a question why are we here. It doesn't have a purpose in the sense that there are goals to be achieved or that there's someone willing you along, wanting you to get there. But if you say do I believe that life presents opportunities that have to be seized or not seized, depending on the inclination of the individual, then obviously it does. I mean life is there for the individual to achieve and to create as much as they possibly can from it. We have this one opportunity. It's finite. We never know when it's going to end: When it has ended, as far as I'm concerned, there is nothing left, at least there's nothing left at a material or a spiritual level, except whatever it is that you have given to the world while you're here and in some cases, and actually, amazingly so in science, and this is one of the things that makes science such an exciting creative enterprise, at least the equal of the creations of the arts, it gives one the capacity to leave an inheritance of knowledge and there is nothing more valuable that human beings have created than the capacity to acquire knowledge. If you've a chance as a scientist to make a small contribution to the catalogue of what it is that we know about the world, for me that's immensely satisfying and quite enough.

CLARE: Were you present when your father died?

BLAKEMORE: Yes, I was. In fact, I was alone with my father when he died. He'd been ill for many years and was in hospital at the time.

CLARE: It sounds from what you said earlier that you really didn't know him, so I wondered was it a painful experience? What was going through your mind when you were there. Regret?

BLAKEMORE: Yes, and it wasn't just when I was there, it was afterwards for several months. This was one of the episodes of depression that I talked about. I was concerned that my father had died and that I felt that I hadn't really ever known him. He was a curious man, very different from other people that I knew and I just felt that we were from different worlds and regretted that intensely when he was gone. Full of self recriminations and doubts and worry and feeling that I'd lost an opportunity ever to make contact with my own father.

CLARE: You blamed yourself for that, did you? You felt that you could have done more?

BLAKEMORE: Yes. I was aware that I had become distanced from my father from maybe even the age of ten or eleven onwards, gradually drifting apart and of course I was partly, at least partly, responsible for that. Maybe entirely.

CLARE: Why? How?

BLAKEMORE: I suppose just being ambitious for a different kind of life from his. It's very difficult to say these things without seeming to be full of hubris, without appearing to be cold and calculating, but I was ambitious. I was ambitious to be successful in a profession but also I was socially ambitious. I wanted to get on. I wanted to escape from the really rather poor conditions in which we lived when I was very young anyway. We lived in a two up, two down rented house in a very poor area of Coventry and I wanted to escape from that. I saw through a chink, as it were, of social experience what the rest of the world was like by going to a grammar school and the world opened up in ways that it didn't for my father. I felt resentful for what the world, or to be more accurate, what the war, had done to him. Maybe that's part of the origin of my intense pacifism. I'm very strongly opposed to violence and to war. And I feel that this had robbed him of opportunities he might have had in his life and, my God, I wasn't going to be robbed of those things, so I detached, wanted desperately to detach myself from the problems that he had been forced into and I think that led to me separating myself from him to too great an extent.

CLARE: Did he ever give you any indication that he resented your moving apart?

BLAKEMORE: No. I think he was embarrassed by his inability to play the role that parents can sometimes play in their children's education, in going through homework, helping with lessons, talking about school, discussing careers. He didn't have that kind of vocabulary or ability. I think he would have done it and perhaps he was shy about even broaching that subject because of perception of his own inability. I mean he was very shy with me, reticent with me in a curious way. I don't know why.

CLARE: Did he keep his emotions under strict control?

BLAKEMORE: Not always. He was a big character, in many respects. A tall man, much taller than I am. He was garrulous, sometimes gregarious, a conversationalist. He loved to talk and chat. He was interest in politics. He could be quite an aggressive man. Not physically aggressive, I never saw him hurt anybody but he could be strong and his eyes could burn. He had dark brown eyes, black hair. He could be a passionate man in his feelings.

CLARE: Was he frightening?

BLAKEMORE: Yes, yes he was. I mean there were many times when I was frightened of him.

CLARE: Did you get an opportunity, when he was dying, to say anything to him or was that impossible?

BLAKEMORE: He couldn't have understood. I don't think he'd understood things that I'd said for a year or so before that because of the dementia, but I did talk to him, yes, of course and, you know, said the things that anyone would say in those circumstances, that I was sorry and said goodbye.

CLARE: What of him is in you?

BLAKEMORE: Do you want the biologist's answer? Half his genes.

Do you want the psychiatrist's answer? Some of his emotions and passions. Yes, I can see elements of me in him. I'm a very different person in the way I present to the world but maybe he was just a little, a little less good at presenting personas, at controlling himself or perhaps to put it another way, perhaps I'm not quite as good at showing what I really feel as he was.

Sir Colin Davis

One of the many interesting things about Sir Colin Davis is that, as he describes it, he appears to have undergone a fairly substantial personality change in the middle of his life. His own portrait of himself as a young man is that of an impatient, idealistic, passionate person given to irritability, 'extraordinarily bad behaviour' and 'seedy bouts of bad temper and rage'. He admits to having suffered fools with difficulty, to riding rough-shod over people and to indulging a tendency toward egomania. He was renowned for his demon temper. In the mid 1960s his life began to disintegrate. He was a hot favourite when the London Symphony Orchestra was looking for a successor to Pierre Montreux but the players voted against him. His marriage to the soprano April Cantelo disintegrated, a breakdown for which now at any rate he appears to take full responsibility. She had been an established artiste, an opera singer in her own right, and had done much to support him in his early struggle to establish himself as a conductor. He left her for their Iranian *au pair*, Ashraf Naini, whom he married in 1964, the same year that his first marriage was formally dissolved. He points to these events as the catalysts for the personality change which he believes has taken place.

It is not too difficult to identify factors in his early life which might explain the origins of some of that demon temper. As a young child and growing adolescent he knew much anxiety and disappointment. His father was one of the millions of young men whose lives were blighted by the ravages of the First World War, a war he had set off for young, handsome and talented and from which he returned four years later pretty well destroyed. Sir Colin, from the vantage point of his own mature years, is now both understanding and forgiving. But as a child he must have raged impotently at the sight of the two fathers – the one competent and attractive, inviting a strong identification and the other damaged and inadequate, who left the caring and upbringing of the seven Davises to his wife. She for her part is idealised as a devoted mother and a highly competent woman. Add the fact that his elder brother sacrificed his own education so that Sir Colin might receive one and then perished in the Second World War, shot down over Belgium, and the end result is a formidable burden of responsibility for any young man – a flawed father, a self-sacrificing mother and a brother who literally dies for you. It is tempting to surmise that the budding musician who entered marriage at the unwise age of twenty-two brought with him the passionate desire, 'an overdose of idealism' to be the powerful and successful man his father had not been and his elder brother could not be, 'to make it right' in Davis's own words.

The marriage that was supposed to make it right lasted fifteen years and produced two children. In the end it came apart amidst a series of personal crises. He was possessed by self-disgust. His career as a conductor was being hindered by his temperament, unpredictability and the fact that, as he revealingly puts it, 'I didn't know how to handle the material which is first of all the human beings in front of me and secondly the music.' He was profoundly at odds with himself. Indeed within the text of Sir Colin's discussion of the psychodynamics of controlling, moulding and leading that great constellation of competing egos and talents which is the modern symphony orchestra there is detectable the reverberating theme of the conflict between the two sides of his own personality, between what might be termed the good father, concerned to bring the best out of his charges, to encourage and cherish them, to make them feel valued rather than denigrated and the authoritarian, powerful father using fear and intimidation to bring about acquiescence and control.

Did conducting attract him as a young man in part at least because it offered him an outlet for his youthful anger with his father, his guilt for his brother? It is, after all, an activity which, within strict limits, permits, indeed encourages, fantasies of omnipotence. The modern stereotype of the orchestral conductor exercises a remarkable fascination for those interested in the nature of power and the manner in which it is exercised. The conductor, baton in hand, standing in front of a hundred or more musicians, in that very moment between the stilling of an audience and the sound of the first note, is the very personification of the power of one man (and it is still almost invariably a man) over the crowd. The very word *maestro* says it all. In his debunking book, *The Maestro Myth*, revealingly subtitled *Great Conductors in Pursuit of Power*, Norman Lebrecht refers to the tendency for powerful political leaders such as Margaret Thatcher, Richard Nixon and Helmut Schmidt to become devoted fans of individual conductors and quotes the philosopher Elias Canetti on the maestro's 'almost godlike authority':

> His eyes hold the whole orchestra. Every player feels that the conductor sees him personally and, still more, hears him . . . He is inside the mind of every player. He knows not only what each *should* be doing but what he is doing. He is the living embodiment of law, both positive and negative. His hands decree and prohibit . . . and since, during the performance, nothing is supposed to exist except this work, for so long is the conductor the ruler of the world.

Fatherlike might be a more accurate description than godlike. Or rather a certain kind of father – the kind that Colin Davis appears to have been in the first part of his incarnation as a conductor and before his personal transformation – the authoritarian, controlling, fearsome father. Many of the most famous conductors have been petty autocrats in the rehearsal hall and the orchestra pit, ruling unchallenged and unrestrained. Today, Sir Colin is dismissive of this stereotype, regarding it as bogus and its appeal as founded on the witless human tendency to admire egomaniacs. To some, his own personal renunciation of power, semi-mystical in its fervour and overtly religious in its origins, might appear understandable in a monk or a missionary, but it raises awkward and intriguing questions in the context of the symphony orchestra. If Sir Colin is not to command the acquiescence and the approval of the London Symphony Orchestra by virtue of a godlike or authoritarian presence, how is he going to do it?

His answer is to challenge the image of the ferocious father with that of the loving father. It is, it has to be said, a courageous answer, given that Sir Colin, when interviewed, had just been appointed the next conductor of one of the world's toughest orchestras. Music critics, not exactly overflowing with the milk of human kindness nor the understanding of the clinical psychotherapist, might be expected to fall with virulent glee on this revelation of Davis as the benign father and the hardy men and women of the LSO as a bunch of sturdy, vigorous children in need of love, understanding and encouragement. Yet, again and again in this interview, Sir Colin Davis endorses the virtues and the influences of persuasion, collaboration, communication. Hence my question concerning the kind of father he has become.

In this context it is worth comparing one of the great exponents of the conductor as dictator, Arturo Toscanini, and Sir Colin. Toscanini was not only a ferocious conductor – his tantrums and verbal abuse were legendary – he was a stern, remote, unforgiving father who never got close to his wife nor to his children. Davis, for his part, has not just changed in a fundamental fashion his manner of relating to the symphony orchestra, he has changed the way he relates to his children.

Sir Colin and Lady Davis have five children. He claims that his approach to them is quite different from the way he related to his two children by his first wife. At one point he declares that he has tried to make it up to the first two children without quite making plain (and to my regret I failed to ask him) just what it was he regretted. What does appear clear from his account is that his second wife has played a crucial role in the transformation of Sir Colin. Shortly after the interview I had the good fortune to meet her and on such a brief acquaintance I did indeed feel that she has played such a crucial role. She insists, for example, that there is more to life than music – heresy and anathema to the Toscaninis and the von Karajans of this world!

Towards the end of the interview with Sir Colin an interesting issue arises. How much does his emphasis on bringing the best out of an orchestra by persuasion and on the superiority of tact over tantrums owe to his admission that, unlike authoritarian conductors such as Toscanini and von Karajan, he himself is not a gifted musician, that he knows his limitations, that he is in touch with imperfection in a way that these other men never were? Is he coaxing and collaborative because he cannot impose his authority by demonstrating his technical supremacy, by making his orchestra acknowledge his superiority as a musician? Is his insistent renunciation of the power that seems part and parcel of the nature and role of the conductor plausible or is it merely a shrewd tactic, reflecting his realisation that he could act like Toscanini and von Karajan and Furtwängler rolled into one but it wouldn't work because he lacks the one element that such infantile omnipotence needs to make it work – namely the ability to match it with high musical talent of one's own? After all, throughout the interview, he manifests vigorous energy, exudes passionate commitment, expresses powerful personal opinions on a wide range of subjects. He lambasts materialism, laments the neglect of music, lauds political and artistic idealism. He projects himself as a powerful presence. He does not embody the calm, unemotional, detached psychotherapist that he so persistently endorses. In fact he is an unashamed romantic. His musical favourites include Sibelius and Berlioz, while his literary tastes cover Blake, Gurdjieff, Karantzakis and Herman Broch (whose *Death of Virgil* he is fond of quoting). Sir Colin is a canny man and knows his orchestra and his audience – and on this occasion I felt from time to time a member of both! He may very well be signalling the kind of person he would like to be rather than is. There is the sense of a lively tension between a furiously passionate and still angry man inside and the whimsical, dry, detached persona projected externally. That is not to say that Sir Colin is not a man more at peace with himself, more contented, more whole than back in his twenties and thirties. He is, but I feel sure if the LSO or one of his seven children warrant a tantrum they will still get one!

Sir Colin Davis has come to terms with his past not by obliterating, denying or projecting it as so many do but by absorbing and making sense of it. He still dreams of abandonment because it is still and will always remain an essential part of him. He is fascinated by death but its constant presence serves not to paralyse but to stimulate him. It is a reality to a greater extent than it is a fear. Sir Colin's interview, more than any other in this particular collection, is a hostage to fortune for his self-analysis and self-description constitute a prognosis which may or may not be fulfilled. At the end of the evening together, I left to return to my life as a psychiatrist. He left to take up the reins of one of the great orchestras of the world. He is poised to put into practice the beliefs and aspirations he so eloquently described in this interview. I wish him well.

CLARE: Sir Colin Davis is, at the age of sixty-seven, a highly acclaimed conductor of international renown. He has occupied some of the most prestigious positions in the musical world, has conducted some of the most famous orchestras in Britain and abroad. He was knighted in 1980 and is the recipient of such foreign accolades as the French, the Italian and the German Order of Merit. In 1995 he will become the first British-born conductor of the London Symphony Orchestra for seventy-four years and indeed, as far as I could discover, only the third. His two predecessors are Sir Edward Elgar and Sir Thomas Beecham.

The orchestral conductor has been described as a mythical hero. Indeed, according to philospher Elias Canetti, 'during the performance, nothing is supposed to exist except the work. For so long is the conductor ruler of the world'. Yet, seemingly, Colin Davis is not a tyrannical ruler but a benign one. His dislike of power and authority, his own as well as other's, is often quoted. Indeed, he has been described as a liberator who talks to players like a psychiatrist talks to patients.

Sir Colin, are you someone who is interested in the process of self examination, who thinks a lot about the motives that drive you?

DAVIS: Certainly, certainly. And I think if I didn't, I wouldn't know what the hell I was doing.

CLARE: And do you?

DAVIS: Know what the hell I'm doing? That's a very good question but whether I do or not, I am able to give myself sometimes the illusion that I do.

CLARE: This process of self reflection, self analysis, a lot of people have said to me apropos of this kind of series, well, people in the arts, artistic people, musical, theatrical, it's expected of them in a sense to be self reflective. It's part of their process. It's going to be very unlikely that you'll find that Sir Colin Davis isn't a thoughtful and reflective, self examining man. Do you think that's true, that all conductors, for example, would be people given to self reflection?

DAVIS: I don't know, but the nature of the work leads one to examine oneself because the minute you come into contact with another human being, and you have to work with him or her, you're in an ethical, moral situation and you have to examine yourself to see how you're going to behave and when you consider that the work of the conductor is about fifteen per cent music and the rest is dealing with human beings, it's small wonder that you compare a conductor to a psychiatrist.

CLARE: You would make it as high as eighty-five per cent?

DAVIS: Well, I mean everything I say is, er, hyperbole, but we've got to entertain the people. (Laughter.)

CLARE: Nonetheless, you're saying that a considerable proportion of your work is involved in influencing, handling, affecting people?

DAVIS: Well, you see, when you're studying a piece of music, that's your problem with yourself. But when you go out to work, and after all, the conductor is not playing one note, it's the others who are playing or they're singing, with a huge piece let's say, like the Berlioz *Te Deum*, you may have as many as 800 people in front of you so it does then become a question of how you are going to behave yourself.

CLARE: What was it about conducting that attracted you? You were a clarinetist.

DAVIS: I was a small boy first.

CLARE: Oh, it was as early as that?

DAVIS: And then I'd had a few gramophone records. My family was interested in music. My father had an interest in music. My brothers and so on, and when I went to Christ's Hospital where my brothers had already been I was given the clarinet. They hadn't played anything so the last Davis brother to turn up there was seized upon by somebody who became a fellow of English at Magdalen, I think, called John Stevens who played the viola, the bassoon and the piano and he said, 'You're going to play,' so I did. And, but it wasn't until I was about thirteen, I think that I went home one holidays and my elder brother had come home with a record and I remember exactly what it was, it was the *Eighth Symphony* of Beethoven conducted by Hans Pfitzner with the Berlin Philharmonic Orchestra and I heard that and it was a revelation. I never heard so much energy concentrated into half an hour before in my life and I wanted to be a musician and I wanted to be conductor. It was the most irrational decision that I've ever made but then, great decisions aren't rational are they?

CLARE: Wanted to be a conductor?

DAVIS: Yes, I wanted, yes, because if you are the conductor you've got to get your hands deep into the stuff of music and that's what I wanted to do. If you play one line and also, I have to admit, if you're an instrumentalist, and if you're a very, very good instrumentalist, you're forever up against the problem of keeping what you have, which is you've got to practise to be as good as you were yesterday. But if you're a conductor, you've got this wonderful opportunity of forever learning more. As Adrian Bolt put it once, in some reply to somebody, his ignorance was profound but not invincible (laughs), which is one of the most beautiful phrases I've ever heard. And that is the life of a conductor. The older I get the more I realise that my ignorance is absolutely impossible because I haven't got enough years to overcome even the smallest part of it.

CLARE: And the family atmosphere wasn't a particularly musical one? You say you were the first and it was largely a school influence.

DAVIS: No, it was music. Music was around. My father liked Elgar and Delius and Debussy. I don't remember any, well, very little Mozart, and there was some, there was a lovely recording of Stokowsky of the *New World Symphony* and so on. And bits of *The Ring*. When I was nine I remember one of my most secret vices was to wait till everybody had gone out and listen to the last scene of Siegfried again. I was so worried about this I didn't want anyone to know.

CLARE: And did you, just as a matter of interest, did you start to do what one does listening to pieces of music like that, did you, in fact, conduct?

DAVIS: No.

CLARE: Had you seen an orchestra being conducted?

DAVIS: No I hadn't.

CLARE: No?

DAVIS: It came later. During the war, I heard, like many other people, all the music from the BBC Symphony Orchestra with Adrian Bolt and they were evacuated to Bedford and they played in The Corn Exchange and that's when I learnt my classics. And he became the kind of hero figure for me, and that's when I wanted to be a conductor. And I bought his book and I read it and I practised what he preached.

CLARE: What was it, do you think, about your own temperament that brought you to being a conductor?

DAVIS: Don't know. I mean, most males between the age of twelve and sixteen suffer the most appalling changes. There's this on-rush of sexual potency and with it goes, occasionally, an immense emotional upheaval. And I think music really rescued me. God knows what I would have done without it. All my emotional excess was drawn into this wonderful world of sounds and I'm still in it, thank God.

CLARE: Were you a very emotional young man?

DAVIS: I still am.

CLARE: But then, can you remember?

DAVIS: Oh, yes, yes. I mean, music was for reality. Nothing else mattered very much.

CLARE: What was your home like? I mean, what did your father do?

DAVIS: Well, he suffered dreadfully, to be fair to him. He was a very handsome young man and he was a very good sportsman and he didn't drink or smoke and along came the first war and he was away for four years and I think that what he saw, what he experienced, what he did, whatever it was, it just pretty well destroyed him really. And when he came back and he got a job and then there was the crash, if you remember. We are too young to remember what happened at the end of the 1920s and then it was difficult to get a job and he had all these children. He didn't take the responsibility that he should have done, I'm sorry to say, for all the children that he had.

CLARE: How many?

DAVIS: We were seven. And we were very lucky because a great uncle who had made money in South Africa became a governor of Christ's Hospital and he was able to get us all into this school, which, in those days and I hope still is, was for people who couldn't afford to pay, but it wasn't so simple in my case. I took a scholarship to Christ's Hospital but I failed it and my elder brother left school so that I could go. This was during the war and he then joined a bank and then he joined the airforce and very sadly he was killed as a very young man. So I owe him, not only my education, probably my love for music and a lot of other things besides.

CLARE: What age would you have been when he died?

DAVIS: About thirteen, fourteen.

CLARE: Did you feel a sense of duty then?

DAVIS: Do you mean to my family?

CLARE: No, to your brother?

DAVIS: Of course, I was a little bit young.

CLARE: In a sense he died for you?

DAVIS: I didn't know, that he would die for me but I knew that he'd left school so that I could go but I wasn't quite old enough as I am now, to appreciate that enormous act of generosity and it was awfully difficult. He also left school, I think, to help our mother who suffered dreadfully the lack of proper housekeeping, to support all these children.

CLARE: What was she like?

DAVIS: She was a really absolutely devoted mother and had a really rough time. But after my father died, really he died rather young at fifty-six, I'm the only surviving male of this brood, she took a typing course, got herself a job and I think that she lived a very happy last twenty-five years of her life.

CLARE: What do you think, in reflection, all of that left you with? What did you carry and did it affect you subsequently when you became a father?

DAVIS: It left me with an overdose of idealism which I think I probably still have and that's why I made such a mess of my first marriage. I was much too young. But I think one of the threads running through all this was to correct all that. I wanted to have a family. I wanted lots of children and I wanted to prove that it was possible to do it as well as go out to work.

CLARE: To make it right?

DAVIS: To make it right, to, so to speak, correct history, in a sense and therefore to make it all right for him and for mother and all the rest. To show that it was possible to do it. And I've been married now for thirty years to my second wife and we have five children and although she says I shouldn't say such a thing because nobody will believe me, I've been faithful to her for thirty years and I must say, I feel an awful lot the better for it. (Laughter.)

CLARE: The descriptions of you, Sir Colin, in the earlier years, suggest someone with a great deal of irritability, impatience, even anger about you?

DAVIS: That's absolutely correct.

CLARE: What do you think that was about?

DAVIS: I think it was the sum of all kinds of things. There was an excess of emotion going in the wrong direction. I mean it was a negative emotion. It was rage at my own unsuitability to be a conductor 'cos I hadn't learnt an instrument as a kid, I hadn't learnt the piano at the age of three or anything of this kind. It was a rage that I was emotionally committed to doing something and I had no idea how to set about it, really. And I felt very much a member of a very poor family who had somehow to make his way. And, you know, impatience as a young man too often gives way to irritability, bad temper, rage and extraordinarily bad behaviour. But I think that I'm trying to make that good now.

CLARE: How, difficult would it have been? How, for example, class-ridden was entering into that kind of world? You say you came from a poor family . . .

DAVIS: I haven't any idea. Probably thought it was class-ridden.

CLARE: You did?

DAVIS: I thought it was but I'm not sure that it was. I don't know. On the other hand, if I had been as unpleasant as we're making out, it's difficult to account for why so many wonderful people helped me. So maybe I was a little bit schizophrenic.

CLARE: You were a passionate man?

DAVIS: A foolish passionate man, as Yeats says somewhere, 'Go to your room that I may die, though I die old, a foolish passionate man.'

CLARE: The reason that I refer to that, you said something like you were idealistic.

DAVIS: Oh, yes.

CLARE: And you linked that with getting married young.

DAVIS: But of course, I was much too young because I hadn't learnt that loving people means being responsible for them. As Hermann Broch says, it's taking somebody else's fate upon your own and that's not so easy for a young man. In fact, it's absolutely impossible but it's going to take a long time to go into all this, but I reached the age of thirty-five and I just didn't like anything about myself at all and I said to myself, I said, 'My boy, this won't do,' and I set out to tame myself and to put all this energy into a more positive form, and to overcome this, these seedy bouts of bad temper and rage and all the rest of it because it brought nothing at all, really. It's just a horrible poison that has to be got rid of.

CLARE: Was there something that was, if you like, the last straw, that said to you, look enough is enough?

DAVIS: Well, yes there was, which was the break up of my first marriage, of course.

CLARE: You took the responsibility for that?

DAVIS: Oh, yes, I mean, certainly. I may not have been entirely responsible but I certainly took it and I began to see all the dreadful things I had done and I shouldn't have done and then I wanted to put that right, and that's what I've been trying to do.

CLARE: Without going into it in complete detail, but when you say dreadful things and allowing for the hyperbole that you warned me about, what sort of dreadful things?

DAVIS: Well, just being such a stupid egomaniac like most old men, riding roughshod over various people that you should be responsible for. Being concerned with your own panic rather than the welfare of other people. It's so obvious I'm sure that when I say these words if anybody's listening they will know exactly what I'm talking about. And so I set out to change myself as far as I could and I'm still on this journey.

CLARE: What did you do?

DAVIS: I was living alone in a basement. It was quite funny actually because shortly after I left this basement the house fell down. Whether I contributed to this disaster or not I don't know but it was a bit gloomy because I went away for a week and I came back and there were mushrooms in my shoes. I mean it's hard living in a basement.

CLARE: Well, yes, Jung I've no doubt would say the collapse of the house signalled a new beginning.

DAVIS: Well, perhaps that was the fall of my old personality you see. It was the crust giving way.

CLARE: And at that stage you were already conducting?

DAVIS: Oh, yes, indeed I was, but I wasn't very good at it and I didn't know how to handle the material which is first of all the human beings in front of me and secondly the music.

CLARE: There seems to be a notion of a conductor that perhaps the early Colin Davis would have matched – tyrannical, imperious, controlling, authoritarian. Indeed, there are stories of conductors being able, almost with a flick of the eyebrow, to quell a collection of toughies like the London Symphony Orchestra. Presumably like many myths, there are conductors who live up to it in a sense – may not be naturally like this but live up to it. If there are such traits in conductors, this would have facilitated that development in you. They would have encouraged it because the conductor has, for a while at any rate, the opportunity to control.

DAVIS: Yeah, that was the image but I turned my back on that because I think it's all bogus.

CLARE: But that was the image?

DAVIS: Yup.

CLARE: And there are other conductors who in the history of conducting, who certainly cultivated that image?

CLARE: Yeah, well I'm sorry for them because I don't think it works really very well.

CLARE: You don't?

DAVIS: No, not really because I don't think human beings

function very well under tyranny, especially if they're artists. If the people are anxious when they play they aren't going to play so well, are they? I mean, the whole point of trying to handle human beings at all in whatever sense you handle them is to free them, is to make them feel relaxed so that they can give what they can.

CLARE: So why has the image of the imperious conductor lasted so long?

DAVIS: Well, because human beings in general only really admire egomaniacs. Why is Napoleon so famous?

CLARE: Is it possible that some orchestras actually prefer that kind of conductor?

DAVIS: Yes, but if they do, then it's no use me going near them.

CLARE: Well, do they? I'm interested. Are there such orchestras?

DAVIS: Fewer and fewer, and few and far between now. I call that a Jehovah complex. The people who want to have an overlord are really the underdogs and they want to think that the man who is in front of them is somehow infallible or he has something, the most incredible talent which makes him almost superhuman. Now that's so ridiculous because we know superhuman men, unless they happen to be Jesus Christ, they're unutterably human and if they pretend not to be it doesn't do them any good. They usually make themselves ridiculous.

CLARE: Is it possible that part of the rise of this stereotype of the conductor as, if you like, tyrant, relates to the times that we lived in – I'm thinking of the twenties and the thirties.

DAVIS: With the rise of fascists?

CLARE: Yes; and of course many of the conductors I'm thinking of were indeed German.

DAVIS: I hadn't thought of that. You mean it was a kind of disease that belonged to that period of history. It's possible. Don't know.

CLARE: I may be putting words into your mouth, but you have to cajole and encourage and support and bring the best out so it's very much a psychotherapeutic venture as distinct from control and authority. We're talking about a shift of style really.

DAVIS: Yes, but you see you're coming back to power, aren't you?

CLARE: I am, yes.

DAVIS: Excuse me, but if you come back to power, we know what happens with power. It's not for me to give a lecture on it because it's so universally known that it wrecks everything. The combination of power and money is enough to wreck any decent human being, isn't it? We've seen it. I mean power wrecked Napoleon. He started off as an amazing guy and then he decked himself out as an emperor and just simply went downhill and this is such an old story and it applies in the tiny little world of music too. But a man who sets out to be powerful is finally trapped in his own isolation in the end. I went, I decided to go the other way which is to try to free myself as much as possible so that when I stand up in front of those people, I feel entirely free and I'm not then hung up about my position, about making a mistake, about anybody calling me this or that or trying to puff myself out, up into some prodigious mushroom that doesn't really exist. It's self evident, isn't it?

CLARE: Yes, it is. The conductor is in control of a symphony orchestra, 130, 140 players of extraordinary individual talents, often quite complicated individuals each and every one of them I can just imagine in my little experience of artists that they are temperamental in many ways and sensitive and they've got expectations of various kinds, high standards, they drive themselves, they're competitive and they've got a great pride in their professionalism. And the conductor in charge of that, it does seem to me, is in one sense a kind of paradigm of power. I can understand why people say it is the ultimate, this man is in control of all those people. I think Ricardo Muti said something like, 'You wave your arm and all this sound comes out,' and it is one of the few wonderfully momentous examples of one man's influence over many.

DAVIS: Well, you can look at it like that.

CLARE: Yes, yes.

DAVIS: But I don't. I look at it as a sharing. It's very, very difficult for 100 people to play together without somebody in front of them who breathes. Now, if you breathe in you have to play.

You've got to breathe out again. If your music-making is tied to the wonderful apparatus that you have, you have a pulse and you have a breath and that is what controls music in the end. The length of your breath is the length of the phrase and there is the pulse and those are the two things that your really need. Now if you have any natural authority, I don't mean a bogus one which you've worked at by prancing around in front of a mirror, but the natural authority of a man who is at home with himself and actually knows what he is talking about and is helpful, you don't need this authority which is imposed on these people because they want to play well anyway. What they want to do is to feel so at home and relaxed that they can give everything they've got, because that's why they became musicians. And they don't need to be, to be hit on the head with a sledge hammer. I'm an old kind of humanist, I don't believe in any of all this. If you like, I'm a Christian, I don't believe in this rubbish. I think that there is a little bit of gold in every man who is sitting in front of me and I'm going to get my hands on it.

CLARE: What is your religous background? Are you Jewish, Christian, what are you?

DAVIS: Davis is a very Jewish name, but I was brought up in the Church of England and I had the wonderful fortune of having to go to chapel every day and twice on Sundays so I'm pretty well at home with the Holy Scriptures, which is a wonderful thing.

CLARE: Davis is a Jewish name. Are you Jewish in origin, do you know?

DAVIS: Davis is a Jewish name. Look at my nose and my short neck. As my daughter says, nobody can behead you, you haven't got a neck and all the rest. And it's true that we do look somewhat Jewish but if I'm Jewish I'm very proud of it. The best Jews are the most tolerant and wonderful people in the world and I've learnt so much from them as musicians it's impossible for me to thank them all.

CLARE: When you were proceeding through that adolescence and into the world of conducting, were you a very introspective person, then? Did you think about such things as what you are and where you came from, where you were going?

DAVIS: Yes, but I was such an emotional chap it wasn't until later that I realised that I had so much feeling I didn't have to worry about my feelings. It's about time I started thinking. And so, I read and read and read and read and I'm still reading like a maniac and I think, because I read for the wrong reasons to begin with, because I felt I had never been to university, I hadn't been educated properly and that meant I was not going to feel inferior to all those people who had, but these kind of foolish reasons for doing things fall away. Now I know I read because I love reading and that's the end of it and I know that every time I read something that I want to read I shall know more than I did before I read it. And all these ideas which I am trying to put over, not very well I'm afraid, have all come to me too from my reading and one of the most important things in my life was when, well you know how it is with books, you read a review somewhere and ten years later you say, there's the damn book on a bookstall and you know that's the book you were supposed to read and you buy it and I bought a book called *The Death of Virgil* by a man called Hermann Broch. He was a Viennese Jew and he ran away from Hitler, he was imprisoned and while he was in prison, he began to think about Virgil and about dying altogether and as I'm sure you know, Virgil on his deathbed thought of destroying his great poem and in this book not only is death examined in a very interesting way but Virgil came to the conclusion that he'd been wasting his time writing pretty verses all his life instead of making one useful human gesture. He was a doctor but he gave it up to write verses and that stuck in my head. That was one of the keys that turned my heart round. Well, the weather turned round, as Thomas says somewhere. And another immense influence was Nichos Kazantzakis who wrote, amongst entertaining books like *Zorba the Greek*, a continuation of *The Odyssey*. I don't know whether you've ever come across it. 33,000 lines picking up where Homer left off which is the kind of examination of human thought up to the point at which he died. And so on, and now I'm reading Stefan Zweig and to have contact with a, with a humanist of that kind and it's, I feel I'm rescuing him because he killed himself in despair, but he shouldn't have despaired because there's still one or two of us left. And so on, I have notions about ideas that enable me to march forward.

CLARE: And is there, for you, a human gesture?

DAVIS: Of course there is.

CLARE: Which would it be?

DAVIS: My human gesture when I stand up in front of that orchestra is to help them to play better than they could if I weren't there. And my human gesture to my family is to try to make the love I bear them something that is also responsible.

CLARE: Are you, then, very different to what you were or is this a constant, if you like, conflict inside Colin Davis?

DAVIS: It isn't. It isn't a conflict any more no, no, no it isn't.

CLARE: There would have been at some stage?

DAVIS: Well, there was and then I came to this conclusion I had to change my life, I dragged my new wife back to where I'd been a child because I wanted to find the child that I was because everybody says, as people generally say about children, that I was one of the most agreeable and jolly things they'd ever met. Well, in that case, it must be still there somewhere and now I think in my tiny way I have, as Goethe would say, won back my childhood and through a greater part of the time, as I said when I met you, I'm invincibly good-natured.

CLARE: I'm stuck for words! It is not often I meet someone who is invincibly good-natured. (Laughter.) It's not my occupational hazard. But if we were to take that view that there is this small Colin Davis child who clearly was benign and loveable and then there was a stormy period and without being too clear about the details, clearly your own family set up and what you've sketched for me already makes its own contribution to that. Has it left you with certain kinds of views that one might have expected? For instance, you said you were an idealist. Would you have idealised women, for example, given that your own father was, I suppose, in adolescent eyes, something of a failure?

DAVIS: Yes, I still think it's possible for people to live together positively and in harmony. And the only way you can start with that, for example, is with your family. Now my wife is a very considerable force.

CLARE: How did you meet her?

DAVIS: I met her in London, then she went back to Persia and she said she wouldn't marry me. She said, 'Anyway, you can't speak my language,' so she went away and for a year I studied Persian and I went and ran after her and she said, 'I'm not going to marry yet,' and so I gave it another chance and finally she did and we've been married four times so it's very difficult to get out of that one.

CLARE: (Laughs.) Again it was a passion.

DAVIS: Absolute passion. She still is, still . . .

CLARE: And would she have known you during this turbulent phase?

DAVIS: Not really, no. No, she wouldn't have known me then. Not in my worst moments. We've had some wonderful and great battles which will not be read about in the history books but they are equal to Leipzig and Lutzen.

CLARE: So in some way that temperament's still there?

DAVIS: Oh, there's plenty of temperament, it's just a question of which direction it goes in. But I wanted to tell you about her because she had a wonderful solution. You see she said, you know music is a mystery. If your children don't learn about music they will hate music and they will hate you because music takes you away, so they're going to learn and you, my boy, are going to practise with them. So, the first two boys were given fiddles, went to Suzuki classes. I took up the fiddle with them at the age of forty-eight or something. It hurt my wrists, not irrevocably, and so we made these terrible, terrible noises but the huge advantage of that is that when you practise with a child you have an absolutely direct and secret relationship with them through this magical thing called music. And so that happened with all five of them and she has made it possible for the children to remain my friends and I don't know how to express my gratitude for that.

CLARE: Did it help that you weren't a master at the violin, as you've described it?

DAVIS: Oh, of course, because nothing pleases a child more than to be better than his dad. I was absolutely hopeless but of course they very, very quickly got much better.

CLARE: But you were a very good clarinetist, I understand?

DAVIS: Yeah, I played quite well.

CLARE: Were you never tempted to continue as a clarinetist? You wanted to be a conductor?

DAVIS: No, because, you know, it's one thing to play a beautiful clarinet quintet but that doesn't give you much chance of getting your hands into a Bruckner symphony, really, does it?

CLARE: This may seem a very obvious question but I'm a bit puzzled by it when I see some of the people I see. When you were talking about this change you decided to make in yourself, the coming to terms with the fact that there were certain aspects of yourself that were unacceptable, and it's interesting that to some extent the way you expressed your emotions was one of them. Did it help to be a musician, because people talk about music enabling people to express their emotions very directly and I wondered whether that has any bearing on it or is that just irrelevant when it comes to trying to control something like impatience, irritability?

DAVIS: No, no, no. What you're saying is absolutely right. In music you are free to express the whole range of emotions from the utmost tenderness to the most violent aggression. The problem with a human being is doing things for the wrong reasons. If you're exploiting the musicians and the music for your own grandeur or for power or for whatever, it's bound to go wrong. It's not what it is. It's the thing itself which matters. If you learn finally to get your damned ego out of the way and you give yourself a chance. This is what I'm always saying to orchestras – hang your ego on the hook with your coat because it isn't any use in an orchestra. Many musicians object to this because they say we lose our personalities. I say, absolutely the opposite. It's the first time you're free because an ego is the greatest hindrance that a human being can have. A musician has this wonderful opportunity to surrender it and take part in something much greater than himself and feel therefore fundamentally refreshed for it.

CLARE: Yet many, many will say that some symphony orchestras at any rate contain a fair amount of talk of a collective ego . . .

DAVIS: Yes, that has to be challenged and with, as I said, invincible good-nature, overcome. There will always be somebody you can't beat but as long as they're in the minority, they won't say a word.

CLARE: How much is it related to insecurity, that you can do this now, because, because you are what you are, there's nobody to argue with?

DAVIS: It's based on the fundamental insecurity of being in a strange world. Being born into a society or an environment where you've got to fight for your life. We have it very comfortably but the majority of the people on this planet don't. It's not the ideal place to live for most people and even those who have it good still have that reserve of insecurity which drives them.

CLARE: When you talk about invincible good-nature and the way you handle an orchestra, you would expect someone from my profession to wholeheartedly agree with you. That's why I suppose in a sense somebody said you are with your players like a psychiatrist with patients. But I'll put to you the awful feeling I sometimes have that, despite my best wishes and perhaps yours, tyranny sometimes works. Now let me give you an example of what I mean. You say to me, look, what can you gain from an orchestra by terrorising them, if you like, or by making them so fearful, and of course you're perfectly right, it's common sense, people perform better when they're not so anxious. And yet your field, perhaps more than any, is full of famous accounts of terrifying conductors I don't want to name any less this may be libellous, I don't know the libel laws of Britain too clearly, they seem to change all the time.

DAVIS: Don't they have any in Ireland?

CLARE: Nothing like as many as yours! Some of the conductors I've seen named as quite terrifying, certainly have brought out of some orchestras some great sounds. And so, when I hear you say what you're saying, I wonder the extent to which you are arguing with some aspect of yourself. You're wishing this were true and in your life you're embodying the humanist principle.

DAVIS: OK, maybe you're right. I said I was an idealist and an idealist I shall die. What I have said doesn't prevent me from taking decisions. If somebody says it is going to be this or that I say it's that. But that's not tyranny, the personal tyranny that you feel. The fear of somebody. I don't think, and here we're back into *The Death of Virgil* that it is permissible to make beautiful music with terror. I don't see what Mozart has to do with scaring the pants off somebody. And I never will and you can talk till next Sunday and I still won't see it because I think it's wrong, I think it's immoral and I don't think it works.

CLARE: But even if it did . . .

DAVIS: If it did . . .

CLARE: The fact that you said it's wrong or immoral . . .

DAVIS: And it works for the wrong reasons.

CLARE: Yes, but you put wrong and immoral first.

DAVIS: Like you get information out of a prisoner by torturing him, that's the wrong way, and you don't always get the right information even then and you've wrecked the man that you wanted the information from and he's useless for anything else anyway.

CLARE: One of the reasons I do these interviews is I wonder how people negotiate moments in their lives that clearly change them. Many of my patients will say, 'Is it possible to change? Can I change? I'm an irritable, aggressive man, my kids can't stand me, my wife can't stand me, I come to you. Is it possible to change?' and it's a very good question because an awful lot of people don't seem to have the capability to change. So when I find someone such as yourself who says yes, I had a demon temper, yes, I was a difficult man, I had all sorts of insecurities and there came a moment in my life. You weren't too old. You were in your mid thirties. There was this change, there was this change over time. So what I'm interested in is what were the factors that were brought to bear on this?

DAVIS: Oh, there are so many. When I read what Gurdjieff said that only if a man carries in front of him every day the idea of his own death will he be ever be able to change anything at all. That was another of the key sentences in my life.

CLARE: Now, let me ask you, were there realities on which that was based?

DAVIS: Yes, because not only my father but very, very many human beings have reached deathbeds wishing they had done it differently and it's such a common thing. I don't want to die like that. I don't want to die like that. I don't want to die thinking, 'You damn fool. If only you'd thought a little bit more, things wouldn't have turned out so badly.' I don't want to do that.

CLARE: And that other death in your life, somebody dying before they could fulfill anything, did that come back in your thirties?

DAVIS: Of course, of course. I'm, in a way, living the life for my brother that he didn't have also.

CLARE: You would have been conscious of that?

DAVIS: Oh yes, of course.

CLARE: And do you think a lot about death?

DAVIS: Oh yes, and I'm so famous for talking about nothing but death that they bawl me out at home. They say, 'There he goes again,' and it got to such a wonderful point where my children actually drew me sitting inside a coffin, smoking my pipe, with a score of Richard Wagner with the worms all dancing around. It was one of the most entertaining drawings I've ever seen. And they drew me what was even better, which was a worm concert. It was like a Hoffnung. There was a great orchestra all being played by these most benevolent worms who were doing a great job for me. But all the same, there's a little worm of truth and going back to worms, there was another saying from the Greeks, from the moment you are born, is also born a worm who sets out to meet you. And sometimes you see him waving from the distance.

CLARE: And when you talk about death, because there are many ways of reflecting on death, what is it you particularly reflect on, what aspect?

DAVIS: I'm not reflecting on death, about which I know nothing and I cannot know until I get there, although there are tales of people who have been so near to death that they've come and tried to explain their experiences. I only know that I do not wish to depart this life having such a list of crimes in front of me that I need not have committed.

CLARE: But that's not what your children when they were sketching, saw. What's interesting about what you told me about the sketch is that it links your musicianship with this concept of death.

DAVIS: Yes.

CLARE: And I just wondered what was that about.

DAVIS: Well, what's that about? Well, if you listen to the greatest composer who has ever lived, which is Mozart, you are confronted with a vision of order which I think is not comparable to anything else we know. You are also confronted with a vision of the Garden of Eden. And I think that is part of my idealism and so far as it has been possible, I have tried, led on by all my heroes dead and alive, to occasionally be able to create that momentary vision of the Garden of Eden. I've got a little way. My children are lovely. This afternoon it was pouring with rain and I was watching out of the window and I saw my daughter come up the path across the fields and she was bending down and I wondered what on earth she's doing. I asked her when she got in and said, 'Did you drop something?' 'No, no, no,' she said, 'we were rescuing the worm.' Now that's how we want it. I taught them, 'If you destroy something and you can't make it yourself, you have no business to do it. If you can make another one of those bumble bees now, OK, you can, you can destroy it.' So, the Garden of Eden begins with the respect for the beasts that are in it.

CLARE: So, is there, side by side with this invincible good nature, tugging away, there's a streak of pessimism too, because, of course, much of what you see around you is not a Garden of Eden?

DAVIS: Oh, yes. My good nature, my idealism, my belief that if I can be free enough, people will come along with me is a protest against the idiotic behaviour of most human beings who get more pleasure out of destroying one another than in cultivating their gardens.

CLARE: Does that make you angry?

DAVIS: It makes me very, very, very depressed. I hate all fanatics. Anybody who knows, thinks he knows better is a criminal. In music especially. (Laughs.)

CLARE: Are you a melancholic person? Do you get low?

DAVIS: I get really down when I contemplate what is happening and the really depressing thing about human misery is to see only what's in front of our noses. And the depressing thing is that they don't think, they don't have these kind of conversations because if they did, they wouldn't be doing what they're doing in Yugoslavia or they wouldn't be making all this money out of drugs and guns and all this stuff, would they?

CLARE: That gets you down?

DAVIS: All of it gets me down and when I think of all the wonderful things that there are in this world, and yet, it's the mud that attracts them. I can't understand it.

CLARE: Looking back over your life, including those periods earlier, did you ever lose heart?

DAVIS: Oh, yes. We go with the pendulum. We have our highs and lows. You'd be the first to admit it, I'm sure, and I don't think any human is immune to that. But the lows, as I was reading in Stefan Zweig, the real lows, only give them in the end more strength to get up the other side of the hill.

CLARE: One of the people you are a great admirer of, a great interpreter of, a great exponent, advocate of, is Michael Tippett who I also was very privileged to interview. His interview very much sticks in my mind. I think of it very often because amongst many things he said was the strength that he derived from being something of an outsider and he described that in a variety of ways, pacifist, homosexual, not quite part of a certain circle. I often notice that when I meet people, they tend to describe themselves like that. Indeed, I sometimes think most people think of themselves as outsiders so it's not necessarily a definitive categorisation. Nonetheless not everybody does. Many people say, 'No, I wouldn't think myself that at all,' and I wondered about you, given your background, what you did with your life, where you are, the extent to which you've made yourself in a way that a lot of other people haven't. But virtually at every step you really made yourself, you made yourself a conductor, you made yourself an international figure and I wonder the extent to which some of the steam that fuelled that came from precisely that aspect that Tippett talked about, being an outsider?

DAVIS: Yeah, the black ball . . .

CLARE: That's why, incidentally, I asked you were you Jewish.

CLARE: Of protest . . . protest which lurks in one's heart. Yes, but we mustn't forget, you say I made myself. I have had the most incredible luck with so many friends who have helped me, some of whom I haven't seen for many years but I've never forgotten them. They were tolerant with me, they thought I was talented. They did everything they could to teach me music, to teach me how to behave and to teach me what I had to do. And not forgetting my children, my wife and all those musicians who have been generous enough to share things with me. It's true there is an immense glee in tackling this job that I do from the other end. Not from the obvious end of saying, 'I'm the greatest and you do what I damn well tell you,' but of turning up without an entourage and saying good morning and saying well let's get on with it. It's a lot of fun that way and I want to prove that it works just as well, if not better.

CLARE: But you used the word 'glee' in the sense that it really is something to be just one of them?

DAVIS: Well, to prove that to be a conductor you can be a perfectly ordinary person at the same time and you don't have to have special status. Because I hate it, you see. That's why I hate authority.

CLARE: So you would be a Boult? You would sit with them and drink tea with them.

DAVIS: Of course, what's the problem?

CLARE: But other conductors don't?

DAVIS: Well, that's their loss. They're not free enough to do it, is all I can say.

CLARE: The reason I'm interested isn't because I disagree with you, because I don't. When you were entering this profession of being a conductor, various people would have said various things to you. Certainly as I work through medicine, I am aware of this kind of expectation that mentors put on you. And there's the mentor who would be Sir Colin Davis. He'd say, 'Be yourself'.

DAVIS: I can say that now but what was said to me when I was young they said, 'My boy, it won't do, you can't do it the way you want'.

CLARE: Well, exactly.

DAVIS: Yes, but they were wrong and I'm going, I proved it. (Laughs.)

CLARE: You would agree with me that there would be conductors out there . . .

DAVIS: No, they're musicians who said, you know, you can't do it like that.

CLARE: And conductors who would have agreed with them, who would have adopted the trappings of power, would have moved around as, as authority figures.

DAVIS: Yes, everybody said that you can't do it like that.

CLARE: Herbert von Karajan certainly didn't do it like that.

DAVIS: Oh, yes, but he was a completely different kind of person. But I tell you, though, which is probably the key to all this, I'm not a supremely gifted musician like von Karajan nor like Toscaninni. I've been very, very lucky to have a balance between my brains and my feelings and my capacity as a musician. The man who is incredibly gifted from a very early age and is admired and adored at a very young age has a much more difficult time than I do because he is so used to this that he stops thinking about it. I know my limitations pretty well. I mean, I know my incapacity. I know that I can't sit down and play the *C Sharp Minor Quartet* on the piano. That doesn't mean to say I don't know it, though, I probably know it quite a lot better than a lot of other people do, but I can't demonstrate my talent as a virtuoso would and that has tamed me. If you haven't got a supreme talent, you can't cavort around as though you had and I thank God, now, that I was only given two talents and not ten.

CLARE: That's very interesting, and if you have a supreme talent, you're saying there's an enormous expectation.

DAVIS: And there's an enormous temptation.

CLARE: To demonstrate it.

DAVIS: To demonstrate it and also an enormous temptation to misuse it because you have power over people by definition. You haven't got to earn it. It's handed to you on a plate at the age of ten.

CLARE: So how would you sum up the nature of your authority over an orchestra? What would you identify as the elements that are the alternative to that other kind of influence?

DAVIS: They know that I'm making an attempt not to kid them by being something I'm not. It doesn't mean they have to like me or that they have to admire my music making or anything of the kind, but they can't say he's bogus and that's already a huge strength. Because what they love to say about us is that he's, you know, he's just pretending, he's not really a conductor, he's just standing up there. You've seen the kind of programmes, you know, it's all, he's a charlatan. I'm not a charlatan. I can't do anything anyway. Come on kids. (Laughter.)

CLARE: One of the delights I had reading about conducting, in preparation for meeting you, was I kept seeing the things said about your profession that are said about mine, and particularly the statement that an imposter could enter it. It's very difficult, as they keep telling me, to be an imposter surgeon, but it's quite easy to be an imposter psychiatrist. And there is some suggestion, likewise, and I'd be interested on your view on this, that it is possible to be an imposter conductor. Maybe that's why you're so alert to the issue of bogus. You're only concerned about the bogus if it's a real risk. It is a real risk?

DAVIS: Yes, and it is very much a real one because it's a real one with anyone who takes a position of authority, whether he's a politician or a churchman or a conductor or a psychiatrist.

CLARE: In my field there is so much public expectation about psychiatrists. In one sense they expect us to be charlatans and bogus and to speak incomprehensibly. But on the other hand there's, there is such an awe that some people can get away with that. Indeed, some patients get better because the expectation they place on their psychiatrist is independent of what the psychiatrist is like. Some orchestras might play better for that reason. That for a brief period anyway, for a brief period . . .

DAVIS: No, they could do it for a long time. But I can't do that. I have no idea how you'd set about that.

CLARE: But you know situations or events or conductors who have big orchestras where that's happened?

DAVIS: Where there have been conductors who simply mesmerised orchestras? Yes.

CLARE: Does it go on working?

DAVIS: But to mesmerise people doesn't mean to say you have to tyrannise them. I was making a moral point here.

CLARE: Yes.

DAVIS: A man who like Mitropoulos wasn't a tyrant but his talent was so incredibly fascinating that everybody played for him. He was a lovely man, actually. He didn't have to play all this rubbish because he simply could do it. Do you see what I mean? He was, he mesmerised them with his talent and the complete absence of bullshit, if such a word is allowed.

CLARE: It is. You've a word that's very psychiatric – 'mesmerise'. Now, some of the elements in the psychological aspects of mesmerising people are bound up with the very presence of the therapist, the very presence. Most people talk about Mesmer's eyes, for example.

DAVIS: Yeah, well they have a radiation, people do have.

CLARE: Yes, they do.

DAVIS: But if he's a bad, bad man like Caliban he can exploit that and then we get into the point when women start dreaming they've been raped by the psychiatrist and all that stuff, and the bad emanations and God know what.

CLARE: Are you conscious of that kind of power with an orchestra?

DAVIS: No, no, because I don't believe I've got it, and if I have it, I don't know I've got it, so much the better. I don't behave as though I have, so I'm all right. I'm saved from that particular sad part of it because I'm not concerned with myself. It's not the point. The point is that as a conductor you don't play any of the notes and the first thing you teach a young man who wants to conduct is, 'Don't forget that you don't do anything and your duty is to enjoy what they do.' And if you can help them by coordinating all this, you're a useful man, and you will die justified. You have grace. (Laughs.)

CLARE: And has that evolution in your character reflected in the way you related to your children? Did you change over time? Would you be a less authoritarian father with the later children than you were with the earlier children?

DAVIS: Completely different. Completely different. I'm afraid you'd have to ask them but I've tried to make that good also with the first two and I've been on very good terms with them but my eldest son of my second marriage is twenty-seven and he says it's impossible. Out there, look you're some kind of public figure and you're just a house teddy bear and that is about how it is.

CLARE: How would I get to the residue of the early Davis? Is there anything that might spark this good nature, not spark it, penetrate it?

DAVIS: Yes, if you could . . .

CLARE: If I use the image of a volcano, how do I waken it, or is it dead?

DAVIS: Try (laughs). We'll see.

CLARE: Well, what . . .

DAVIS: (Laughs.) Give me the keys of the kingdom, yeah, all right.

CLARE: That's right, give me a hint.

DAVIS: No, I'm not going to.

CLARE: But it does occasionally erupt. What is the phrase you used about your good nature?

DAVIS: Invincible.

CLARE: Invincible. Does that mean omnipresent?

DAVIS: I'm sending myself up terribly (laughter). I mean I don't know what the English word is, but in German it's *selbstpersiflage* which is sending yourself up really, because the moment in which you take yourself too seriously you're pretty well lost. You've lost the battle. They've got you. You have to watch out. It's a juggling act. Go on, and you know it too. If you stopped, if you suddenly take yourself seriously as a psychiatrist, don't you feel the ground slipping away?

CLARE: Yes but . . .

DAVIS: You've got to keep a distance.

CLARE: Yes, but I know that I do occasionally take myself seriously as a psychiatrist, too seriously, and I wondered when you say invincible good nature, what I was trying to get at was the extent to which this is a state in which you now feel comfortable or whether this is a state where sometimes you have to work at it, that there's a temptation that occasionally you regress.

DAVIS: Always, always, the shadow of regression is behind you, like Satan and . . .

CLARE: So if I talked to your wife or your children they'd say, 'Here, he's not always an invincible good-natured bugger, he can be very difficult.'

DAVIS: Yes, but they wouldn't mind that much. I have to work very hard at controlling my temper professionally, when I think people are not behaving as professional musicians or the whole system is completely crazy. I'm not going to go into details there but I have had to speak and I find, you see, it comes from experience, I find that if I am, as I absurdly put it, invincibly good-natured, things work better. That's the thing that works for me. Not to go in there and throw the chairs about. King Billy Bombles as Yeats put it. (Laughter.)

CLARE: One of the more public examples, it seems to me, of a collision between a certain kind of expectation and the sort of person you feel you were, was the whole issue of the Last Night of the Proms. That curious British institution that baffles me, but then I'm not British. And I wondered the extent to which your temperament as much as your intellectual judgement about the musicanship involved in the Last Night was not suited.

DAVIS: Yes, you're not British but you're an inhabitant of the British Isles.

CLARE: Quite.

DAVIS: Come on . . .

CLARE: So I do know a fair bit about the Last Night of the Proms. (Laughs.)

DAVIS: And we know, all know that these people who claim to be

Irish write better English than the English and all that and all
our famous heroes from Swift onwards, so don't try all that.
The Last Night of the Proms ceased to me to be about music
and I always had fantasies that somebody would break in there
with a machine gun and there would be a terrible massacre. It
could have been one of those British from over the way, from
Ireland.

CLARE: You got me (laughter). Yes but you . . .

DAVIS: But seriously, that's why I didn't want to do it any more. It
wasn't about music. I'm a musician.

CLARE: You felt it was political with a small 'p' or a big 'p'?

DAVIS: Yes, and it's not for me. People said, 'Well, why did you
give it up?' Because it made me famous. People saw me on
television. What a price to pay for doing something that you
don't really think is your job.

CLARE: Would you have had fantasies that you might have been
the one to reform it?

DAVIS: I couldn't reform it.

CLARE: You tried?

DAVIS: I tried, I tried here and there to make it a more musical
thing, make it more fun, but they didn't want it.

CLARE: No?

DAVIS: But it wasn't failure that made me run away, in that sense.
It was that I was asked to go on with it, even after I'd left the
BBC Symphony. I think it was Robert Ponsonby who followed
William Glock, but I didn't want to do it. It wasn't my thing
and that was part of my change, of course. As a young man I'd
have done it but I didn't want to do that. People thought I was
crazy.

CLARE: Did they?

DAVIS: Well, you know, to be in the public eye is everybody's
ambition. It's not mine any more. I keep out of it, really.

CLARE: And yet you're taking over the London Symphony?

DAVIS: Well, that's the basic conflict in me, probably, which is
what gives the spark, is the conflict between wanting my
private life and having to be a public figure. But taking over the
London Symphony Orchestra is really because they're a
wonderful orchestra and we can make wonderful music. I

don't want any of the rest of it. That's what I said: there's one condition upon which I'll take it and that is that I have no power.

CLARE: The rest of it being?

DAVIS: Auditions, choosing the players, choosing the conductors, choosing, you know, who else is going to conduct it, getting into all that. I didn't want anything to do with it. It's their orchestra. It's the London Symphony Orchestra Limited. Let them do it. They've done a wonderful job, I couldn't do it better. Why, for the sake of the feeling of power, should I get into things which are quite unnecessary? The music is hard enough.

CLARE: Yes, that's very interesting because it's so difficult now, almost at every level, the highest levels that one gets to there are all these administrative elements as part of the job.

DAVIS: That's right.

CLARE: Being a principal conductor would have involved all your predecessors in those kinds of things.

DAVIS: I did all that kind of stuff at Covent Garden and also in Munich with the Bavarian Radio and I realised that's not for me either. It's throwing things away. Throw away. Keep the good cards and . . .

CLARE: Someone else can do it.

DAVIS: Of course, much better and if the thing that you really want to concentrate on is music and not shaming your old age, it's better to get rid of the things that don't suit you.

CLARE: Are there things that you want to do?

DAVIS: No, no, not really.

CLARE: That would be a general ambition, the one you mentioned to me, which is to make good music.

DAVIS: Well, I take each day as it comes now. I haven't got so many left and they go by at a repulsive rate. (Laughs.)

CLARE: You've been a physically very healthy man.

DAVIS: Very lucky but who knows when one's health is going to crack up? That's another thing, so long as you're healthy you're all right but then don't, I was going to use a very coarse phrase but I won't, don't overdo it my boy, you know. Give yourself time, give yourself intervals when you don't work.

And so over the last fifteen or sixteen years I've taken all the school holidays off to be with my family, so that's great. So it's a couple of weeks at Christmas and three weeks at Easter and five or six weeks in the summer as a basic kind of thing. It's wonderful. That means giving up all kinds of things you might do. It means going to no festivals, not doing the operas that are available at Christmas and all this kind of thing. Never mind, you can't have everything. You want your family, you've got to sacrifice and it's so easy to lose a family in this profession just in a couple of weeks if you do the wrong thing. And that was the great fight between myself and my wife, how on earth are we going to get this right? But we must have got it right because we're still there. And after all, it's the survivors that count in this horrible world. Don't know why I got on to that, but you talked about the conflict, the conflict between family and profession is something that many actors and musicians or artists don't solve.

CLARE: But you also mention the word 'sacrifice', that to solve it involves some kind of sacrifice.

DAVIS: Of course it does. Any responsibility involves sacrifice.

CLARE: Now I'm again intrigued because one of the similarities I've noticed between medicine and music, medicine and the arts, is that there are powerful figures in both who say they demand the ultimate sacrifice.

DAVIS: You mean from their families?

CLARE: Yes.

DAVIS: Yeah, that's right. OK.

CLARE: The artist too. It almost becomes a religious value.

DAVIS: I think that's absurd because I think it only damages their artistry. You don't do that. If you love somebody, why do you have to murder them? It's the whole Oedipus thing, isn't it? It's God and Jesus and Abraham and Isaac and Jethro and his daughter.

CLARE: It's also the notion that there has to be a sort of one hundred per cent commitment. In that sense, human relationships are almost seen as a distraction.

DAVIS: Yes, I think that is totally wrong. It has to be a one hundred per cent commitment for what you do as an artist but why it involves sacrificing those people for whom you're responsible, I can't understand. Of course, it's difficult because inadvertently, you've planned this or that and you don't think and now you've got to change it, you've got to cancel it, it's not going to work. I've been through all that. But, as a young man said to me, do you mean to say you cancelled things, or you didn't go. I said the places I haven't been to are probably far greater in number than the places I have. But he said you're still there. I said, yes, you don't have to do all this.

CLARE: That took some nerve, though.

CLARE: It took some nerve and it took a lot of juice out of me but I accepted it. It's difficult.

CLARE: Are you a man who has profound fears, or are you fatalistic. Do you say quite regularly, 'I'll take what comes, each day as it comes?'

DAVIS: I have to.

CLARE: Are you a worrier?

DAVIS: Not in my better moments now.

CLARE: You sleep well at night?

DAVIS: I do. Not like a murderer. (Laughs.)

CLARE: So there are no significant anxieties?

DAVIS: I have terrible dreams of abandonment and like everybody else, when my wife's been particularly horrible to me or my best friend had his head chopped off or there are lions in the wardrobe. These are perfectly normal, I wouldn't worry too much about them if you have them (laughs). But if you'd like to consult me. (Laughs.)

CLARE: Well, it may come to that, Sir Colin (laughs). So that when you do look back, because you've been talking about your early life and your musicianship and your family life and the changes, and you've been pulling my leg a bit as well. Are you surprised at what has happened to you?

DAVIS: Yes, it seems a pretty unlikely position to be in when I look back on my beginnings. Certainly does (sighs), but I must have had some talent for taking good advice. I think probably that's a very important thing. I would put it another way. When you hear something you're supposed to hear, you're not absent. You know what you're supposed to be, you recognise immediately when you have to know that, whether you're reading it or when, whether somebody says it. Do you understand what I mean there?

CLARE: Give me an example.

DAVIS: Well, I've given you some examples from literature.

CLARE: No, but from your life.

DAVIS: Yes, well, when having planned too many weeks away from home and my wife said but that's not on, it took some digesting, but I knew she was right. And it's that. Otherwise I couldn't have my family, you see. There has to be a margin which is flexible at the edge of every ideal, there has to be the ability to compromise between human beings, otherwise I can't see how you get anything done at all.

CLARE: And you've said in that example you give that there have been times when you've sacrificed the music for the family.

DAVIS: Certainly, or ambition I would say. You haven't sacrificed the music because you haven't made it.

CLARE: No, no.

DAVIS: At no point has my family demanded that I sacrifice the music, so to speak, for them, but to sacrifice your family for greed or ambition or power is actually not on.

CLARE: Just one last question, you referred to humanist values, do you think much of what comes after death? You said you think of death and you talked about that caricature, a cartoon that they drew. What about after death?

DAVIS: Well, I haven't the faintest idea and neither have you. There are so many intriguing theories, but I'm waiting my turn with an open mind. If there is a hellfire, perhaps I won't burn too long in it. If there's rebirth, maybe I'll come back either as a hamster or a better musician than I am now. I mean, I don't know.

CLARE: But why would you burn, with your invincible good nature?

DAVIS: Well, that is the most irritating thing to the devil, that can possibly exist!

CLARE: Do you find paradoxically that your invincible good nature can be irritating to others?

DAVIS: No, not to the people with whom I work, no. It gives them confidence and relaxation. It gives the impression of being a master of yourself, which you probably aren't at all. And that gives people confidence, wouldn't you say? I mean, if you're marching up and down chain-smoking and scratching your head and looking furtively behind you're not going to give your patients much confidence, are you?

CLARE: No. You really are at peace then?

DAVIS: I think as far as it's possible for me to be at peace, I am at the beginning of what that might be like.

CLARE: So Freud was right, in a way, when it comes to you, because in so far as he could identify what gave people happiness and satisfaction, he identifed two areas. He said to love and to work, and you've laid great emphasis on those elements in your life.

DAVIS: Yes, but he wasn't alone. I think Jesus would have said much the same and Mozart demonstrated it. The only other question I think is to occupy yourself in a positive way, however humble that may be, like what we do, for the good of other people. It can only increase your capacity to love because you feel you are useful and to feel that you are useful and you are contributing to your fellow human beings and, and their well being is the most you can expect from this life. And also, I'm going to be a bit more arrogant than that. I think that when we make music we demonstrate not only that it's possible to put your ego on one side for a little, but it also shows that human beings can, and very readily will, cooperate with one another. You wouldn't think so from politics but it's quite clearly possible. And in our tiny little way we're demonstrating against chaos, too. More organisation is where music is. Less organisation where politics is. (Laughs.) Here endeth the lesson.

CLARE: No dominance?

DAVIS: No man may think that he knows better than his neighbour. This is the problem of war and, of couse, while the music is going on nobody may speak. It's been extraordinarily difficult to declare war with a Mozart symphony. You have to have words to misuse, which brings me back to something which may entertain you. Of course, in the beginning was not the word, in the beginning were the notes, because God knew about the word but he'd shut away the books. And it was Lucifer stole the books and brought them, and, of course, for that he was thrown out and he brought them down here so that we could make war for him because with the notes it was quite impossible to start a war.

CLARE: So, for you, in the best sense, music is political but the political statement it is making is a statement about human collaboration.

DAVIS: Yes.

CLARE: And a lack of competition.

DAVIS: Yes, for the thing you are doing which is, in our case, making the most beautiful music we can, cannot in any sense be a negative ambition.

CLARE: So in short you would describe yourself as a fortunate man?

DAVIS: Unbelievably fortunate and I try to deserve my fortune.

CLARE: Sir Colin Davis, thank you very much indeed.

DAVIS: Thank you.

Les Dawson

On Thursday, June 3rd I met Les Dawson for the first time. It was a warm summer evening in Manchester and he had driven down from his home near Blackpool with his second wife, Tracy, to record our interview. He did not look very well. He perspired excessively, breathed at times with some effort and his skin colour was pasty. He was having a heart check-up, he told me, later that week. (He had had several heart attacks.) But he was in tremendous good humour and talked, joked, clowned and recalled memories of his life and times with an energy and gusto that was infectious. Tracy sat with my producer, Michael Ember, and from time to time Les would nod to her through the glass panel, grin and after he had delivered one of his more teasingly chauvinistic opinions on womanhood glance conspiratorially at her and wink. He was immensely proud of baby Charlotte and, meeting head-on the criticism of a man of his age having a child, declared, 'I want to be here long enough to see her happy and settled and then I'll go,' and then added, characteristically, 'Well I won't. I'll struggle a bit,' and we both laughed. And then we did something which rarely happens at the end of an *In the Psychiatrist's Chair* interview – we exchanged addresses. I told him that I wanted him to come to Dublin and if he did I would arrange for him to meet and sit with a group of my patients and talk as he had done with me of his life and his experiences, what had helped him through the bad times of heavy drink and depression, his philosophy of life and his simple faith – 'No matter how bad things are, and there are some terrible things, there's always a light side. Most people I know who've gone through very bad times and have had a sense of humour always come through.' Whether he would have convinced those patients, many of whom have been through terrible times, I do not know. I know he would have given them laughter and, for a brief moment anyway, brought them close to joy.

One week later, sitting in my car in a Dublin traffic jam, I turned on the six o'clock news to hear that Les Dawson was dead. The interview he had given me and I had at the time felt so privileged to have been given, was his last. While attending a check-up of his heart, he had collapsed and died. The interview had not yet been broadcast. Listening to it in the aftermath of his death it had the feel of a valedictory summing up, a personal reflection of a full and varied life, lived exuberantly, even defiantly. Michael Ember and I discussed it and decided to send the full version – Les had sat and talked for nearly two hours to me – to Tracy Dawson for her decision as to whether it should be broadcast. A few days later she told us that she wanted it broadcast; indeed hearing Les so happy and so funny and so honest had helped her, had moved her to tears, that for her it was the best interview he had ever given. And so we broadcast it and for Michael and myself and all our colleagues at the BBC it became part of the tribute to a very funny, generous, wise and happy man.

I use the adjective 'happy' with a certain diffidence. Recently I was asked to deliver the Thomas Baggs lecture on happiness at the University of Birmingham. Baggs, an alumnus of the university around the end of World War One, had made his fortune in the US and then left some money to the university to endow an annual lecture on the subject. A descendant of his told me that from what she knew of him he had been a driving, successful, ambitious and distinctly unhappy man whose bequest, she suspected, reflected a feeling that at least one useful thing that might come of university research might be an answer to the riddle of happiness – how come we all pursue it and yet so little is known about it? When the distinguished Vice-Chancellor of the university, Sir Michael Thompson, extended the invitation to me to be the 1994 lecturer, I pointed out to him that asking a psychiatrist to talk about happiness was a little like asking a publican to discuss the merits of sobriety or a politician consistency! My work, for the most part, brings me into contact not with happiness but with unhappiness, not with joy but sadness, not with contentment but discontent. Psychiatric textbooks bulge with references to melancholy, depression, anxiety. They swell with analyses of the negative impact of bereavement, separation, loss, the detrimental consequences of stress, dependence, addiction, the pathological effects of deprivation, isolation and neglect. You will search in vain for any reference to happiness, joy, contentment or the dozen or more synonyms for that state of mind which for Alexander Pope was 'our being's end and aim'.

In my professional experience as a psychiatrist I do not encounter too many people who I would describe as happy. The people I meet outside the psychiatric clinic, however, are equally reluctant to describe themselves in this way. Perhaps there is some truth in George Bernard Shaw's observation that 'men who are unhappy, like men who sleep badly, are always proud of the fact'! Happy people may feel a certain shame and guilt and admit their peccadillo with difficulty. Confessing to being happy suggests remarkably good fortune, a life devoid of set-back and failure, a degree of insensitivity to Auden's 'dreadful shuffle of a murderous year', those miseries and misfortunes of mankind detailed day by day in newspapers, on radio and television. To be happy suggests an inpaired ability to understand and empathise with those whose lives are plainly miserable and unfulfilling. Perhaps that is why during the course of nearly one hundred radio interviews only a handful of interviewees have spontaneously described themselves as generally happy people.

What do the majority of ordinary people regard as of importance to psychological well-being and happiness? A few years ago, there was a government-backed drive to persuade young people to stay clear of illicit drugs which was focused on the exhortation, 'Say yes to life.' Two Oxford researchers enquired of a pilot group of subjects as to whether there are any characteristics which people regard as life-affirming. Five life-affirming and five life-denying characteristics were mentioned by more than ten per cent of the sample. Of the life-affirming characteristics, drive, sociability, happiness and optimism were significantly endorsed. The respondents seemed to be saying that people who believe in being happy and work at it end up happy people. Other studies of the factors in physical as well as psychological well-being suggest that having strong social and personal relationships, a solid sense of personal worth and a lively interest in life are all reliable predictors of being happy.

The psychotherapist and guru Carl Jung was once asked what he considered to be the basic factors for happiness in the human mind. He responded with the following list and in the following order:

- Good physical and mental health
- Good personal and intimate relationships, such as those of marriage, family, and friendships
- The faculty for perceiving beauty in art and nature
- Reasonable standards of living and satisfactory work
- A philosophic or religious point of view, capable of coping successfully with the vicissitudes of life.

When I apply Jung's dicta to Les Dawson I find that they make an impressive fit. He had reasonable physical health until the heart disease that killed his own mother at the early age of forty-three years began to affect him. Like many people who rarely suffer pain he had a marked fear of it – it was the fear of dying rather than of death that worried him. His psychological health, however, was somewhat more complicated. The early poverty, family difficulties, his father's drinking took their toll particularly of Les's self-confidence. He was not then the confident nor the philosophical man that, bolstered by success as a comedian, he was to become. And even then, as is clear in the interview, he never could shake off the insecurity and self-doubt acquired during his formative years. He did, however, stumble on a most remarkable talent and a formidable truth, namely that the one thing he could excel at was failure and he could turn that failure into comedy. But, paradoxically, his success as a comic could only be guaranteed by his encountering failure again and again.

He did make a successful first marriage and his wife and children sustained him through difficult times. I suspect that like many men he came to the realisation that it is these relationships and not the public adulation and fame which ultimately matter – I would not be surprised to be told that as a father he took more direct interest and was more immediately involved in baby Charlotte than in the two daughters and a son by his first wife,

Meg. But, as his own account makes plain, he could not survive the loss of Meg – he, like so many men, could not survive on his own. I recall a former research colleague of my own, Monica Briscoe, when we were working together at the Institute of Psychiatry in London, showing that married men are psychologically healthier than married women and single men. Her studies, supported by many others, lent support to her conclusion that 'women need jobs in the same way that men need wives' – to sustain self-belief, self-confidence and self respect. Dawson's personal account of his relationship with both of his wives certainly reflects the extent to which his ability to survive and sustain his own life crucially depended on having a wife to sustain and support him. His work did provide him with a reasonable standard of living and with great personal satisfaction too – another of Jung's factors – and he would often point out to himself and anyone else who happened to be there, 'You've not done bad for a slum kid.' And he was always preoccupied by the central religious question of human existence – what is the point?

When asked if he was religious, his answer echoes that of many: 'I can embrace Christ but not the Church.' He was drawn to Buddhism – his approach, in the words of one critic, Robert Chalmers, 'is characterised by the kind of naive enthusiasm which a formal education would have smothered at an early age'. The lack of formal education did not leave him bereft of one of Jung's other factors in happiness – a faculty for perceiving beauty in art and nature. Dawson loved literature and he adored words, playing with them, subverting them, sabotaging them. He was exeedingly well read and quite capable of disconcerting a patronising critic with a sudden burst of Wordsworth or Shelley. He cultivated literary ambitions too – indeed he had published quite a few books, most of which had sunk without trace, although one, a rambling, discursive futuristic novel set in Huddersfield entitled *A Time Before Genesis*, deserves a read.

When I re-read the Les Dawson interview I noticed an interesting thing. Whenever we began to talk about the dark side of his life, the miseries and conflicts of his early childhood, the separation from his father, the lack of a formal education which he forever resented, the struggle to survive and make a name, the drinking and the womanising and the periods of bleak despair, we ended up contemplating what he insisted on calling 'the credit side' – the feeling of community when he was growing up, the sense of an extended and warm family, the love of his wives and children, the satisfaction and enjoyment in his work as a comedian. I do not believe that it is simply an example of denial at work – Dawson readily acknowledges that his life has not been roses and he has not been a stable individual – but rather an implicit acknowledgement on both our parts that a life was being summed up, that an account was being constructed and a judgement was being made. When he is tempted by me to be a little gloomy, a touch pessimistic, he begins to succumb and then there is a humourous flash and the cloud lifts. I ask Dawson if he is a pessimist and he thinks he is. A Sad Man? Well, yes perhaps but this then leads on to reflections on cowardice, the inability to say no to people and the role that first Meg and then Tracy have in helping him control his urge to take on too much. There is a link between all of this and it is, I suggest, the sense that Dawson had of life's chance and mercurial nature. Time and again, he muses on the arbitrariness of his life. His mother's death, his father's reaction to it, and then his own wife's death fuel his belief that life is a cosmic joke but not one to render us impotent and despairing but to encourage us to laugh through our suffering. His humour is not the humour of gags and punchlines but a humour of images shrewdly painted with lovingly selected words. The message is that life is a bitch and can be bleak and unforgiving but it is to be lived and enthusiastically enjoyed at a pace because you never can tell when death strikes.

'I want to be there long enough to see her happy and settled and then I'll go.' That was his answer to my question about the criticisms that some people expressed when they heard that this man in his sixties was going to become a father again. His own mother would almost certainly have expressed the same hopes for her Les – to be happy and settled. Sadly he won't see Charlotte settled. She may, however, one day take a close look at the life led by this extraordinary man with the facial appearance of a 'bulldog chewing a wasp' and the gloomy ruminative comic skills reminiscent of the great W.C. Fields, and may find consolation in the fact that her father looked loss and deprivation and death in the face, glowered and grimaced in a manner that endeared him to millions and then got on with it and said a very emphatic 'Yes' to life indeed. The interview helped Tracy Dawson in the conviction that Les was still very much alive in the minds and hearts of all those privileged to have known and loved him and who he made laugh. It was Martin Luther who reportedly said, 'If you're not allowed to laugh in Heaven I don't want to go there.' I believe you are and Les is there.

CLARE: Les Dawson, the rubber-faced comedian of morose countenance with a seemingly inexhaustible supply of mother-in-law jokes, was born on February 2nd, 1931 in a slum district of Manchester. When in work, his father was a labourer in the building trade and the Dawson family lived in extreme poverty. The young Les left school at fourteen and after a series of menial jobs, was called up for National Service. After the army he went to Paris with £30 in his pocket, to write, but after several months of trying to keep body and soul together by playing the piano in a house of ill-repute, he returned home and started the long and often dispiriting journey through northern clubs and pubs to television and stage stardom.

His comic talent has made him one of Britain's greatest pantomime dames. He's also tried his hand as a straight actor, most recently on BBC television when he played the part of a 100-year-old woman in the black comedy *Nona*, about life in Argentina after the Falklands War. He has appeared in a number of Royal Variety performances and is said to be a favourite of the Queen and Prince Phillip.

Les has two daughters and a son by his first marriage to Margaret Plant, who died in 1986 of cancer. Last year he became a father again at the age of sixty following his marriage to his second wife, Tracy, who is seventeen years his junior. Apart from two volumes of his autobiography, *A Clown Too Many* and *No Tears for the Clown*, the authorship of more than a dozen other published books testifies to his continued literary ambition.

Les Dawson, how do you feel about talking about yourself?

DAWSON: You know more about me than I know about myself. How do I feel?

CLARE: About talking about yourself?

DAWSON: I don't know. It's like sitting back and seeing somebody else. You don't relate that closely. Talking about me, I feel very detached from it.

CLARE: When you were writing the two volumes of your autobiography, having read both of them, I sense that you're continually surprised at where you've got to. That you contrast continually the earliest years of your life and where you are now, the poverty, the simplicity of life, the lack of material goods, really being born into a fairly basic situation and now where you are – success, well known, recognised everywhere. Is there that element continually in you? Are you continually at odds, in a sense, with these two aspects of Les Dawson?

DAWSON: Oh, constantly. I can't forget the past. I've always said to most of my contemporaries that the future, only the future matters, which it does of course, you must go on. But the past of course is still the basic layer which your persona develops on and I think that those days still leave a mental scar. A small point putting it a little better, when the children were younger, if I saw them waste food it used to really annoy me. I could fly into a real temper over that.

CLARE: Your own kids.

DAWSON: Yes, because we hadn't got any. We were very lucky. The only way mother could feed us was by throwing a tin of soup in a pan, it was almost at that level! So I hated waste because we couldn't afford to have waste. If I left a meal at home, and I didn't eat it, that meal would be there the following day. My father would say, 'You either eat it or you don't and that's it.' So it worries me sometimes.

CLARE: You've mentioned that, a kind of irritation with your children when they take for granted things that you just wouldn't have dreamt of. Is there a more fundamental scar? What would you say has been the single greatest impact on your formation of those early years? What do you think its done to you?

DAWSON: When I say 'mental scar' I don't mean in the sense of an ugly mark that left me with a traumatic experience. It's just in some ways a very nostalgic scar, for want of a better phrase because also on the credit side of all this past, there was a warmth, there was the love, comradeship which you had in those days. Every street was sort of its own mentor.

CLARE: That would have been true would it? Just say a little bit about that. In your own street would you have known all the neighbours?

DAWSON: Oh yes, there was no child ever left to want. There was always somebody to fend. There was always an amateur undertaker. There was always somebody to knock you up in the morning for work if there was any. There was always somebody who knew how to deal with coughs and colds or something. There was always a doctor. So the whole street was a community within itself and it was like a small nucleus of people who were different from the next street, but collectively it was a great social pattern. So there was a lot of affection in Collyhurst in those days.

CLARE: Were you an only child?

DAWSON: I had a brother but he died, he died when he was very young.

CLARE: What age were you? Was he older or younger than you?

DAWSON: No, he was younger than me. I was about six or seven when he died.

CLARE: Do you remember that?

DAWSON: I can only remember people rushing in the house and, you know, holding my mother down and all the rest of the house in a turmoil.

CLARE: He was just a baby when he died?

DAWSON: Yes, just a baby when he died. Yeah, more or less.

CLARE: Do you remember him being born? Do you remember the fuss about him coming?

DAWSON: Just about, barely. That was in those days all the street knew. Everybody was there to dance attendance on the pregnancy so I only know it barely, I would be a liar if I said I could go into any depth on it.

CLARE: What about the fact of being an only child? You don't dwell on it much. I wonder, had it much significance? In those days one tended to see families with larger families.

DAWSON: Oh good God, in Collyhurst some of the families! There were so many kids in one family they had lifeboat drill. It was ridiculous. There was that many wet nappies there was a rainbow in the lobby. Big families were the norm because that was the sense of power, remember. And it still is in most tribal areas and ethnic groups. There's a sense of family and so it was strange to be the only child but it never actually affected me because my parents were very protective of me despite the fact that my father was out of work so often the insurance stamp was no more than a penny black! There was very little work. I think one of the poignant things I do remember is listening to him groan as he sat near the fire and my mother rubbing oil into his back because he was a hod carrier in the building trade. He used to set the bricks up on it and he was in terrible pain with his back and I always remember that and the sense of despair which was tempered by this closeness which was nice. So I grew up with a liking for family life, a love of it.

CLARE: Were your parents affectionate?

DAWSON: Oh, yes.

CLARE: Physically?

DAWSON: Oh, yes.

CLARE: How close would you have been to your father?

DAWSON: I was quite close actually until I was about ten or eleven, oh no, younger than that, when the war broke out and of course, he went to war and never came back for about four and a half years. And a stranger knocked on the back door, I'm now about thirteen or fourteen, and I've missed those vital years. So there was a tension between us because this wasn't the man I pictured who went. He was a taller man that went and a much younger man, a vibrant man. The man who came was smaller and I thought, 'This isn't the dad I had,' and of course it was, but of course, I'd grown up.

CLARE: Where had he served?

DAWSON: Yes, he was in the Middle East. For four and a half years I never saw him.

CLARE: And during those four and a half years where did you live? Were you still in the family home? Were you evacuated?

DAWSON: No, we did a mysterious move from Collyhurst. I vaguely remember being propped up on the back of a cart with my few belongings as we pushed away from Collyhurst. We got this corporation flat and then from there we moved to a corporation house in Blakeley, Manchester. And he just knocked on the back door the night he came home and there was his kit bag on his shoulder and I somehow had to find a new relationship with him.

CLARE: And had he changed? He'd physically changed, but had he changed?

DAWSON: Well, it's hard to say because it's a different man who went away obviously, you know, and it was a bit difficult for a while to adjust to him.

CLARE: Were you closer to your mother?

CLARE: Oh yes, extremely so. We'd been sort of in rest centres when the war was on because the house was bombed and everything, so there'd always been this closeness together which lasted, well, until she died.

CLARE: What sort of woman was she?

DAWSON: Small, fiery, full of good humour and I think if I've inherited any sense of humour at all it's from her.

CLARE: Really?

DAWSON: More than my father.

CLARE: Were either of them performers in the sense of entertaining others or being humorous?

DAWSON: No, but she was marvellous, she was a great mimic, my mother.

CLARE: Was she?

DAWSON: Oh, a tremendous mimic. The only one in the family with anything of a comic was my grandfather.

CLARE: That's her father?

DAWSON: Yes, her father, who was a great pub wit. A great one, he could reel off James Joyce, you know, with his great Irish brogue and he was quite a wit.

CLARE: He lived with you? Your mother's parents lived with you?

DAWSON: In the early days in Collyhurst. Well, there was nowhere else to go. There was this sense of community which overruled the fact that we were living in sort of very small premises. When a family gets together it can overcome anything. It creates its own space, oddly enough, in its own way.

CLARE: Was there much sickness?

DAWSON: No, I don't remember a lot of sickness, no. What they had is little things I remember. The old fashioned back-to-back ovens, those marvellous great things, there was always a fire, there was always the oven on, there was always a pot on the hob and everything went in there, flies, potatoes, whatever there was. I always remember that because coming home from school I'd have a dip of this stuff and it did you a world of good, it was a panacea for all ills. God knows what was in it. I shudder to think these days, but there we go.

CLARE: Were you a skinny or a chubby child, can you remember?

DAWSON: Well, I've always been sturdy!

CLARE: Sturdy!

DAWSON: Sturdy. You see I like that phrase, I strongly object to chubby. It's not fat. I've got broad shoulders and a deep chest but most of its behind me now. But the thing is, I was always fairly stiff. That was a phrase they used to use, 'He's a stiff little fella'.

CLARE: What was going to school like for the first time? Was leaving home and going to school a wrench for you? Can you remember much about your early childhood?

DAWSON: No, not really, not really, no. I mean to go to school was just a reason to get out of the house, I suppose. It was lovely to get in a room. No, not really, but the schools in those days of course were so bad that even the headmaster went barefoot. Any type of education was nominal, you know. Having said that it was a three Rs education which I think wouldn't be a bad idea today. I think they put too much into children's curricula.

CLARE: So you learnt to read and you developed an interest in reading.

DAWSON: Read and write and arithmetic. Learn the three basic Rs to get you through life and the rest comes easy.

CLARE: Were either of your parents ambitious for you? You were an only son and you were living in a working-class area. Did they have hopes that you would do something that they'd been unable to do?

DAWSON: Funnily enough my mother's idea of a successful life was security at all costs and the only thing that ever seemed secure to our very small and limited lives was the Co-op, Balloon Street, Manchester. You hold your breath when you say this, there was a pension at the end of it so most of us were committed at the age of fourteen. If we could get in the Co-op that represented security with a capital S. I went to the Co-op, pulling skips which was a dead-end job, mind you today it would be considered an artisan's job and from there, mainly to please my mother, I went as an electrical engineer which was totally not me. I can't look at a fuse without bursting into tears so that was no good to me. So I had various jobs, you know, but you see I hate the word 'security'. I think security nullifies ambition because once you get that terrible label, security, then you're finished, you're incarcerated.

CLARE: But your mother would have wanted that. It didn't cause you to be insecure, a worrier, an anxious person about your future. You would have been pretty easy going?

DAWSON: Oh, yes.

CLARE: Even though we're talking about the post war years now?

DAWSON: Oh, yeah.

CLARE: There wasn't a great deal of work around?

DAWSON: Oh, good God, no, no, very little.

CLARE: But you didn't worry about things?

DAWSON: No, I never did, funnily enough. I've never been a great worrier I must admit. I worry over some of the totally inconsequential, the silly things.

CLARE: But failure?

DAWSON: Well, I'd been a failure in any case. I felt like a failure because I wasn't very good at anything. I could put together words, I loved the English language. I love the prolific backcloth of the English language but of course to talk about poetry in the area I was brought up in meant of course you were wearing nylon stockings and a blouse. You didn't talk about things like that.

CLARE: You were what, a hard man?

DAWSON: Well, you had to appear hard, you see.

CLARE: Though your grandfather talked.

DAWSON: Oh, yes.

CLARE: He talked.

DAWSON: I think probably from him I've inherited it and he had a lovely phrase, he was once, he was once referred to as wild Irish, which I thought was a lovely phrase.

CLARE: Was he Irish?'

DAWSON: Oh, yes, yes.

CLARE: Yes, I see. When would you have had a sense that you had an ability to make people laugh or for people to notice you?

DAWSON: I think at school, maybe at school.

CLARE: Why, what was it about?

DAWSON: Well, the classroom jungle is a very profound one and you form into several little groups for want of a better phrase. There's the quiet ones, there's the hard ones, there's the ruthless ones and there's the ones who are always flitting from group to group and they are the funny ones. They're accepted in any social strata because they make you laugh. So, if a fella threatened you, you'd pull a face and he'd go, 'Hah hah.' So, it's an acceptance and I think it was probably so with many comics. It enables you to go from group to group because if you're that way, the extrovert, which I suppose is in all of us, you don't want to stay with one group. You get a bit bored with that one group, and to be able to make them laugh and to be accepted there, there and there, it was great and I think it sort of broadens you out.

CLARE: That's an interesting aspect of you. I sense that actually you relate to large numbers of people.

DAWSON: Yes I do.

CLARE: Rather than close groups.

DAWSON: Yes, yeah. I think you can get too close. It can be very claustrophobic in a relationship. I like to have more acquaintances than three or four close friends.

CLARE: And is that the way it is?

DAWSON: Oh yes, exactly. We have some very close friends but we have a lot of very good acquaintances which other people would call friends. We might not see them for twelve months, but they're there if we need them. I like to have a very broad net, to be honest with you, I prefer that. Maybe that's because of an insecurity in me that doesn't want to get too close. I just find that once that starts then it colours your own characterisations of things. But then, if you're meeting people in different groups or whatever, and different levels of society, then it gives you a much broader outlook on life.

CLARE: You can actually identify the origins of your life as a comedian. It would be that it enabled you to survive in a kind of jungle. It was your skill.

DAWSON: Exactly, it was my way of surviving.

CLARE: You wouldn't have been too analytic about it. It would have been some years before you realised that you actually got some kind of physical kick out of it, I presume, making people laugh.

DAWSON: Oh, yeah. At the time it was a great way to make friends, to hop from group to group. You're quite right.

CLARE: There's a strange process involved in it. Linking it at the moment with your mother's preoccupation, her understandable preoccupation with security – but actually being a comic, the process of actually making a joke itself, teeters on security and failure. Once it comes off it's fantastic but when it doesn't! This kind of risk element, is there something physical about that for you? Do you actually feel charged up when you're performing and then, depending on how it breaks . . .

DAWSON: Well, what I tried to do, before I started to get recognised, was to try to make a word picture. For instance, I used to use a thing in the opening of the act, to give you a rough idea, I used say, 'The ashen-faced mourners hunched closer together as a cold grey fog embraced its clammy shroud, the wind howled like a lost soul in dire torment and from beyond the dark, brooding rain-sodden hills, a demented dwarf strangled his pet racoon' – one two three, 'On a wonderful day like today' – which, looking back, it's a wonder I ever got out of these clubs alive, but I tried to create pictures. I found that after a while, people were listening. The problem with today's comedy, just to digress a little bit, is it relies too much on smart material. Good comedy comes from inside. That's the difference. Not the words.

CLARE: So when you say, 'it comes from inside', it's like the distinction often made about acting. Some actors build it from outside, and some do it from inside. So you would classify yourself as that it's you really that's funny. It's you. It's not so much the material. What is it about you that you'd say is funny? Forget the jokes for a minute. What is it about you that you think people are laughing with?

DAWSON: I think, what they identify with is you, everything you say. I mean not just the mother-in-law jokes but what I relate in the act is exactly what's happened to them, like income tax, the wife, problems in bringing up kids, only on a much more 'serious' basis. Plus the fact that the face is one of those faces you can't do much about. Never be a matinée idol. Probably helps, I don't know.

CLARE: Just sticking with the face, because you said as a school boy you pulled a face, you made people laugh with your face. That's something you were born with. That face as you know is very funny but it was then too, was it?

DAWSON: It was once described as a bulldog chewing a wasp, awful.

CLARE: And further back, as a child?

DAWSON: Yes, as a kid, I mean in every photograph I was pulling faces. When I had my photograph my mother used to go absolutely mad when we had a family photograph taken.

CLARE: She didn't like it?

DAWSON: Oh, no. Well, no mother wants to see a son making this grimace.

CLARE: What did she make of you going on stage?

DAWSON: In the early days she said, 'Oh, he's funny, he does make me laugh, our Les.' And there came a talent show in Manchester, oddly enough where we used to do radio shows years after, it was called *Talk of the Town*. It was a sort of talent show between Salford and Manchester, to give you some idea. I devised this act which I thought was hysterical. Thinking back on it now, it's a wonder I wasn't taken away into an institution with a bag of biscuits, quite frankly. The idea was – I had a ginger wig secreted in the piano and I'd sit at the piano and I played this ridiculous ditty and I said, 'I must have, oh what is this,' and I poured this little glass of something out, drank it, pulled a face, put the wig on and crawled up the piano you see, which I thought was hysterical. Apparently the silence was like a forgotten tomb but I was so full of myself I didn't realise it. Now, I'd invited my mother and father, I was so full of this act. Course, they disappeared. I thought, 'That's a bit off,' so I go home and I thought, my mother's going to come out and say, bless you my son because you have talent. But she dragged me and she said, 'Get in before any bugger sees you,' she was so ashamed of me. So I said, 'What's wrong with you?' 'You were awful, rubbish.' So she was my first critic.

CLARE: If we see your kind of humour as coping with a world, as a way you have of making your mark, of holding off all these other kids who are rough and tough and clever and miserable, the usual bunch, then it could be said that the aspect of your humour that is most potent is its ability to make a kind of triumph out of disaster or make people laugh at a certain kind of lugubrious misery. There is an element of all of that in you.

DAWSON: Well, yes, I think a lot of it is based on a terrible pessimism.

CLARE: But are you?

DAWSON: A pessimist? Yes, I think I am.

CLARE: Are you a sad man?

DAWSON: Well, yes . . . yes, sad, I am.

CLARE: Are you?

DAWSON: Well it's a good question. Tony Hancock was always a sad clown but there was always a note of optimism in everything he did and I'm the opposite 'cos I'm a coward you see. I can't face reality if I'm going to be honest with myself, because if I'm a pessimist and things turn out as bad as I imagined, then I can say, well there you are and I feel mollified. You could say it's a streak of cowardice, moral and physical cowardice if you like.

CLARE: You mention that a lot in what you write about yourself, cowardice.

DAWSON: Oh, I've often said I'm a terrible coward.

CLARE: Why do you say that?

DAWSON: I just feel it. I always remember an incident in the army. They used to call it blind boxing. It was some sergeant, some idiot, the idea was everybody was blindfolded and you milled around in the middle of the ring, knocking seven bells out of each other. Well, I just walked out of the ring. I took the bandage off and walked away 'cos I thought, this is ridiculous. But I thought afterwards, is that the mark of a coward?

CLARE: Was it the physical pain that you . . .?

DAWSON: No, I don't know. It might have been that. To me it just didn't seem right. It seemed a bit stupid actually. I could never see the sense of the thing, you see, but maybe that was my cynicism, trying to escape the fact, the feeling of being a coward.

CLARE: But you see to be a comic some people would say is an act of heroic bravery.

DAWSON: With my act it is, I think I've exonerated myself now. When I thought back at some of the things I used to do and some of the clubs I've played in – if they liked your act they didn't clap, they let you live.

CLARE: But let me stick with this because when you say cowardice, there's physical cowardice when you talk about yourself with kids, you actually used your humour and your face to keep a lot of these kids, other kids at bay. Then there is moral cowardice, I can't see how you could be accused of that. There is something extraordinarily outrageous about being a comic because you put yourself on and if you're a disaster you've only got yourself to answer.

DAWSON: Oh, true, yes. Maybe it's my way of trying to recompense for this feeling I have. I was a boxer, amateur boxer for quite a time.

CLARE: For how long?

DAWSON: Oh, about eighteen months. It was my father's idea. My father was firmly convinced that I could punch very hard, and I'd one or two wins, which made me cry. I knocked one fellow down and went down and picked him up and the referee said, 'You don't do that,' and I thought actually, I can't see the sense in physical pain. I'm not a martyr. I don't believe in the church's edict that pain is good, I think pain is awful and it should be stamped out as quickly as possible. So, maybe it's that, maybe it's the feeling of not wanting to be in pain. I don't know what it's a throwback to, I really don't know.

CLARE: There wasn't all that much pain?

DAWSON: Oh no, that's the whole point of it. We had fights at school and all the rest of it, you know, I remember fighting one kid who was at the top of the school and for a week I was physically sick; then, when we had a fight he hit me and a red mist came down and I knocked, and the next thing he's on the floor. But I mean, that, now, that horrified me that I could do that, you see. So I'm a mass of contradictions, that's the trouble with me.

CLARE: Was there much violence in your home?

DAWSON: Not really, I'd a wonderful upbringing. Oh, no, my dad was marvellous, you know, every time I had a bath, to keep me warm, he used to throw the electric fire in it. You know, we used to play wonderful games, like blind man's bluff on the M1.

CLARE: I can see that this was a fairly healthy upbringing!

DAWSON: Oh, yes I'm a mass of contradictions, and I don't really understand myself, that's what I'm saying.

CLARE: But are you underneath it all, a sad man? Do you, from time to time, feel quite melancholic, sad? Do you ever get depressed?

DAWSON: Oh no, no, no, no. I don't get depressed. I'm extremely happy in my life. It's very happy with Tracy and the baby and everything. We have a wonderful life. It's just that I look at things sometimes and I think, and I get, no not depressed, that's the wrong phrase to use because depression is an illness, I think 'What are we doing with the world? I think that it's such a great world we live in, that there's so much that we could create. But it is awful to read about the Serbian business.

Again, the past creeping into all these ridiculous hatreds and ethnic problems and that's what saddens me. I think that humour generally in this country has taken a downward turn. The British, particularly the British, we are exponents of laughing at ourselves. It's been our greatest weapon throughout history. We are the only people who made Dunkirk a victory. The only people who could do that are the British. Nobody else would. The French would say, 'Eh, eh, we have lost,' which they do, frequently. But the thing is with us, we can laugh at ourselves which is our greatest weapon. It kept the Jewish faith alive for years, laughing at themselves. If you can do that . . .

CLARE: And you do do that?

DAWSON: Yes, exactly, I'm laughing at myself. In today's world there's a pomposity about people – 'Don't you laugh at me,' and 'You're driving too fast, don't you come close to me, how dare you.' We're living in this stressful insularity which is destroying us, you see. I think that in ten years to twenty years' time most organic diseases will have an antidote but the mind is going to be under pressure. That's when you're going to be in plenty of work.

CLARE: But you wouldn't see your mind as having been under great pressure. You've been fairly resilient.

DAWSON: Yeah, I do have an ability, I suppose, to sit back and let it waft over me. I just have a very stoic view I suppose. Performers who are backstage and get terribly nervous backstage which is understandable, particularly at a Command Performance, but I have a blankness come on, I sit there and I think to myself, I sometimes talk to myself, unashamedly and say, 'What does it matter, if it's to be, it's to be.' So there's this stoic fatalism which I think helps. Maybe that's the pessimism I'm talking about. We're not making this a very interesting interview are we, really? I'd like to stride forward manfully and say, yes, I know exactly what I'm doing. I don't.

CLARE: No?

DAWSON: Every day to me is another challenge. What I have got is a great back-up, for want of a better phrase, with the wife and a wonderful, great relationship with the baby. Marvellous.

CLARE: But you have had setbacks. There was the loss of your first wife.

DAWSON: Oh yes, oh yeah. As far as I was concerned that was my life over and then . . .

CLARE: Now when you say that, if you were a truly melancholic person, that might really have opened up that side of you quite a bit. Now, did it?

DAWSON: Well, there were two things that really, I suppose, helped. One was the fact that I knew she was desperately ill for a long time but I couldn't tell anybody because I didn't want the media to get hold of it 'cos it's nothing to do with anybody else and naturally I didn't want the children to know.

CLARE: Did she know?

DAWSON: No, she didn't know.

CLARE: She didn't know?

DAWSON: No, only when she went in the wheelchair at the end was the thought, I could see it in her eyes, as much as to say, 'Is this it?'

CLARE: Did she ever ask you?

DAWSON: Yes, and I lied. I lied. Anyway, apart from that, after she died, I thought, 'Well, that's the end of my life in that sense. I'll sell the house, get a flat,' because the kids were grown-up by this time and doing their own thing. And then somebody up there smiled on me and this grubby little man simply found this great girl, Tracy, and she's been magic. But you don't go out to get married. I didn't go out with a sign on my back saying, 'I want to get married again.' The odd thing was, I did find that some women that we had known as personal friends suddenly became predators. You know, whether they thought I had a mass of shillings in a bag somewhere under the floorboards, I don't know but . . .

CLARE: Do you?

DAWSON: Oh yes, doesn't everybody!

CLARE: That's a relief. But just going back a little bit, you said it very rapidly, it took me aback really. You said, when I asked you when she asked you, you lied. Was that protecting you or her?

DAWSON: Probably protecting myself because, you see, you put it at the back of your head. You put it at the back of your mind. You don't really want to know. It's that awful moment of truth when I was wheeling her down to Christie's in Manchester, who were absolutely wonderful, and we'd made several trips in all and with such a dreadful disease there are times when it seems arrested, there are times when almost a miraculous change comes over the person and her face was fine, she was full of it, she was marvellous. I took her in the wheelchair.

CLARE: And this had gone on for how long?

DAWSON: Oh, eight years.

CLARE: Cancer, yes?

DAWSON: Eight years. And I said to the doctor, 'How is she?' laughingly and he said, 'Can I just have a word with you?' and we went in the other room and he said, 'She's got about three weeks,' and you suddenly look at the walls and you hear his words but you don't really hear those words. They're coming from a long tunnel. Three weeks for what? And then it hits you like a ton of bricks and I had to tell the children, of course. So there was that awful period but then, as I say, I must have done something right because Tracy, she pulled me out of the doldrums and we've got a new life now and she's wonderful.

CLARE: You were in the doldrums?

DAWSON: Oh yes, to a certain extent, because, well, you've got to look at yourself, you know, and you're not exactly the stuff of dreams that a young girl conjures up. You're built like a back end of a bull terrier with a face to match. And the first time I dated Tracy she wouldn't go out with me for the simple reason I'd got these denims and I looked well, a denim wall. I looked so awful that if I'd have bent down we'd have lost an hour's daylight. So, quite rightly, she sent me packing. She said, 'I'm not going out with you, go and get changed.' But I won her hand and that's a new life.

CLARE: We talked about intimacy and close friends and large audiences, but the truth is, you wouldn't have found it easy to live on your own?

DAWSON: Oh, no, oh, dreadful.

CLARE: Tell me about that, why?

DAWSON: Dreadful. I need to give to somebody. I need to give affection and love because without that I wither.

CLARE: You're a very physical man?

DAWSON: Yes, but also, it's the poet in me. I love that film with Robin Williams – *Dead Poets Society* – in which he said something that I've always said. He said, 'What do we have language for?' and this boy said, 'To communicate.' No, it's to woo a woman, it's to fight off dragons. That's what language is about. You should know, being Irish. The Irish are poets and bards and will be until the end of time. But I need to give that love to somebody. I need to have it. Without that I'm lost. I'm rudderless.

CLARE: One of the things I was very struck by with your first volume, your autobiography, was that you were very unabashed about how physical you were, how sexual you were, how you enjoyed sex. It's quite unusual in books by Englishmen of a certain period. I was quite taken by that. I mean you said very straight – there were these relationships, you screwed around, there were some terrific women, you had a good time. You actually are a rather sensual man.

DAWSON: Yeah, providing that there's love with it. I think there's got to be love with it. I can't see sex for the sake of it. Never could, to be honest with you. I mean when you're seventy, eighty or ninety then I mean it's a totally different thing, isn't it, but, I think the biggest tragedy of today's world, particularly with our children, is they're maturing so quickly yet the mental level isn't, so we're producing a nation of morons if we're not careful. They're huge physically, their physical appetite's far in advance of their years. Opening a newspaper or anything, everything's about sex, a sex guide, a sex position, nobody mentions the word love, because, rather like the devil in religion, we keep it away now. That's, 'Don't be silly, don't talk about that.' I mean that's what's slowly strangling the church, the fact that we don't renounce the devil, we just say he doesn't exist any more, but he does.

CLARE: But there isn't much element of the devil in you.

DAWSON: Oh, I think we've all got the dark side, all of us. This is what you're a psychiatrist for.

CLARE: Yeah, but I don't find much evidence of a dark side in you.

DAWSON: Well, that's very nice of you to say so. You might do when I get the cheque for this (laughs.) No, there's no doubt you're right there . . .

CLARE: Let me put it this way. What do you think would be the commonest critisism people make of you.

DAWSON: That's a good one. That's a good question. Simply to say the jokes are too old, which they are. There was a rather punishing thing happened the other day, I was on one of the TV shows *The Swinging Sixties*, with Lulu, and that was taken thirty years ago and although I looked very much the same facially, the body obviously was a lot thinner, the jokes were the same. That hurt. So I think people would say, now here's a strange thing, some people would say I'm coarse, but vulgarity was always comedy and today's world with the alternative comedians, people are unabashed about it, they say, well, that's fine. But they're dirty. Good comedy was never dirty. It's vulgar, of course it is, like Chaucer's plays are vulgar.

CLARE: Right, so they might say that. What would they say about you as a person?

DAWSON: I don't know, I don't know about that. I wouldn't honestly know.

CLARE: What would be the aspect of you you least like?

DAWSON: Now, we really get down to the nitty gritty now, and the wife's out there, she's clocking all this, you know that, don't you? I think the worst part of me, I would like occasionally to have the guts to say 'no'. I'm too fond of trying to please everybody which causes a degree of dissatisfaction in my dear spouse. I try to be a man for all seasons and it doesn't work so I would rather like to just for once to say to somebody, 'No,' but I haven't got the courage. I want to please.

CLARE: You do?

DAWSON: That's my trouble.

CLARE: Is that what you mean about the coward?

DAWSON: I think that's probably what it is. Yes. I like to think that I need, I need warmth, I need people. I can't understand people who buy lovely homes and they put themselves behind twelve foot walls. People is what life's about. Without people there's no life, no point in living.

CLARE: But do you wish you could say no?

DAWSON: I'd like to be able to turn around and be really strong. At present it's Tracy who's the strong one. I do honestly tend to be a bit weak there.

CLARE: And was Meg strong, your previous wife? Did she play that role as well?

DAWSON: Yes, pretty much so, yes. She used to get fed up with me as well.

CLARE: Because you take on too much?

DAWSON: No, I try to please people.

CLARE: So how would it come out?

DAWSON: Well, suppose you're on the phone to me saying, 'Look, I've got this bit of a do in Dublin, it means you'll have to catch the night ferry and we haven't got a cabin so you'll be wet through but it's going to be a great do if you're there,' and I say, 'Yeah, fine,' because I want to please you. Now, Tracy would be very sensible and say, 'Don't be stupid, with no cabin on the night ferry, you hardly know the guy, and why worry about saying no?' So there you go, you have a chance to meet somebody interesting and that's where it starts, and that's my problem, weakness. Terrifying, isn't it. I tell you there's a case history here for you. Adler would have had a joy with me and I don't mean Larry Adler either!

CLARE: But when you say you wish you were able to say no, is that because other people wish it or you genuinely feel bad about yourself that you don't say no?

DAWSON: I don't like to upset people.

CLARE: Why is that?

DAWSON: I don't know.

CLARE: Did you ever upset people?

DAWSON: Oh, I think I upset a lot of people. I upset people by trying not to upset them so, I mean, it's a Catch-22 situation.

CLARE: Why, because you have to cancel things or say no after you've said yes?

DAWSON: Well, supposing you and I were to go on to O'Connell Street to a pub which we'd both enjoy enormously, just the two of us and we'd talk about the world, we'd talk about psychiatry, we'd talk about philosophy, reincarnation, whatever you like. I wouldn't want that night to end so I will keep you there as long as possible, till the whole of the Liffy and O'Connell Street is empty and dawn's rising. I don't want that night to end because I will never reproduce it or recreate that night again. That's the trouble. So I get Tracy pulling my sleeve and saying, 'It's about time we went,' and you look round and there's only the janitor left. So I'm always the last at the party but it's just that, it's a lovely night, I don't want it to end. It's a very basic thing really, I suppose. So I'd like to be able to be forthright and say, 'Thank you very much, it's been a wonderful evening, it's been wonderful meeting you, goodnight.' Couldn't do it. Couldn't do it. I'd have to find the Mrs!

CLARE: Even though you yourself might at times want to do it?

DAWSON: Well, yeah, yes, even so, exactly.

CLARE: Let's take that example you gave me earlier. When you put down the phone after having said yes to the chap in Dublin who wants you to go on the night ferry and so on and you've said yes, you put it down. You don't need Tracy to tell you, God, that's the last thing I need. So there must be in you, though she tells you, she articulates it, but there must be in you a feeling, blast it, I should have said no.

DAWSON: Well, I tell you exactly what I do say. 'Yes, that would be great,' and she'll say, 'What are you saying that for?' I say, 'Well, I don't want to upset the guy,' I mean, you never know, we might need him. So I always find an outlet and that is a basic character flaw in my view.

CLARE: How much of a burden is it being a comedian? For example, the tendency of other people to expect you to be funny all the time.

DAWSON: Never bothers me, I think it's nice.

CLARE: Do you?

DAWSON: Well, everywhere we go people smile and, you know, say 'All right, Les?' You've never met them before. I don't mind in the slightest.

CLARE: Or in social situations, where maybe you don't feel like being particularly funny?

DAWSON: Well, now you're going back to the small group thing. If you go to, say, a cocktail party, you always get somebody who'll totter over with a glass and a flushed expression and a watery eye and say, 'Is it true that so-and-so's so and so?' They all want the inside gossip 'cos they think I know it all, you see, all the gossip. And there was one of these, this fella, was impugning somebody's ability to be masculine, so he said, 'Is he, is he a poof?' so I said, 'I don't know but I will give you a bit of gossip.' The fella went, 'What's that?' and I said, 'Shirley Bassey is effeminate.' He said, 'She's not?' and he waltzed off to tell his mates. That sort of thing I hate because there's always a view that if you're in showbusiness therefore you're at orgies, you smoke pot. I wouldn't know an orgy if I fell over one, to be honest. Nobody's every invited me to an orgy.

CLARE: You say that with regret.

DAWSON: In total regret. Do you note in the voice the timbre.

CLARE: I did.

DAWSON: When we first moved to where we are now, it's a little quiet road in the middle of the woods and it's quite nice, and there was one lady and she said to me, 'Do you know, Mr Dawson, when I heard that you were coming to live here, I sent a round robin to the neighbours seeing if we could thwart your occupancy.' So I asked, 'Why?' She said, 'Well, I had this mental picture of you going about the lawn naked at three o'clock in the morning.' She said it with that sort of regret in her voice. She said, 'But you're really quite ordinary, aren't you?' And I think there was a sense of regret in her voice. So you do get that but on the broader basis, no, it's nice because, let's be fair, it opens some doors to theatres and things like that. It's hard work, our business, and there are some very bad points to it but there's that side which is very nice and I find people basically all right. And I find that people are very nice towards you which I think is great. We have a daughter, eight-months-old daughter, and she's doing my faces already, I'm teaching her to pull faces. That's the key to it. Never mind your O-levels, pull a funny face.

CLARE: What about class? You emphasise in the first book you write, you precede every chapter with a little clip about the

Queen at a Royal Variety Performance coming towards you, going down the line of very distinguished performers, she's coming towards you and at the beginning of each chapter she's getting nearer you and you think about the contrast between the person she has seen perform and will meet and where you come from. It's a contrast between a public achievement, a dazzling kind of glamourous setting and an image of working-class poverty, struggle, an otherwise unremarkable little boy in short pants, grimy, struggling really to make something of himself.

DAWSON: Were we in the same class at school? You seem to know me!

CLARE: But in British society, some feel marked by a sense of inferiority.

DAWSON: Oh, not at all, no. The only reason I commented on the diverse sides to the character was the fact that it was great for me to be there and to think that I'd actually made it. I must admit, I thought of my dad, 'cos they died tragically young and my mother died when she was only forty-three so they never saw me get anywhere.

CLARE: They didn't?

DAWSON: No, I just thought, 'Here I am, it's the Palladium or Buck House or wherever we go and here's the top lady of the land, talking to a guy who was born in the backstreets' and the first thing that came to mind is, to quote the Americans that anyone can do it, that is the great thing of democracy which if you take away all the trappings of it, the fact that you can go from there to there. I don't think in many societies you can do that. That was the main thing I was trying to say in the book that, you know, don't matter where you come from, come on. In other words, the human spirit is capable of going anywhere it wants.

CLARE: Now, interestingly enough, of the kids at your school, you might, however, be the only one who made it, and you made it on a kind of innate talent that pays no homage to class, or education or Oxbridge or whatever.

DAWSON: That's exactly what I'm saying about the educational system.

CLARE: So, I wouldn't like you to misunderstand what I mean when I say this. You were fortunate, you were given something.

DAWSON: A talent, oh yes, something, oh yes. But I also think that everybody has a gift. One of the problems with the economic climate that we live in, there may be people who could have been great artists or painters but because of the class structure, they had to earn a living and therefore that had to be a hobby and it takes a very bold spirit to break away from all that but you have to do it, that's what I had to do.

CLARE: You could have been in the Co-op.

DAWSON: I could still be at the Co-op.

CLARE: What is it that got you out of that? You said it takes a very bold spirit and yet you talked about cowardice. There is that kind of bravery. You didn't say, I better settle for 1.6d a week and then plod up the ladder. You took lots of risks and did all sorts of strange things.

DAWSON: Oh, sure, sure. I'll tell you what happened. I decided it was no good for me, so to extricate myself from all this I got away from pulling these skips which was driving me up the wall. I had a rope rash on my hands, I mean it was ridiculous for a kid of fourteen. So I went as an electrical engineer apprentice. I was useless at that. I can't stand electricity. I still can't wire a plug. But fortunately, National Service reared its ugly head and that was my escape route. So everybody said, get a deferment until you're twenty-one. No, said I. I want to go now and get it over with and some thought that's a sensible idea. It wasn't that sensible, I just wanted to get away from what I saw as a crushing social net, you see.

CLARE: Yeah. And in the army, did you develop?

DAWSON: Hated it, hated it.

CLARE: But did you develop as a performer?

DAWSON: Oh, yes, yes.

CLARE: You did. Did anybody spot it? Outside your parents and your family and so on, did anybody say, 'You know, Dawson, you've got a talent?'

DAWSON: Only when I got out of the army, when I came out of the army.

CLARE: What age would you have been then?

DAWSON: Twenty-one, I came out of the army.

CLARE: And who was it?

DAWSON: Max Wall. He was doing a series of auditions and I auditioned for him in Manchester, the old Manchester Hippodrome, as it was, and he said to me, to quote, to use the voice, to paraphrase, 'I think you've got a talent.' In them days I was playing the piano and singing, you know, and getting a few laughs, particularly when I played the piano. So that's how it started. He was the first one. But in the army, the only thing that brought it to light was that we went AWOL for some reason or other and they put me in the guardhouse ready to be sentenced. I was in the tanks, the Cavalry Regiment and they needed somebody to play the piano and the only one who could knock a tune out was me. So I was marched briskly from my cell to the sergeant's mess where I entertained them royally and I never went back in the cell. They put me on open arrest and dropped the charge, so that was the end of that, and I used to entertain the lads. I hated the army, loathed it. Couldn't see the sense in military discipline at all. I mean they used to play the bugle while I was alseep. You know, silly things like that.

CLARE: Are you a worrier? Do you worry about things?

DAWSON: No, no.

CLARE: Death?

DAWSON: Pardon.

CLARE: Death.

DAWSON: No, death, no, I mean death doesn't bother anybody. It's the method of death that worries people.

CLARE: Well, dying?

DAWSON: Dying itself no. It's only an extension of life.

CLARE: You've seen people die?

DAWSON: Oh yes, yes.

CLARE: So what about pain?

DAWSON: Well, that's it. We're all cowards when it comes to pain. It's surprising what you can put up with. I suppose there have been occasions when I took ill with pain.

CLARE: If you had cancer would you want to be told?

DAWSON: Oh, that's a good one. I think, yes.

CLARE: You would?

DAWSON: Because if I had anything to do with cancer or to help in any way I would say, be angry with it. I think one of the problems is with the word, it's the word, cancer, that's a problem. It is a dead cell which eats up the cells, that's basically what's wrong with cancer and it also throws the pain elsewhere. So it's a very difficult thing to track down but I think if you're told and you can face it, it takes a hell of a lot of facing, I think in the long run it's better because then you can fight it. There are groups at Christie's where they actually get angry with it, angry with themselves and it seems to cause some sort of change in the andrenalin or the blood that helps to fight it, because it can be beaten, as any ills can be beaten.

CLARE: So do you think about that in relation to your first wife? Did she fight it? She didn't know though.

DAWSON: Well, she had breast cancer, she knew about the breast cancer of course. What happened was when that about a year or two later, she fell. I never knew about this and she fell in the square, St Annes Square, and of course it flared up again and began spiralling all over the place. But that was treated as something else and it was only when I saw the specialist's face that I thought this is more serious, you know. But then I was in a quandary becaue if you want to know the truth, to a certain extent, now comes the selfish side of me, I don't want the press to get hold of this story because then, 'I'm going to be lambasted with it,' you know, his wife's dying, how could he go on there? I still had to work, you know, and go out there and be funny which is the most difficult thing, of course, in the world. Like a friend of ours, Roy Castle, and I said this, I said the very thing to Roy on the phone, I said, 'Fight this, you know, fight it, be angry, be angry with God because He can take it, He's big enough, be angry, don't be afraid.'

CLARE: When you are sad, perhaps your kind of comedy would be better.

DAWSON: Let's hope to God it improves, with the laughs I'm getting lately.

CLARE: But, seriously, but seriously, when you're feeling pretty low . . .

DAWSON: Pardon.

CLARE: When you're feeling pretty low? Comedians talk about going on when something disastrous has happened immediately around them but it's their job and they've got to go on the same way as a surgeon has got to operate and a pilot has got to fly a plane, or whatever. With your style of humour, I just wonder sometimes whether when you're not feeling so good, it is actually funnier?

DAWSON: That's it, that's right, exactly. I mean if I go on there and say, 'It's been a rotten day today,' they go ho-ho, 'So this fellow dropped dead in front of me.' You can also go on there say hi everybody – nothing.

CLARE: When did you realise that your particular brand of comedy, your skill, was this kind of morbid, not morbid, gloomy, lugubrious kind of humour, about the blackness of life and you inching your way along, commenting on it. The character of Ada, too, this extraordinary woman who mouths silently the latest disasters. When did you discover that that was what made people laugh?

DAWSON: Well, the lugubrious aspect you put so very nicely, started in Hull. I was playing the clubs up there and it was difficult to describe them but they used to throw drunks in, you see. You laughed then, didn't you, I count that as a major breakthrough. And I was, to quote the showbusiness phraseology, I was dying where I stood. And it was on a Thursday night, and I always remember this. It was there in the land of green ginger where the slave markets used to be and there was a very good pub there with excellent beer, excellent, and I sipped mightily of yon malt to the extent I couldn't get up hardly, I was stoned, to put it in a nice phrase. So I went on to the club that night and there was a makeshift curtain keeping me away from that seething mass of humanity out there who were baying for my blood. And I sat at the piano and when they announced me I couldn't get up. So I looked at them bleary-eyed, fed up with them, fed up with myself, and just told them what I thought about them and what I thought about myself and they roared. As daylight's bars crept through the window and the head had stopped pounding, I thought 'What happened last night?' and I did remember getting laughs, which was an alien sound to me, laughter. I mean silence, you know, you could chew a lozenger and hear it rattle like a musket when I was on stage. Suddenly I'd got a laugh so then I worked at it and then I began to think. And, slowly, that's how it started. Then I started doing television work. I used to work around the great love of the Lancashire mill woman, because my mother-in-law, first mother-in-law, was one and she had a face like a bear trap, to be honest, but they had this lovely majesty of morality, northern women. So if there was anything to do at all with the private parts of the female anatomy they would never say one word. They would pantomime it, they'd mouth it. They'd say, 'Is it true that (whispers) I believe she had a show?' Now you knew instantly what had happened. She didn't have to say two words. She said more by not saying anything. And I used to like these women, I thought, 'This is great,' and so we started doing them, this partner of mine, Roy Barraclough, and they became an instant hit because they were just genuine. That's exactly what they were and we developed things so he would always be slightly better class although they lived in the same street, she was better than me, better than she was. So we used to do lovely things like we went to a seance, it was one of my favourites and I said to him, 'What does she do, does she contact the dead?' and he would say, 'Oh, yes, Mrs Prendergast is wonderful, she speaks through her widgee,' and you don't have to say another word, all you have to say is, 'Fancy,' that's all you had to say. And that's what made them funny. Because now the ball's in their court.

CLARE: What's happening to those kind of women?

DAWSON: We're bringing them back, we're doing a show at Christmas.

CLARE: But the women themselves that they're based on?

DAWSON: They love them, oh, we have a great following.

CLARE: You like women?

DAWSON: Yes, very much so, very, very much so. I've got a lot of time for women. I was disliked by a lot of women until another character years ago called Cosmo Smallpiece. I based this character on a fellow who had thick glasses and we thought he was a pervert. He never did anything wrong but he just looked. So I got these thick glasses. He could make sex out of everything. We're talking about strawberries, and of course he would make strawberries and the planting of strawberries very important. 'We must have strawberries sown far apart at the borders because strawberies do tend to go in the same bed. Ooh, ooh, strawberries, they're always at it, you see.' He was that type of character. Now I sat back and thought, this will open the portals to the most virulent criticism and I never got any. In fact, on one occasion at the Savoy Hotel a very carefully coiffured ladey drifted by and she said, 'Oh, you, it's you isn't it?' I thought, well here we go, she said 'That little man, that Cosmo,' she said, 'I think he's wonderful.' So I said, 'Why?' She said, 'Because he's honest.' And I thought, well, looking at it I suppose in a way, he never touched or did anything, but, and that got me funnily enough liked by women more than ever before. Strange. That's women, isn't it?

CLARE: The mother-in-law jokes referred to in the intro?

DAWSON: I'm still in trouble with certain factions.

CLARE: Yes, that's right. What is your explanation for that kind of genre. It's very British.

DAWSON: Of course it is.

CLARE: And what is it about? What do you think it's about?

DAWSON: Well, in most families the mother-in-law had been the building blocks of any family, the crucible of the family. The mother-in-law is the most powerful because you've got two points where you want to get the fun. If she has a daughter, no man on earth would ever be good enough for her daughter. If she has a son, there'll be no woman ever good enough for her son. So whatever you do, you could be the next Pope, you'll still be in line for criticism from the mother-in-law and so they became very powerful. If the grandchildren came round Nana or Grandma is a very powerful figure.

CLARE: It seems to me there's no father-in-law joke really.

DAWSON: Well, there's nothing funny about fathers-in-law. They would have to have permission to breathe, most of the poor buggers, you know.

CLARE: You lived in a family where your mother's parents were there. How did your father get on with your mother's mother?

DAWSON: Oh, not too bad actually. Yeah, not too bad. His face always lit up when he saw her, she used to put his nose in a lamp socket. No, they didn't do too badly actually.

CLARE: She was a tough little lady?

DAWSON: Oh, she was tough, oh, she was tough lady, aye, she were tough that . . .

CLARE: Was your father around all that much?

DAWSON: Well, that was his shape, he was round.

CLARE: I mean would he have been out of the home much?

DAWSON: No, I think because it was so claustrophobic, we were all sort of pent up together, we didn't really see much of them when we left.

CLARE: What I'm getting at really is the role of a father in this culture. You're a father now, twice, several times over. It's always struck me there are these powerful women and your act is about a powerful woman, Ada.

DAWSON: Oh, yes, yes.

CLARE: Powerful women, there's no questioning the role of women in northern British life. Strong, castrating sometimes. Sometimes pretty ugly or repulsive, that's how you imitate them, or indeed extremely nubile and attractive. But the men are either shadowy or rather pathetic or rather innocuous or rather inferior or just absent. Now, what about you as a man, as a father, what sort of father do you think you are?

DAWSON: Well, I'll put it very bluntly and Tracy's out there now, but I'll put it very bluntly. I wear the pants in our house, you can see them from under my apron. And the thing is, we're not being emasculated. I disagree with Havelock Ellis who quotes penis envy and all that rubbish. Women by their very nature are nest makers. That is their function, I don't care about careers or whatever they call them. The average woman wants a family, she wants a home. And having said that, then she becomes very important in building that home. You forage for the scraps to build that home. So that puts you in a secondary position because by being the homemaker she is the most important. And I've said it, and there you go and I think women are very nice, I think they are lovely creatures.

CLARE: And your role as father?

DAWSON: My role is to look after them as father, is to be there, benign, wise. You know I enjoy family life.

CLARE: You do?

DAWSON: I don't thing there's anything better. I can't think of a kibbutz system, I like family life, I think it's great, I think it's marvellous. I think the more you can shroud your kids in affection and love they'll grow up better citizens.

CLARE: Are you an ambitious man?

DAWSON: Yes.

CLARE: What are you ambitions?

DAWSON: I don't know, I just don't know. I do anything, anything. If anything crops up, like, I'm not being disrespectful, this. When my agent first approached me about this, you know, I was first inclined unto him to say the biblical phrase, 'Go forth and multiply thyself,' but to be perfectly honest, I wanted to do it because it's different. My ambition is to do, is to travail anywhere that's different. I think that's what keeps a human being's brain active, I think it keeps us alive. And we are by our very nature spiritual explorers, for want of a better phrase. We like to do different things, and once we're cosseted in something that's secure, then we are failures.

CLARE: Now, when you compare yourself with the little boy growing up in working-class Manchester, obviously there are things that are quite different. Certainly the external things are different. Do you think you're a very different person?

DAWSON: No, not particularly, not particularly.

CLARE: You don't think you've changed much?

DAWSON: No, my eating habits are still as bad.

CLARE: What about your drinking habits?

DAWSON: Oh, they improved. Oh, you mean, not in quantity, not after tonight that's for sure. No, I used to drink. I was never a hard drinker because I found it easy, but now I've got much more sensible about it. I mean I used to wake up quite close to where I lived at one time but now I'm better.

CLARE: Did you drink ever because it made you feel any different, made you feel better?

DAWSON: No, I used it to forget to be honest, and I used to forget what I was trying to remember!

CLARE: Forget what?

DAWSON: Well, I couldn't remember what I was trying to forget, then I forgot what I was trying to remember and I tried to forget it, so I gave up. (Laughter.) I drank because I liked it, it's as simple as that.

CLARE: Did you?

DAWSON: Yes, I loved it.

CLARE: Your grandfather drank fairly heavily.

DAWSON: Yes, he died through drink and I'm getting revenge. No, he did actually, he died through drink.

CLARE: Did he?

DAWSON: A barrel fell on his head.

CLARE: (Laughs.) Did your father drink much?

DAWSON: Yes, father drank, yeah, they all drank.

CLARE: They were heavy drinkers in those days.

DAWSON: Well, to give an example, when my father was buried three weeks after he was, when he was buried you could smell his breath at the inquest.

CLARE: I can see that . . .

DAWSON: The flowers that grew on his grave were hops. But I like drink, I admit it freely. I don't drink now as I did, I don't smoke and I'm so happy I could kick this microphone. (Laughter.)

CLARE: Are you a religious person?

DAWSON: I can embrace Christ but not the Church.

CLARE: Why is that?

DAWSON: Because the Church is built in homage to a person who never used the Church so I don't see the point in having these great purple colours and ermine robes for a man who was very simple. I can embrace his edicts but I can't embrace the Church.

CLARE: Does that mean that you believe that death isn't the end?

DAWSON: Oh, no, no, scientifically death can't be the end because nothing, nothing dies. You can't create or destroy matter.

CLARE: So what's going to happen to Les Dawson?

DAWSON: Cosmic life force like all of us. That's God. Cosmic life force.

CLARE: Will it have a persona? Will you be around again?

DAWSON: No, I doubt it. One religion that attracts me is Buddhism, to a certain extent. But certainly nothing dies in this world. When you bury somebody, for instance, you're only burying his empty skin, that's all, a discarded lump.

CLARE: Would you translate that into your relationship with your first wife? Would she still be alive in one sense for you?

DAWSON: Oh, oh yes. It's in the heart, you never forget. I have a strange feeling that, although I might sound daft, she actually helped to put Tracy and I together. Now that might sound absolutely ridiculous but sometimes I wonder because, I don't know, we seemed to be guided, Tracy and I, to each other.

CLARE: Did your wife ever talk to you, when she was ill, you know sometimes people suddenly apropos of nothing at all, talk about should anything ever happen to her what she would like to happen to you. Did she ever say that? Did you ever talk about you as somebody who needed somebody around?

DAWSON: Oh, I always said to her, 'If anything happens to me, you know, if you find somebody who's right for you, you know, for God's sake don't live a life alone because that's only purely physical.'

CLARE: You would say that to Meg?

DAWSON: Yeah, and she would say the same to me.

CLARE: She would, would she? You referred to your marriage to Tracy almost like beauty and the beast.

DAWSON: I beg your pardon?

CLARE: In the sense that . . .

DAWSON: How dare you call her a beast. (Laughter.)

CLARE: You often refer to yourself in this way, as a sort of oddity, a sort of physical oddity.

DAWSON: I wouldn't go that far. I mean, I'm not exactly the elephant man but I don't think I'm very attractive, I'm not a very good-looking fella, let's face it. A character face, probably lived in but I wouldn't say anything else. I mean, it's not the stuff, as I say, of a young girl's dreams.

CLARE: Would you like to be?

DAWSON: No, no I wouldn't change it.

CLARE: Why?

DAWSON: Well, I think it's nicer to laugh a woman into bed. It's got more depth to it.

CLARE: Takes longer.

DAWSON: Takes longer, of course, you've got to have a lot of patience, but the Richard Geres of this world may fundamentally get the first shot but after that, I think they go downhill a bit. Whereas I can, I can keep my missus.

CLARE: Was that what attracted Tracy to you, the fact that you made her laugh?

DAWSON: Yes, I think it was, I think it was.

CLARE: Had she been sad?

DAWSON: Oh, she's had a rough life herself, very, very bad life, with a lot of unhappiness. She lost her parents, she lost her dad in a car crash. Lost her mother in the same way as I lost mine and so we were two really unhappy people, to be honest.

CLARE: How did you lose your mother?

DAWSON: Heart attack, very severe heart attack.

CLARE: Very sudden?

DAWSON: Oh, yeah.

CLARE: Were you there?

DAWSON: Yes, yeah, yea. She was only forty-three, you see.

CLARE: What age were you?

DAWSON: Twenty, about twenty. I think I'd just got out of the army, something like that. Very difficult to go back in time. So my father and I then we tried to carry on together but it wasn't quite the same, 'cos again, she was the very nub, a cog in the wheel.

CLARE: She held it together. What happened to your father after she died?

DAWSON: He never got over her death, he never got over her death. He did look after himself. Then when I got married I begged him to come and live with us. We lived with him for a while, but then we got our own place and, well, he stayed on his own and I think he made up his mind to join her. Thirty years later he did. But that's the way they are. I don't like that attitude. I think life is very, very precious. As I say, regarding religion, I have friends that are Church people, we've a great friend who's a priest, but I can't come to grips with the cant and hypocrisy of man-made religions 'cos the very man that they endear themselves to stood on a bloody hillside. If you want to make a cathedral, let it be the sky.

CLARE: I know you were very worried over that the media would make a lot of the age difference between you and your second wife, between you and Tracy.

DAWSON: Well, she's older but that doesn't bother me, it's just one of those things! I don't think that honestly matters. There's too much made of this again. It's like dieting. It's like all these ridiculous impositions we place on ourselves. Yes, there are a few years difference between us but I think age is in the mind anyway, to be perfectly honest. I think some people are very old at twenty-five. I think it depends on how you look at life again. I think you must always look at life through a child's eyes, that's why I love having kids around.

CLARE: Nonetheless, when we're faced with it ourselves, we have to work with these anxieties. When you leave aside what other people say, did you yourself find yourself thinking, worrying about the age thing, thinking was this right?

DAWSON: Never once, never once. Never once entered into it. Never once.

CLARE: You were confident that this would work.

DAWSON: Well, I knew we were great together. It's obviously on the cards I'll go before she does but the point is whilst we're here, it's going to be a very happy time, and that's what it's all about. And having the baby of course, I mean, if anybody said to me what is the answer to stave off the encroachment of age, it's have a baby, because there's no doubt about it, everything changes, your metabolism, your lifestyle, it jolts you out of any rut you might be in. Somebody faced with a 9lb thing that's bawling it's head off at 2 o'clock in the morning and he's got to remember all the nursery rhymes and do all the things, and suddenly, your back in time, it's great.

CLARE: What age is your baby?

DAWSON: Thirty-two. No. Eight months.

CLARE: Eight months?

DAWSON: Eight months old, yeah. Gorgeous.

CLARE: I know the kind of things people write. There are people who say, 'This is dreadful, this man is in his sixties, he's got an eight-month-old baby, when he is eighty the baby will be just about twenty.' What do you say to that?

DAWSON: That is enough, the baby doesn't want me around all that time. Surely one of the biggest problems with any family is the fact that the parents sometimes outlive the kids. Oh no, let them have their own life. I want to be there long enough to see her happy and settled and then I'll go. Well I won't, I'll struggle a bit. (Laughter.) There's too much of this age factor. Nobody wants to live forever, for God's sake. Exhaust yourself.

CLARE: I sense you won't want to die, ever.

DAWSON: Oh, no, and I won't, I'll refuse to go. I'll scrabble at the shroud, I won't go. If I drank some more of this wine I might be half-way there. (Laughter.)

CLARE: But you (laughs) you will.

DAWSON: Put in the back of a motorbike you'd do twenty miles to the gallon.

CLARE: You really enjoy living.

DAWSON: I love life.

CLARE: So you are a real counter to the notion of the Pagliacci, of the melancholic clown.

DAWSON: Oh, no, I don't want to be a Hamlet, for God's sake.

CLARE: You're not a melancholic clown?

DAWSON: No, no.

CLARE: You're as happy inside as outside?

DAWSON: Oh, yeah. I'm a happy person, yeah.

CLARE: Do you ever madden people by being happy? Does your wife ever say, 'Oh for God's sake, lay off the humour, I'm not in the mood?'

DAWSON: She never laughs at anything I say anyway.

CLARE: She doesn't?

DAWSON: No.

CLARE: She's a struggle to make laugh?

DAWSON: Oh, a poker face.

CLARE: Seriously?

DAWSON: Oh, a struggle. It's a hard life, I'm filling up now (laughter). No, she's marvellous.

CLARE: I'm getting a bit overwhelmed myself.

DAWSON: We have a lot of laughs, don't we? She's out there, you can see. We have a great life together. She saved me, she saved my life, actually.

CLARE: Go on, say more about that. Why do you say that? What would have happened to your life? Should your father have married again, do you think?

DAWSON: No, I tried to encourage him to marry again.

CLARE: That's what I mean, do you think it would have made a difference to him?

DAWSON: Oh, I'm sure, yes.

CLARE: You talk about him wasting away, is that what would have happened to you?

DAWSON: I think so, yes, yes.

CLARE: You don't like your own company?

DAWSON: Well, does anybody, honestly? You'd have to be a terrible egotist to like your own company.

CLARE: Well, hang on, let me give you an example. Some people can spend hours, days, on their own, in their own company, walking moors, going on holidays on their own, going on vacation on their own. There are such people.

DAWSON: Well, they must be a very special breed. I couldn't do that.

CLARE: You couldn't do that?

DAWSON: I have to relate to other people to exist, that's the fabric of society.

CLARE: Have you ever spent a lengthy period of your time in your own company?

DAWSON: No.

CLARE: Never?

DAWSON: No, 'cos I've heard all the jokes anyway. What am I to do, look in the mirror and mouth inanities to myself? To me there's something sadly wrong about people who can cut themselves off from society, there really is. I find it very strange to become almost reclusive.

CLARE: So it was inevitable that when your wife died, and it was a very good relationship I understand from the way you've recorded it and your children seem to agree with that, it would be inconceivable really for Les Dawson not to remarry. Or if you didn't there would be trouble, really, becaue you would have found yourself lacking that kind of close relationship that makes life for you.

DAWSON: Yeah, I've got to have a cause to live by after a while and Tracy became my *cause célèbre* because she was great. I needed her.

CLARE: What about your children?

DAWSON: Well, I couldn't have married them, it's against . . .

CLARE: What age were they, when your wife died?

DAWSON: About twenty-one, twenty-two, the eldest, something like that. I forget, though, to be honest.

CLARE: But again that wouldn't have been enough? They were, what, living their own lives?

DAWSON: Oh, no, no, that wouldn't have been enough, no.

CLARE: How close are you to your children?

DAWSON: Oh, we're fairly close. They live their own lives and have got their own lives now but we're still close.

CLARE: What did they make of you?

DAWSON: I really don't know sometimes, because there's often the feeling that maybe it's the worst thing to have sombody in the family who's a so-called celebrity because it presupposes they're going to get some stick at school, for want of a better phrase, which I think they did. I've got two smashing step-kids as well now and I know they got a lot of stick. But, of the five of them that we've got, I'm not counting Charlotte, my step-kids have come to grips with it better than my own kids, I think, in a strange way. Maybe because they were more detached.

CLARE: And it came later for them?

DAWSON: Yeah, yeah, they've come to grips with it much better, I must admit.

CLARE: Would the others, by and large, prefer to stay out of your shadow? There's the problem of being Les Dawson's kids.

DAWSON: Yes, this is the problem you see, and I saw the problem. Like if they mention that Stuart, my son, they might say, 'Oh, he is Les Dawson's son.' I always remember, what's his name, Rex Harrison's son, Noel Harrison, who always seemed to be there under his father's shadow. That's why Stuart is a motor mechanic, and a very good one. And I wouldn't like them to follow me into this business because of that. Not that I'm against showbusiness itself. If they want to go into it it's up to them but there would always be that, oh, his father helped because jealousy is a, is a killer of all the social fabrics. God, I've never talked so much like this for ages. You're good at this, you know.

CLARE: (Laughs.) Do you talk about yourself much to other people?

DAWSON: Not a lot, no. That's another fault. I repeat myself.

CLARE: Do you?

DAWSON: Oh, totally. I'm not saying I'm boring but I once sent a glass eye to sleep.

CLARE: (Laughs.) Do you think you're boring sometimes?

DAWSON: Yes, I do.

CLARE: You worry about that?

DAWSON: No, no, it doesn't bother me.

CLARE: It bothers other people?

DAWSON: Yes.

CLARE: Do you worry about money?

DAWSON: Yes. Again, this is probably a hang-up from the past when you hadn't got any, you know. I think the only thing that money does for me is give me confidence to be able to wake up and say, 'Well, you're not working this week but, however, we're not going to be desperate.' I used to go to the pawnbrokers with my father's suits, so I don't want them days to come back again. So there is a feeling of insecurity, yes.

CLARE: Do you worry about waste then? Are you a hoarder? Do you keep things?

DAWSON: Yes, yes, I think we do, yeah.

CLARE: What sort of things?

DAWSON: Clothes, anything, I've got clothes there that, you know, from the Elizabethan period.

CLARE: You don't throw things away?

DAWSON: Not if I can avoid it, no. We do have an occasional purge, it's usually my stuff that goes. Yes I'm a bit of a hoarder and a bit of a miser in some ways.

CLARE: Are you?

DAWSON: Yes, yeah. I mean just a small point, Tracy, and she's quite right, she said she couldn't manage the house-keeping on £5 a week. Now I didn't hesitate, I doubled it, now she gets £5 a fortnight. A rotten gag but it illustrates just how miserable I am.

CLARE: But there is a seriousness behind that.

DAWSON: I don't like money wasted, I'll be honest because I don't. It goes back to the old days if we haven't got anything. First time I saw a butcher's shop I thought there'd been an accident when I was a kid.

CLARE: Would Tracy argue a bit with you about this?

DAWSON: No, because she was brought up in exactly the same circumstances, she's great on that. She's a good manager.

CLARE: Do you . . .

DAWSON: In fact the baby said its first word the other day, Harrods.

CLARE: Do you have any regrets?

DAWSON: No, oddly enough, no. With all its ups and downs, with all its trauma, call it silliness, and the awful mistakes and the stupidity I've done, no, no regrets.

CLARE: And during this life of yours, has there ever been a moment when you felt despair, where you felt you couldn't go on, that you were near losing control?

DAWSON: No. I've been sad about things, stupid things, being away from home in terrible digs. You know yeah, but never, never to that extent. Because I, my philosophy was you've got to know failure before you know success. I tell you what, I've had that many failures I could recognise success. People used to say, you know, that success is just around the corner but I lived on the M1.

CLARE: The people I see are people who feel that life has dealt them a bad hand or they've had catastrophes and it's taken its toll and they have teetered on the edge of disaster. And they're interested in people like you who've gone through life and put yourself on the line. You've had tough times and so on, so they're interested to know, well, what is it about you that sees you through these things and you keep bouncing along?

DAWSON: A sense of the ridiculous.

CLARE: Well, say a bit more.

DAWSON: No matter how bad a thing is, there's always another side to it. When Meg died, I used to do the shopping at the local shops, just a small point, and when you've lost somebody, when somebody's deceased, people are very nice but they tend to talk up your nose, they bend their head forward and say, 'Are you managing all right,' so you even get an element of farce in a tragedy, because that's all comedy is, a reverse coin to tragedy, and I found in everything there's still a sense of the ridiculous. Old ladies used to take me round the back of the supermarket and say, 'Just give you a tip on prices,' and it'd be a tin of peas there for 10p. They'd say, 'Don't take the top tin, take the one at the bottom because that'll be 9p, you've saved a penny,' and they spend all day saving sixpence which to them, they've beaten the system. So there was always in everything an element of farce. To recognise that and say, yeah, that's what it's all about. If you ask why there's so many jokes about death – tragedy and comedy are hand in hand. We laugh at a person slipping on a banana skin because it isn't us, that's the only reason.

CLARE: And that would be . . .

DAWSON: We couldn't even afford a banana!

CLARE: That would be your particular recipe for what's kept you going?

DAWSON: I do a silly thing, Trace will bear me up on this. A silly thing. No matter how bad things are, look in a mirror and pull a face. Funnily enough, it seems to be a panacea of youth because if you take life like that with a sort of good-natured resignation, no matter how bad things are, and there are some terrible things, there's always a light side. Most people I know who've gone through very bad times and have had a sense of humour always come through it. And it's very vital to the human race. I think half the trouble today is there's no sense of humour anywhere. That's my theory and God forbid we should ever lose it altogether.

CLARE: Les Dawson, thank you very much.

DAWSON: It's been a pleasure, any time.

Bernie Grant

In 1990, according to statistics obtained from the UK Office of Population Censuses and Surveys (OPCS), there were over two and a half million people in Britain whose ethnic origins were the New Commonwealth. People from ethnic minorities living in Britain, particularly if they are black, experience a variety of practical disadvantages and difficulties, particularly in such areas as housing, education, health and employment. They can also be subject, in numerous everyday contexts, to overt racism and prejudice. There is, surprisingly, little reliable information as to their general psychological adjustment although there is much controversy concerning seemingly elevated rates of severe forms of mental illness. However, according to the British psychiatrist, Roland Littlewood, who for many years has been a powerful and influential voice concerning the complexity of the relationship between culture and mental health, there is ample evidence available 'that to be black in Britain today is to be exposed to a variety of adverse stimuli which can add up to a quite serious hazard to mental health.' (Littlewood, 1992)

Bernie Grant is one of those two and a half million. He is that rarity in Britain, namely a black member of parliament. There are still only a handful. Amongst the variety of adverse stimuli to which he has been exposed are taunts and accusations concerning his own mental stability. His alleged membership of that curious political sub-group known disparagingly as 'the loony left' attracts the disagreeable attentions of tabloid hacks and right-wing blimps. Simultaneously, prejudice against blacks and the mentally ill is obnoxiously expressed. Not even the most rabid journalist these days would use the term 'leprous' to describe the extreme left nor 'spastic', even 'senile'. But epithets of a psychiatric nature – 'psycho', 'schizo', 'loony' – are still considered acceptable and fair game.

Coming, as Bernie Grant does, out of a colonised corner of the Caribbean, he has a first-hand knowledge of what it means to be a black immigrant to Britain. A singular challenge from the outset is the question of identity. For Grant's pugnacious fellow-MP, Norman Tebbit, the issue is simply resolved. What country do you support at cricket? Responding to that particular test, Bernie Grant, along with many cricket lovers, is a West Indian! Actually, he is very clear indeed as to where he comes from because he has, like many of his contemporaries, made strenuous efforts to trace his roots. Grant speaks persuasively of the profound, restless yearning of contemporary blacks to find their home, their origins, 'to know that one thing, where their parents were from, or where their grandparents were from, which part of Africa.' His own great-grandparents came from the Congo, Sierra Leone and West Africa, and it is Africa, not Britain nor the Caribbean either, where he finds his spirtual home. Grant's emphasis on the importance of knowing your family tree, your ancestry and inheritance is interesting to set beside the discussion later in this collection with Professor Robert Winston, one of the pioneers of *in vitro* fertilisation.

An orthodox psychoanalytic examination of the psychology of Bernie Grant would lay considerable emphasis on his relationship with his father and his mother. Freud argued with his customary intransigence that the Oedipus Complex, the alleged desire of the male child to kill his father and possess his mother, was a universal neurosis. Upon it rests Freud's overall interpretation of individual psychology and social organisation. Grant's youthful radicalism, his fiery political activisim, his visceral anger expressed in actual physical terms – 'my heart starts hurting . . . I get very, very burnt up inside' – would be conventionally interpreted by Freudian psychoanalysts as the conscious expression of unconscious hostile impulses directed against his weak, ineffectual father, a man prepared to suffer and endure rather than confront discrimination and exploitation. In contrast, Grant's mother is idealised, a mother capable of caring for her own five children while teaching other people's, a guide and a mentor who turns him in the direction of political ideology and action and provides the passion and the power to take him to the top.

The problem with such an analysis is that it ignores the role of culture and the social context. It sees Bernie Grant's conflict, the black man's alienation within European society and culture, as an individual question. Class and culture-bound conflicts become reduced to inescapable human predicaments while the human individual is envisaged as little more than a bundle of primitive impulses. One black psychiatrist who took particular exception to Freudian psychoanalysis on these very grounds was Frantz Fanon who was born in Martinique, died of leukaemia in Bethesda, Maryland and who in his brief span of thirty-six years provided one of the most uncompromising and illuminating expositions on the psychology of racism that has yet appeared. Fanon was particularly critical of the Oedipus Complex. In his remarkable book, *Black Skin, White Masks*, published in 1967, he contested Freud's thesis that neurosis was an inescapable consequence of all cultures and thus inherent in the human condition – 'Every neurosis, every abnormal manifestation . . . is the product of the cultural situation' (Fanon, 1967).

In fact, Grant's early childhood and family atmosphere seem relatively normal but, if Fanon is right, this only complicates the issue further. As he put it, 'A normal (black) child having grown up within a normal family will become abnormal in the slightest contact with the white world.' The nature of life in Guyana when Bernie Grant was growing up meant that contact with the white world was unavoidable. He was christened with the name of a white British field-marshal. He spoke in his Caribbean home the King's English. His secondary education was at the hands of religious whites. Yet it is clear that even in childhood Grant experienced a personal discomfort in the world that was Guyana. The stimulus for the development of a conscious awareness of racial stereotyping in Grant was the rigid hierarchy of racial prejudice in his college – the whites at the top, followed by the Portuguese, then the Chinese and the Indians and so on down to the blacks. Interestingly, it was a somewhat similar experience that awakened the adolescent Fanon to entrenched alienation. His biographer, Hussein Abdilahi Bulhan, describes how Fanon, in the presence of an acquaintance, was uttering a disparaging remark about Italians when, suddenly, he realised his listener was himself of Italian extraction. The incident,

Bulhan argues, underscored for Fanon the force of stereotypes inculcated in him because of France's 'cultural imposition' on Martiniqueans (Bulhan, 1985). In Grant's case, the conflict provoked by Britain's cultural imposition was fanned by an influential mentor, his mother's brother. By the time he comes to Britain, the source of the culture which provokes the inner tension in the first place, he is a young adult, still struggling to establish a clear identity in terms of his race, his politics and his origins.

The Grant I interviewed, however, is a mature man, just turning fifty, who has struggled reasonably successfully to resolve the inner tensions generated by such an upbringing. He sounds more urbane and serene than his public persona would suggest. He has come to terms with many of the contradictions inherent in his life story yet surely the issue of cultural identity is not so easily resolved? By becoming a member of parliament and entering the outer circles of the Establishment Grant has risked his identity as a spokesperson for his own community. But by marrying a white woman he has risked being accused of a consuming desire to be white by proxy, of unconsciously distrusting his own blackness, a process of assimilation that has been called 'lactification'.

What is interesting about Grant is that it has been through an almost mystical relationship with Africa, an emotional identification with the idea of the continent from which, over a century ago, his ancestors were ripped and transported to the Caribbean, that he has come to terms with the psychological conflict that working as an MP in the stately chambers of the House of Commons constantly aggravates. Bernie Grant's sense of a communion with Africa might seem to strike a Jungian rather than a Freudian chord. Though he himself only went there for the first time as an adult, he instinctively feels it is like he has been there before. 'I get a very, very peculiar feeling . . . I certainly feel as though there is something there that is pulling me.' Jung would have rubbed his hands with satisfaction for his concept of the collective unconscious, that reservoir of primordial images inherited from the ancestral past, would seem to explain Grant's powerful inner sense of oneness with the continent of his ancestors. However, Jung's credentials to speak with authority on issues of ethnicity and race appear with hindsight to be even more compromised than Freud's. Frantz Fanon was particularly scornful and his attack highlights the vulnerability to social and political circumstances and events of the supposedly intrinsic and innate collective unconscious.

> Coming to take stock of reality, endeavouring to ascertain the instant of symbolic crystallisation, I very naturally found myself on the threshold of Jungian psychology. European civilisation is characterised by the presence of what Jung calls the collective unconscious, of an archetype, an expression of the bad instinct, of the darkness inherent in every ego, of the uncivilised savage, the Negro who slumbers in every white man. And Jung claims to have found in uncivilised peoples the same psychic structure that his diagram portrays. *Personally I think that Jung has deceived himself.* Moreover, all the peoples he has known – whether the Pueblo Indians of Arizona or the Negroes of Kenya in British East Africa – have had more or less traumatic contacts with the white man.

Jung was in no doubt about the uncivilising influences of the negro. In an article he published in 1930 he warned that living in close proximity with 'primitive peoples' was hazardous culturally and psychologically.

> Now what is more contagious than to live side by side with a rather primitive people? Go to Africa and see what happens . . . The inferior man exercises a tremendous pull upon civilised beings who are forced to live with him . . . To our subconscious mind contact with primitives recalls not only our childhood, but also our prehistory.

Bernie Grant is a man with a profound sense of destiny, of a mission of some kind that he may be privileged to undertake and fulfil and which is connected with the fierce battle against the kind of Fascism that Jung's statement embodies. His mission, however, does not seem to be connected with Britain. Time and place, what poet Louis MacNeice called 'our bridgeheads into reality, but also its concealment', may well be, for Grant, the future and Africa. In the meantime he soldiers on, identifying with and fighting for the marginal, the displaced, the disabled, the disenfranchised of Haringey, London, Britain; fighting too the severe form of diabetes which afflicts him and which he suffers with an impressive resignation.

CLARE: Bernie Grant is one of the true mavericks of British political life. He was born Bernard Alexander Montgomery Grant on February 17th, 1944 in what was then British Guyana. He was educated by the Jesuits in Georgetown and he came to Britain at the age of nineteen. He became Britain's first black council leader and for years one of Fleet Street's favourite targets, a loony lefty with a nickname of Barmy Bernie. In the aftermath of the Broadwater Farm Estate riots Douglas Hurd, then home secretary was moved to describe him as the high priest of racial conflict and even called the Labour Party to disown him as a prospective parliamentary candidate. But the call went unheeded and in 1987 Bernie Grant became member of parliament for Tottenham. Indeed, in the 1992 general election he almost trebled his majority.

His image as a hard left, anti-police militant has undergone considerable change since last year when he helped to defuse a potentially explosive situation caused by the death of Joy Gardener when the police tried to arrest and to deport her to Jamaica. As a result he has been hailed as the new voice of moderation by some and called a patsy for the Establishment by others.

Bernie Grant, do you feel there's a major discrepancy between how other people see you and how you see yourself.
GRANT: I think that that's correct because when I read the newspapers or I hear commentators on radio describing me, I don't recognise the person they are describing and I might tend to feel that they're talking about someone who's totally different, so, to some extent what they say doesn't affect me because I know within myself that that's not the person that they're describing.

CLARE: What is the factor that you think is most irritating, the feature that they appear to apply to you that you think really misses the point?

GRANT: Well, I think that I'm misunderstood. I think that what people tend to do is that they tend to associate me with various things or they tend to read into something that I'm saying that isn't there. And, you know, as a result they get it totally wrong. You know, I come from a long line of people who are story tellers, who are quite capable of telling stories and the culture that I come from, which is a very oral culture, particularly amongst people of African descent in the Caribbean. I think that that culture is one where you tell a story, you embellish it, you bring in a whole number of extraneous matters, and people expect it of you almost. And sometimes I find that when I say something they, the press and the media, they take what they want out of it. They don't give the whole context of it, so therefore it turns out to be totally different to what I'm saying.

CLARE: Do you find this a very literal culture in comparison, that's to say one that doesn't regard words in quite the same way as the culture from which you come?

GRANT: Well, that's right. Well, I think that there are two things. I think that we have different associations with words. Our words mean different things. That's one thing. But secondly, even on the basis of normal English grammar, I have found that when I say something, when I mention a word, that word might have three or four meanings and I might just pick one of those meanings and an English reporter, a white reporter, would take another meaning out of that word. If I can give you an example. Last year I had a meeting with the Metropolitan Police Commissioner, Mr Condon, during the Joy Gardener situation when we were trying to keep things calm and so on. And I came out of the meeting with Mr Condon and I was standing outside Scotland Yard and I thought, oh, well, let me make things a bit lighter, right, so I said, 'You know I've just been to see Mr Condon. We've had a very good meeting and I'm calling for a cessation of hostilities.' Now, the reporters thought that, you know, this guy is crazy because I mean, you only use that term if you're talking about a war or something that's going on. But I remember I checked carefully in the dictionary and hostilities mean any acts and so on, and I used it in the typical, in the literal, in the sort of open sense. But they sort of said, 'Oh, this guy must be a bit crazy because he is using a term like this.' That to me, you know, is an example of the kind of things where there is jut a total non-meeting of cultures and of people.

CLARE: There are others. You're very well placed in one sense to comment on them because you've come from a rich alternative culture. You come here but by immersing yourself in the politics of Britain, you've had to straddle the divide. You've had to cope with both cultures and you've got often to negotiate the flash points that occur between the two of them. In terms of your life here since you were nineteen, has that strengthened your sense of identity in terms of the first nineteen years of your life or has it altered it?

GRANT: Well, I think that the first nineteen years of my life set the foundation for me that I can't change one way or the other and coming to Britain to a different culture, although it's not that different because we knew what to expect as colonials. I keep telling people that I'm the product of a colonial educational system and so don't blame me, blame the colonialists. I think that what has happened is that I have been forced, as you say, into a position of being a go-between, between those various cultures. Now, I have no intention of getting rid of my own basic culture because I think it's superior quite frankly to a lot of other cultures that are around. And secondly, I have to try and bridge this divide so that when I'm with people who are white, I can't say English because black people are English as well, and when I'm with people who are white, I think that I have to try to moderate my sort of exuberance that I would normally sort of display. When I'm with black people, I'm able to be more open and I'm able to speak in a language that's different. So that I find that when I'm giving speeches, I have to tailor my speech accordingly to the audience I'm dealing with. So if I'm speaking to white working-class people up in Huddersfield in Yorkshire or something, I have to speak differently to when I'm speaking to a black audience. But sometimes I get confused. I get mixed-up because of the response of the audience and you tend to go a bit further. You sort of have to pull yourself back. I mean it's quite difficult, I think, to do this sort of balancing act or to act as a go-between between those various cultures and the various peoples.

CLARE: Do you think of yourself as Guyanese or English?

GRANT: I think I have to think of myself as Guyanese. Not necesarily Guyanese but Caribbean more particularly, because I'm not one of those people who is sort of tied up in the country that one grew up in. I think that's just, you know, an accident that I was born in Guyana as opposed to Trinidad or Barbados, particularly if one studies the history of enslavement. We could be anywhere, I mean we could be from anywhere but I see myself as a Caribbean person more so than I do an English person. You know, I think that's quite fair.

CLARE: And let's just take a look at the influences that you feel were most crucial in those formative nineteen years, I pick them as the years before you left. Your parents were both teachers, I was struck by that. Were they ambitious for you?

GRANT: Oh, yes. My parents always told us that we had to first of all speak the Queen's, the King's English I think it was at that time, very, very well indeed. And my mother was particularly strong on English grammar and syntax; and I remember she drilled these parts of speech into me and things like that. She was very good at English, an excellent English teacher, even when she came to Britain, you know, her talents were appreciated here. And my father was very much of the old school. He was very historic and he kept going into the history of not only the Caribbean and of Africa but also England. I took him to the House of Commons the other day and he saw all these pictures of James VI and so on and he would give you, even today, a whole spiel about, you know, the different kings and queens. So I grew up in an atmosphere that was very sort of academic in that sense.

CLARE: I sense by virtue of your name, that you were called after a prominent British General, Bernard Montgomery, that your parents would have admired Britain. Is that true?

GRANT: I think so. I was born during the war, which was why I had all these names. As a matter of fact, I was called Monty at home. It was only when I came to Britain, they started calling me Bernie.

CLARE: Do people still call you Monty?

GRANT: Oh, yes, if I go back to Guyana, they all call me Monty. When I came to Britain first, I was called Monty and our next door neighbour who was a white woman, she obviously thought that Monty didn't suit, you know, I mean, El Alamein and all that sort of thing, this is not the person. So she said, 'Why don't you try Bernie, it's a much nicer name,' (laughs) and they started calling me Bernie. I never thought of that, you jogged my memory. But, as you said, they were very British in that sense in that they were very straight-laced. We had a lot of moral guidance and they had a lot of respect for the king and this type of thing. They were brought up as real, proper colonial people with a lot of values.

CLARE: And how many Grants were there, how many children?

GRANT: There were five children. I've got an elder brother. I'm the second then I have three sisters.

CLARE: Of your parents, which do you think was the more influential with you?

GRANT: I think my mother. I think she was the more influential with all of us because to some extent we spent more time with my mother. She was a sort of career person in that when, you know, whenever she had a baby she didn't stop working, she had people in to look after the kids and she went, she kept on teaching because she saw teaching as something that was very important to her. Because she always said that for us in the colonies and for black people generally to make their way in the world they had to have a proper education. She saw it as her duty to teach not only her own children but everybody else's children, and she was always a teacher. She just seemed to do that. And I think that she had the larger effect on my life. My father is a Protestant but my mother's a Catholic and you know, we were brought up as Catholics and she the person who sort of guided us in that sense. So we started off with a kindergarten school run by the Carmelite nuns and that sort of thing and went on to the Jesuit school and so on.

CLARE: How did your father feel about that?

GRANT: He didn't seem particularly worried, to be frank, because I think that his sort of religion was very open and loose, but, you know, Catholicism is very tight, but he seemed quite happy. Another thing was that my father, he went into the interior of Guyana a lot and so we spent more time with our mother than with our father. As a matter of fact, he used to turn up at three or four in the morning and, you know, we'd just hear a whistle or something or a knock on the door and our father would appear and he kept doing this. When I was eight, I said, 'Look, why don't you take me with you because I'm fed up, you know, you keep turning up at these hours?' and he took me away with him right into the interior and I spent many happy years in primary school there with The Amerindian because I used to go out into the rainforests. The school that he taught at had a lot of Amerindian, you know, the native Guyanese and, you know, we befriended some of them and sometimes I'd go and spend days in the forest with them. That was quite an exciting part of my career.

CLARE: And then you went to a Jesuit school?

GRANT: Yes, I passed the sort of eleven-plus exam because we had that sort of schooling at that time. I went to a Jesuit secondary school, St Stanislas College and then I met a whole different sort of situation than the one I'd been accustomed to from being up in the countryside.

CLARE: Was that a mixed school?

GRANT: Yes, it was the main school for expatriates as a matter of fact. There were whites and blacks and Asians and Chinese and a few Amerindians. The other school which was its equivalent was called Queen's College. That was a government school and that mainly had black boys. These were boys schools, black boys and Asian boys, but the one I grew up in was very multi-racial.

CLARE: And the Jesuits themselves, where did they come from?

GRANT: The Jesuits came mainly from Ireland and from Scotland and a few English but the majority were from Ireland. You know, they told us all sorts of tales about Ireland. I suppose that's where my love of Irish folk music and rebel songs comes from because they used to tell us, you know. *The Boys of Wexford* and all this type of thing so that I picked up a lot of Irish history from the Irish Jesuits who taught me.

CLARE: It's intriguing. Here you are in a British colony, being educated in this school by Irish Jesuits who presumably would have, to some extent at any rate, passed on some of the Irish, anti-colonial history and tradition. Would that be so?

GRANT: That was right, and we detected, even as boys, the difference and some animosity between the Irish Jesuits and the English Jesuits in particular.

CLARE: In the school?

GRANT: In the school. And they of course taught us about life back in Ireland and about the potato famine and stuff and they talked about the fact that they were a colony of England and so Irish nationalism was coming through to me even at that very early age.

CLARE: And would you have made explicit connections between the Irish experience say, and the Caribbean experience?

GRANT: They didn't go that far, I have to say. Later on, when I was in sixth form and I started talking to some of them privately, they would then say that. But I suppose they felt that they had to keep a sort of air going that, you know, they're all in it together. So they didn't explicitly come out and talk about the differences between the English and the Irish.

CLARE: Did you develop a radical sense of your past and your experience during adolescence? There were your parents, loyal and committed to a variety of good British ideals and standards and values, and many of them are excellent. And then you were going through adolescence in this school. Did you start to see your destiny and your identity in somewhat different terms to how your parents had seen theirs?

GRANT: I think so because whilst I was growing up there were a number of things happening in the world. It was the beginning of the anti-colonial struggle, in places like Kenya. We used to hear about Mau-Mau in Kenya, Kenyatta, Nkrumah in Ghana. Of course very close to us we had the Cuban revolution with Fidel Castro and Che Guevara and so on and it was a period that was second to none in terms of political upheaval, you know, in history. I think that certainly for us these were very, very important times. As we were growing up, all these things were happening. We kept going to the Jesuits and asking them and because they were a radical order, they would put the best possible motives on those events so that we came out feeling, you know, very radical and very sort of rebellious and, of course, they encouraged a lot of political thinking. We had a lot of debates. The debating society was very important. And because we didn't have distractions like televisions and all those types of things, we found ourselves very involved in the political situation that was going on at the time.

CLARE: Did this worry your parents?

GRANT: It worried my father I think, because he was more cautious on these matters but my mother, she was very odd. As far as she was concerned, anything the Catholics did was OK anyway, but apart from that she was a bit, she was quite a bit radical herself in how she dealt with people and so on, so I think that she wasn't worried but I think my father was a bit worried about it.

CLARE: People here, as you've probably noted, in England that's to say, tend to see the Jesuits somewhat differently to the way you've just described them and certainly to the way that I experienced them. Because in Ireland the Jesuits likewise were seen, perhaps not to be radical but certainly liberal and had a tendency to make you think. They didn't deliver a given ideology. It sounds something similar there. They made you think about Nkrumah and Ghana and the political conflict and turmoil. Is that right?

GRANT: That's right. I think you hit the nail on the head when you said they made you think. I think that when I go back when I think about maths and Latin and all these things that I did I begin to realise what they were actually doing. They were actually making us unravel the things for ourselves so that they wouldn't just teach you something by a rule. They took you to the roots of everything, whether it be maths, whether it be Catholicism, whether it be politics, we always had to get to the roots of it and then we had to try to unravel it for ourselves and I think that this is what the Jesuits did, that I think was all superb. There was another element to when I was growing up. Guyana was British Guyana and it was a colony and you know in Guyana itself there was a struggle for liberation against the British at one stage; the British had suspended the constitution of Guyana, sent in a lot of troops, the Royal Highland Fusiliers, the Blackwatch and so on and there was political upheaval in Guyana. They shot a few people and so on. We were also caught up in that internal struggle. What was going on in Guyana against the British was, again, like the Irish and so the Irish were seen as like allies in the struggle against the English because the English were certainly identified, I think, as the real baddies.

CLARE: They were?

GRANT: In all this, yeah.

CLARE: Now, you did your O-levels in this school but then you dropped out.

GRANT: Mm.

CLARE: What happened?

GRANT: Well, I think that they tried to slow me down because by this time I mean I was getting a bit rebellious really.

CLARE: Were you fiery?

GRANT: I was quite fiery, I think, at that time and some say I still am! But I was quite fiery and they wouldn't put me into sixth form because I'd done my O-levels. I'd got ten O-levels and they said that I couldn't go into sixth form because I couldn't be a prefect because, you know, I was too rebellious. All the sixth formers were prefects and they didn't want to make me prefect so they said I had to go into this thing called fifth remove or something where I just sort of basically hung around for a year doing the things that I'd done before in order so that my discipline could get up to scratch.

CLARE: And that's what it was, it was about discipline.

GRANT: Yes it was about discipline.

CLARE: Controlling yourself.

GRANT: And controlling me so that in the end I got fed up and left.

CLARE: What were the things that would have happened that would have caused trouble?

GRANT: Well, I used to argue a lot with the teachers and so on, you know, pick them up on all sorts of points of history and that type of thing and with the politics, with the political situation going on, we used to listen to the BBC news. I remember seven o'clock in the morning and seven in the evening and we kept hearing about all these things that were happening around the world and I think it began to affect me probably more than most. And they thought that I was a bit unruly and a bit too troublesome, not because I was bad, you know, fighting and all that, but I think that the questions that I was posing to them I think that they couldn't deal with it and they couldn't deal with those questions. So I think that they felt that they best put me into a safe haven for a year to cool off.

CLARE: Did they see you as a bad influence?

GRANT: I think so, yes. I think I was seen perhaps, probably, as a bad influence, yes.

CLARE: Did you sense that you had leadership qualities, that people listened to you? I wondered whether you got a sense that maybe you had the ability to lead?

GRANT: Well, I think so. There were four or five of us used to go round, young fellows who were at college and that type of thing and they always used to congregate at my house, you know. It always seemed to be the central place and people used to keep getting attracted to it. So I suspected that perhaps people came here to hear what I had to say.

CLARE: Was it very male, I mean was it an all-male school?

GRANT: It was very male, yes.

CLARE: Did girls figure much in your adolescence?

GRANT: Not that much, to be frank with you. We tried our best to pull the odd girl so we weren't very good at it. I used to live near to the convent which was the girls school which was sort of opposite to our college, St Joseph's High School. And, you know, we used to try but I don't think we really succeeded very much, so that was one of my failures I'm quick to admit.

CLARE: So you went into this fifth year. But did you ever get into sixth year or was that when you came shortly after to the UK?

GRANT: Well, what happened is I was in this fifth remove and I stayed about a term there and then I got fed up with it and I left altogether and I went and worked sixty-five miles up the Demerara River in a bogside town called McKenzie and I got a job in the lab as an analyst. I used to analyse these bogside samples to see how much iron ore they contained, how much aluminium and so on and I worked up there for a couple of years and so I just left my studies and I went up there. I got involved in the trade union movement up there as well.

CLARE: You did?

GRANT: That was important. Whilst this was going on my uncle was head of the Guyana TUC and he was also the head of the teacher's union.

CLARE: Was this your mother's side or your father's side?

GRANT: My mother's brother, and he was very, very fiery, he was my hero and he'd been involved in politics locally and he'd been involved as well in trade unionism and he used to play bridge and he was a bit of a swashbuckling type, used to sing, had a great voice and so on, and so I was very attracted to him and he seemed to like me. So he took me around a lot and I began to pick up a whole number of trade union and political issues.

CLARE: So, how come you then came to the UK? You could have become a great political leader in Guyana.

GRANT: Well, in fact, you know, I could have done something politically in Guyana certainly because I'd joined the youth organisation. I was quite prominent. But my parents, my mother came to England because she had high blood pressure and had to have a temperate climate. My father and mother decided that I would best come to England to complete my studies, rather than stay in Guyana, so I came over here at the age of nineteen.

CLARE: Did the rest of the Grant family come too?

GRANT: Yes, my sisters came before me. My brother went to university in the West Indies and he joined us later on, about ten years later. And my father, he stayed in Guyana, working in Guyana, he was head of the teacher's training college and that type of thing and then later on he came up to join us.

CLARE: Now, you arrived in Britain in the early sixties. What was it like?

GRANT: Ooh, terrible. I came here in February, and everything was very grey and at that time we used to have all these fogs and smogs at Christmas, at winter time and I thought that the place was amazingly drab because everyone had these grey coats and there wasn't much colour around and the houses were all joined on to each other whereas where I came from, the houses had been separated. Everything you touched was cold because you never had central heating in those days and everything was cold. The plates were cold and I just couldn't handle it. For the first few months I thought it was terrible. And the other thing is that I found that Britain seemed to be behind what I had left in Guyana because being close to America, we had all the American influences so that all the films, the American films, and all the American styles and all that, you know, we were quite accustomed to in Guyana. And we came to England and we found that those things hadn't arrived here as yet and in fact, some of the films and stuff that we had seen didn't come up to Britain until six months or a year later. So I thought it was a bit of a backward place.

CLARE: Did you encounter different reactions in terms of your colour than you had anticipated? I don't know quite how it was in Guyana. Clearly there must have been, as there was in most colonies, a white Establishment and I don't know the sense in which your rebellion fed off that. But certainly coming to England you would have been immediately conscious of the fact that you were black. Just let's stay with Guyana for a second. When would you have been conscious that there was a black/white issue?

GRANT: I think when I went to secondary school, when I came back from the interior with my father and with the Amerindians and I came to college with the white boys and the Portuguese and so on, and there quite clearly, there was a colour code, with the whites being at the top. We talked about the whites, we talked about the English, the Scottish and the French and so on and we called the Portuguese non-white, you see, they were like the second rung on the ladder. Then we had Chinese and Indians and so on and I began to feel it then because, you know, boys would tell you all sorts of things, you couldn't go to their houses or they said you couldn't go, or if you went to their houses you had to stay outside, you couldn't come inside because you are black and that type of thing. And I began to get the feeling then and we had one or two racist incidents from one or two of the priests, who, you know, said a few things to some of the black boys and so I began even more to associate myself with what was happening in Kenya and what was happening in the rest of the world. So that from the age of twelve I think I began to feel it in Guyana.

CLARE: So when you came here would you have been already, if you like, sensitised to discrimination?

GRANT: Well, I think that I was to some extent but not as much as when I got here because although there was this quite clear division on the basis of colour, you know that everyone in the bank was going to be white or because they even had a division if you are light skinned black, then you were of course better because you're closer to the whites than if you were black. So, we had all those things but we still had the feeling that we were, you know, we were moving and that we were going to get self-government and the black people who were in the ascendency would take over and that type of thing. So, we thought it was just a matter of time. When I came to Britain I found that the racism here was very overt. I remember walking down the streets in Hornsey on a Saturday evening, and a car would pull up and a lot of white boys would just pile out and start calling you names and rush to attack you and so on. We never got that type of thing in Guyana and, you know, at those times, you know, the only thing that you had to do was run like hell to get out of it. I also found that when I tried to get jobs and so on, people used race against me. I remember at that time, I thought I was fairly bright and I took a test to become a counter clerk with the post office and it was a maths test and English test and it was very elementary stuff and I got through it very quickly and he started asking me all sorts of questions, trying to trap me, and I got through all of them. But then he asked me what was a tanner and I said , 'Oh, a ten pound note.' I thought he said what was a tenner and I know his face lit up and he said, 'Ah, how could you be a post office counter clerk if you don't know the difference between a tanner and a tenner.' And on that one thing he failed me, you know, even though I'd spent about two hours passing everything else. So, I got the feeling that this country was, you know, it was pretty racist.

CLARE: And what did you do?

GRANT: Well, I went to Tottenham College for a couple of years to do my A-levels. I started off doing it part-time because I was working in the civil engineer's office of British Rail at Kings Cross as a clerk. I then did the A-levels and left and went to university where I was doing mine engineering for a couple of years and the race thing seemed to follow me because there was a lot of racism on the course and in connection with the placement of the engineers as students, because the white students were able to go to South Africa and to Zambia during the long holiday, and they worked in supervisory positions, even in places like Zambia, you know, we weren't allowed to go . . . So I got thoroughly fed up with it because I told the professor I was getting a second-class education, I wasn't prepared to stand for it and basically I dropped out of the university after a couple of years and I got a job in the summer working in the post office as a telephonist, an overseas telephonist. I got involved in the trade union movement there and stayed there for about ten years. I was supposed to come back to university, I was still deciding whether I should or not, but eventually, I thought that I'd better stay and work in the exchange. I got involved in the trade union movement, people were depending on me because they hadn't had anybody that knew so much about life generally, I suppose, or had such academic qualifications, so I stayed behind . . .

CLARE: Just remind me, at that time, was it unusual for someone from the Caribbean and Afro-Caribbean to be active in the British trade union movement? One thinks of the Irish, of course, and the Scottish, strong elements of working-class

Irish and Scots in the British trade union movement. What about Afro-Caribbean?

GRANT: It wasn't unusual, but people were at very low levels, because the black people from the Caribbean and from Africa always knew that organs like the trade union movement were organs that we needed to work with to get anywhere, but we were never given an opportunity of coming through the ranks. We were there in positions like shop stewards and that type of thing, but we never got very high up the union ladder. But there was quite a lot of participation at the grass roots level. Mind you, there was a lot of racism amongst trade unionists as well.

CLARE: What was that affect on you? What did it do to you, being exposed to that level of overt racism. Did you become a very angry man?

GRANT: Oh, yes, I was constantly angry because, you see, I was brought up by my uncle in the trade union movement and he was always singing the praises of the trade union movement because they were affiliated to the TUC over here. He came here, they went over there and so on and he talked about brotherhood of trade unionists and so on and I was very firmly committed to the trade union movement. And when I saw the racism, at that time the dockers marched with Enoch Powell, we had a lot of racism in terms of British Rail and some of the unions saying that blacks could only get certain positions, certain jobs, and that type of thing. I was fairly sickened by it all but I still knew that it was the only hope really for black working-class people, so I stuck with the trade union movement.

CLARE: What about revolution? Would you have been drawn into that?

GRANT: Sure. The post office had the forty-one-day strike in 1971 and I got approached by people from the Socialist Labour League which was a Trotsky organisation. We were very militant and, you know, we were sold out, I believe, by Tom Jackson at that time who was the general secretary, so we were all feeling a bit discouraged and that was the time when they approached us, a group of us and said, 'Why don't you come here?' and they started talking about Marxism and dialectical materialism and so on. So I got drawn into that and for about three or four years I was very active in the Socialist Labour League and, you know, went and did a lot of Marxist schools. I went to Marxist school and we talked about a different approach to the way things were happening in the world and being brought up as a Catholic, I was, you know, I was constantly taught that everything was done by God and this and that and the other and what they did was, they gave me· an alternative view of the world which made sense. It made sense logically and I think that I was very attracted to that and because I'd lost my faith, basically, in Catholicism, and I'd lost faith in the West, and the way in which they were treating people, the Americans in Vietnam, et cetera, I think that this was an alternative that grabbed and so I spent about four years with the Socialist Labour League as a Trotskyist.

CLARE: And what changed you?

GRANT: Well, I changed because I found that what they were saying wasn't actually coming through. Because they kept saying constantly that the revolution's around the corner and that type of thing and when things happened, I remember when Rolls Royce collapsed, they said, 'Oh, well, this is it and something else will crash in the stock exchange.' They said this was it and it didn't actually quite work out. Gradually I got disillusioned and I faded away and came back and joined the Labour Party in 1975.

CLARE: And yet, of course, the Labour Party would pose its own problems in terms of someone such as yourself joining it. The trade union movement was very strongly allied to the Labour Party so the kind of racism you would have found in one, you would have found in the other.

GRANT: I actually didn't find a lot of racism in the Labour Party in Tottenham. I remember there was racism in other Labour parties yes, but certainly in Tottenham I didn't find that and, in fact, we set up an organisation called the Haringey Labour Movement Anti-Racist Anti-Fascist Campaign. It's the longest name of any organisation I've been associated with, and the object of that was to try and combat the growing threat from the National Front and other fascist organisations around 1977. And what we did was, we actually organised ourselves with the trade union movement locally in order to ensure that no fascist had a platform within Haringey and we organised in that way and up until today, you know, the fascists leave Haringey alone. They don't come to Haringey very much.

CLARE: So, you really were becoming a political figure during the late sixties, early seventies. What about your personal life at this stage? Had you married? Did you have children?

GRANT: Yeah, I had kids around 1975. I think my first son was born in 1975 and I was married, you know, at the time. She is someone of Italian parentage and we met in the post office. She used to work for the post office as a telephonist so we met and we had a son. And then later on we had twins. In this time I was married and doing a lot of work in terms of community groups and the trade union movement.

CLARE: How long would it have lasted, because it did break up didn't it?

GRANT: Yeah, it lasted until 1985, so it lasted about ten years and then we split up.

CLARE: And you're now in a long-standing relationship?

GRANT: Sure.

CLARE: And that relationship itself has been the source of considerable interest because you're living with a white woman?

GRANT: Yes, yes.

CLARE: Has that caused you any difficulties in terms of your own cultural group? I ask that because of this problem which all of us have who, in a sense, marry across a cultural divide but it is particularly sharp, isn't it, when it becomes a colour issue in a society such as Britain? And I wondered how you've experienced that?

GRANT: Yes, it does cause some difficulty and I know that there are some groups and some black people who avoid me like the plague.

CLARE: They would unite on that issue, would they?

GRANT: Yes, yes, they'd say I'm not a wholly black person because I've got a white partner. It's something that comes up and also some very militant and black feminists, you know, they throw this at you and sometimes they use it to test you out. Sometimes in the United States of America as well . . .

CLARE: Test you in what sense?

GRANT: They test you to see whether you are truly 'black' in quotes or whether you're just a sell-out.

CLARE: An Uncle Tom?

GRANT: Yes, that type of thing. So there is that and sometimes I feel that in certain sections in the black community I'm not fully, it's quite clear that I'm not fully accepted because when I'm a politician, even though they might think that I'm not a bad politician, but I'm a politician so that I'm somewhat a sort of Establishment figure and then secondly because I've got a white, you know, I've got a white partner, then they think also that that's a problem.

CLARE: How do you cope with that, because it must be painful sometimes?

GRANT: Well, sometimes it hurts but I just say to them, 'Well, I'm sorry but you know I met my partner at a time when I met her.' I didn't become famous and then go out and look for a white partner in order to establish my fame or anything like that. I met her before I became nationally known so that what am I supposed to do? Am I supposed to say, 'Well, hang on, now I'm nationally known I'm going to kick her out and get on and get a black partner just for the sake of appearances.' I don't think that that's on.

CLARE: You've put your finger on it yourself, there is a sense that now that you're a famous man, that in some way being involved with a white woman says something denigratory about black women.

GRANT: Well, yes, that's the impression and that's what some people try to say. It's a difficult argument to argue against sometimes. Sometimes when people want to get at me, when I get up and talk about Africa and about African origin and I talk about the good things about Africa and our heritage and so on and then someone points a finger and says, 'Yeah, well, if it's so good about Africa, why is it that you're with a white woman,' you know. So, you know, that's a bit of a problem but

I think that what I try to do is I try to let people know that this is not a problem for me. I think now people have accepted it because I think that I've been through a lot of tests and I think that people say that that's just one thing that we hold against him but the rest of him is OK so I think that I've got this kind of arrangement with the community.

CLARE: But has it changed you? Let me explain why I ask. It's to do with the fact that by virtue of my work I'm interested in the way the private, the personal, influences the public and I wondered whether becoming involved with your partner – we'd better give her name – it's Sharon, isn't it?

GRANT: Sharon, yes.

CLARE: Becoming involved, falling in love with this woman, and sharing your life with her, whether that itself changed you? Whether you might have gone a different direction about the issue of race and culture on a political public stage but for what is a personal and largely private experience, that's what interests me.

GRANT: Yes, I think that it must change me. I mean I'd be crazy if, you know, you'd been with someone for many years and that person doesn't change your life and I hope that I've changed her as well. It has changed me in that it has made me realise that, well, like you know, all white people aren't bad. I knew that but it reinforced it because it's very easy at a time when you know, people are getting killed and murdered and racism is rampant for people to quite easily forget the good people and just concentrate on the bad people and say well, these people are the cause of all our problems.

CLARE: And did you occasionally find yourself in that position, in that emotional position?

GRANT: Oh, yes, quite often.

CLARE: Had I met you at certain stages you might have expressed that kind of view to me?

GRANT: Yes, yes, yeah, quite often. And I think that what Sharon has done is she's helped me to temper that. I think that she's done a lot anyway in terms of organisational things and dealing with the press and so on and I think that she's given me a kind of stickability that I think, you know, as a person of

African origin, I didn't have. I tended to be very sort of bright but like a butterfly, flitting from thing to thing, from one thing to the other and I think that she's a stabiliser. But I think what it has given to me is a different view of the world. There's no way that I could have a view that I hate all white people and all this type of thing, you know, because of the relationship, that's quite clear.

CLARE: And of course, in a sense, that's what some of your critics fear. They would fear you mellowing in a sense, of taking a broader vision. Isn't this the great conflict for a politician? That if you develop a broader view the purists see you selling out. If, on the other hand, you remain a purist, you're locked into a small, no doubt reassuringly, pure idea but it doesn't take you very far.

GRANT: Yes, again you've hit the nail on the head, because if you stay a purist in that sense, you don't advance the cause that you're fighting for because you're locked in, you're isolated and so on. If you move too far the other way, then of course you're in danger of selling out but you have to move in order to break the deadlock because, you know, in order for there to be advance in terms of race, racial equality, blacks have to concede something and whites have to concede, both sides have to concede, so people have to make the first approach. The problem is taking people with you so that sometimes I'm forced to make more militant statements than I would perhaps want to make but I have to do that because I know that there is a constituency out there that I have to bring with me and that if I allow them to push me aside, or if I'm allowed to become isolated from them, then there's going to be no hope for those people, and a lot of them are some of the young black people.

CLARE: Do you encounter, yourself and Sharon, do you encounter much practical problems? What's it like to be a mixed couple in Britain in the 1990s?

GRANT: It's not too bad. I think that perhaps I'm a special case and maybe not the right person to ask because I'm easily recognisable and so on and people know us and people accept us or they don't, you know, but there's no big deal?

CLARE: Do you have children?

GRANT: Yes, yes I've got three boys but not with Sharon but my previous wife.

CLARE: Yes, I meant with Sharon.

GRANT: No.

CLARE: Would you have any anxieties about having a child of a mixed marriage in Britain at the present time?

GRANT: No . . .

CLARE: Do you feel it's society that's genuinely changing?

GRANT: I think that it is possible to change this society. I think it was changing quite quickly, but I think in recent years that the change has stopped and that concerns me. I've got kids who are of mixed race, they're very sensible and the thing that encourages me, I think, is that they believe that they can cope and they don't have huge hang-ups because the sort of people they go around with, the people that they meet, the young white people and so on and other people, they act very naturally to each other and they are accepted and they accept and so there's no big problem in that sense. The problem comes when they try to get jobs and when the instituionalised racism begins to come down on them and when they're picked up by the police doing nothing and that type of thing. That's when the problems appear. But in terms of the relationships with their peers, they don't have a problem with that at all. I think that certainly from the inner city areas, Haringey and so on, how the races, the young people mix, they should be an example for the older people, but unfortunately, you know, they aren't. But the young people have no problems at all.

CLARE: Do you feel that the Afro-Caribbean in Britain has the kind of pride and confidence you clearly did have? It came across in the early sixties as a kind of fiery racialism and you were an angry man, I suspect, but you were projecting a lot of your feelings outward. I doubt if you were depressed, we'll come back to that in a moment as to whether you ever became so, but, that wouldn't have been the picture of you. You would have been animated by projecting your feelings outwards and being determined to do something about various things. What about the extent to which Afro-Caribbeans in this culture, by virtue of their experience, are depressed?

GRANT: I think that a lot of them aren't able to be as outgoing as I was. First of all because they haven't grown up in a country which they can feel belongs to them and that they're free in that country.

CLARE: That was important to you.

GRANT: Most important, because it gave me an outlook on life that was totally different and it also gave me the feeling that if anything happens, I can go back there or go home, where I'll be safe.

CLARE: Would you still have that back there, at the back of your mind?

GRANT: Yes, yes, yeah. I still don't feel as though I belong totally to Britain. I still feel as though I belong in the Caribbean or in Africa as opposed to Britain and it's nothing to do with the climate or anything like that. It's to do with how people perceive you and how black people fit into this society here. And I think that one of the other things that a lot of black people in Britain don't have is they don't have the education, educational background. They don't have the knowlege of geography, they don't have the knowledge of history that we had. And they don't have the struggle that we had when I came here. When I came in '63, you know, we had to struggle, we really had to struggle, but our children and our children's children, they don't have, they don't come into the same situation. They come into a situation where they are able to go wherever they want to go because of the Race Relations Act that we fought for and that type of thing. So that our experiences are totally different to theirs and I really regret the fact that a lot of these kids nowadays are brought up in a way that doesn't equip them with the tools of being able to express themselves properly and to fight for their own rights and to feel as though they belong to this country. So that's why I'm arguing that, you know, we should retain our links with Africa, the African culture and those things, because they strengthen those kids and they will inevitbly strengthen British society. There are people who argue, 'No, let's cut off all those links and let's have a monolithic, monocultural society which is purely white,' and that's wrong.

CLARE: But of course, in addition, what you had in Guyana was, you personally had a very strong family with parents who invested a considerable amount in education. I was struck by that comment that you made, that they saw that as really the ticket to making yourself something in this world and the Jesuits, for all their faults, gave you a good education.

GRANT: Sure, that is right. And of course, there is no equivalent. I haven't been able to find an equivalent.

CLARE: Here?

GRANT: Here, in this country, and that's regrettable. A lot of people of African origin in Britain know this, and this is why people try to set up supplementary schools and try to bring in additional education. Unfortunately, a lot of local education authorities don't see the value of these instruments, these different Saturday schools and so on and that creates a problem for us.

CLARE: In comparison to the education you got, the education that's here isn't all that great, is it?

GRANT: No, it's very substandard really. Give me a colonial type education any time to what's happening here. It happens in reality, a lot of kids who go back to the Caribbean have to go two or three classes lower than their peers, you know, when they arrive there because the educational standard here is so much lower that it's unbelievable. I remember in 1981 we took a group of kids from Tottenham, bright kids from Tottenham, to Grenada and Trinidad and we had them mixing with their age group in those countries and those kids were miles ahead of them.

CLARE: The kids in Trinidad?

GRANT: In Trinidad and Grenada and so on. They were miles ahead of the Tottenham boys, and a part of that was because those kids were in their own country. They were confident, they knew what they were about and they were able to learn and they just exuded confidence and our kids in Tottenham couldn't match it.

CLARE: The extent to which that troubles you, do you ever get depressed to the extent that you feel the problems that you see around you, particularly in terms of your own people here in

Britain, are so gargantuan that it'll grind on, that there'll be no great change? Do you ever get depressed about how little you can do?

GRANT: Yes, oh, yes, I get depressed but depression doesn't last long, you know, with me because I've invariably got so much to do that I don't have time to sit and meditate and, you know, feel sorry for myself.

CLARE: You're a doer.

GRANT: Yes, I think so. I've always been very active but sometimes you think, 'Oh, there's no way out,' but a part of that is because of the sort of Marxist teachings as well, because one of the things we learnt in dialectical materialism is that things change into their opposites. So that, OK, depression will change into joy or whatever and, of course, joy changes into depression as well, so that if you believe that, then you believe that you know this state that you're in can't last for long and the position that we're in can't remain the same for long because things are constantly changing. So therefore there is hope. And I think that it is that more than, over and above, everything else that makes me carry on, because I believe that, OK, things might be bleak today but tomorrow is a new day and anything can happen and anything is possible.

CLARE: So if you do get depressed, it doesn't last very long?

GRANT: No, it doesn't last very long.

CLARE: Have you ever been at the stage where you felt like throwing everything in and doing something else?

GRANT: No, not really. I've got a very strong sense of history. It's almost as if I'm being guided by some force that I can't really come to terms with because you know, sometimes I feel that I have to go down a certain road or I have to say something and it's almost as if it's not speaking, as if something has taken hold of me. I don't know why, I can't understand it and I can't explain it. I haven't asked anybody about it.

CLARE: Would it happen in the middle of a meeting or sometimes before it?

GRANT: It will usually happen in the middle of something?

CLARE: That you feel almost seized by something?

GRANT: Yeah, you know, at a moment when there's a moment of

confusion, you know, before there is clarity there is a moment of confusion and it can go in several different directions. And then something would sort of say, well right, this is the road, some sort of guidance would come. I don't know where it comes from. I'm not a religious person.

CLARE: You're not?

GRANT: No, because I don't believe in a God and all this type of thing but I certainly think that I'm quite a spiritual person and I sort of have a feeling and an empathy with certain things that I believe could be responsible, somehow, for this but I just feel as though I'm a part of some kind of history and that I'm just playing my part in it.

CLARE: Do you ever feel that you might have a major part to play in it?

GRANT: Yes.

CLARE: A sense of destiny?

GRANT: Yes, sometimes I feel that but I don't think the moment has arrived just yet. I just keep thinking that there is always something that isn't quite right so that I think that I haven't reached the pinnacle of whatever it is.

CLARE: And would it be here in Britain?

GRANT: That's a good question. That's a good question. I don't know. I've been going to Africa and going to the Caribbean and certainly in Africa I get a very, very strong feeling of some kind of destiny that's linked with Africa in some way. I don't know what it is but I know that whatever it is it's going to be linked with Africa and certainly when I go to the continent of various countries I get this very, very strong feeling.

CLARE: What is it like for you to go to Africa? What is it like?

GRANT: Well, I can't say that it's like I've been there before but it is like I've been there before. To me it's like a home that has been kept away from me for a long time. It's almost as if I'm going back in time. And when I get there I get a very, very peculiar feeling, particularly in Southern Africa, in places like Zimbabwe and in South Africa. I certainly feel as though there is something that is pulling me and when I go there you know, I give really great speeches and things. I really get moved. So that I think there is some destiny linked with Africa but I don't know what it is.

CLARE: Do you know much about your background, about where your parents and so on came from?

GRANT: Sure. My father told us that his grandfather was one of three brothers, and that they came from the Congo, right, which was Zaire and all those places were a part of the Congo at that time and that they split them up, they put one into each of the counties in Guyana in order to split up the family and my father said that my great grandmother came from Sierra Leone. On my mother's side, I think that they came from West Africa. I think we've traced it back through the sorts of songs that they sing and that type of thing. It's traced back somewhere around Nigeria, Ghana area. So it's a mixture.

CLARE: And yet you feel, if anything, more at home further south?

GRANT: Further south, yeah. I feel it very strong.

CLARE: No idea why?

GRANT: I have no idea why. I went once to meet one of these people called, oh, I can't remember what it's called, it's sort of like a native doctor who cures you and everything and he threw you know, sticks and stuff, and he said that I came from Zimbabwe as one of a particular tribe. And, in fact, when I was in Zimbabwe a number of people came up to me as if they knew me and when I said that I didn't know them and everything, they were very shocked and that type of thing. So I think that there is some link there that I haven't been able to establish. Because this is one of the things, you know, where people come from that is constantly eating away at people of African origin. I mean we need to know where we are from. You know, people, the greatest, you know, African people who were slaves or taken away, they always want to know that one thing, where their parents were from or where their grandparents were from, which part of Africa.

CLARE: And you're the same?

GRANT: I'm the same. This yearning that's in you, that you can't get rid of, I don't know why, but every single black person has that yearning and people don't understand it, white people don't understand it. So that when we call for reparations and all these things, it is as if something inside us is saying, 'Please let us have the truth about the situation, we want to know.'

CLARE: And you've really located yourself in three places. There is Guyana itself, there's Britain, then there's Africa. But is it fair to ask you, where do you feel at home?

GRANT: I (sighs), I think that I feel most at home in Guyana. But that is probably because I haven't spent a long time in Africa. I think that I would feel most at home in Africa if I were able to spend, you know, spend three or four months there. I think I'd feel most at home there because when you go there you just fit into the place in a way that I don't even in Guyana. I suspect because with Guyana it's very westernised and so on but when you go, particularly into the rural areas of Africa, there is a feeling there that I can't describe anyway.

CLARE: So how do you cope with the dissonances, with the angles of living and working here and right in the centre of the British Establishment and power centre, the House of Commons? Do you have a sense of detachment as well as involvement?

GRANT: I have that but I think that I'm doing a job, I think that I'm here to do a job and that much as I would love to go and live in Africa or in the Caribbean or wherever, that it's a sacrifice that I feel that I am making in actually being in the House of Commons and I think that I'm there because at this moment in time, it's necessary for there to be somebody like me in the House of Commons in order to represent people, in order, perhaps to find out something from the past in terms of what's in the records of the House of Commons library or whatever. But I feel that I'm there for a purpose. So that I can rationalise my being in the House of Commons but it's pretty hard sometimes, you know, when I feel that I would really want to give it up and, you know, just go and live an ordinary life or just to get rid of Britain. If I didn't have this sense of responsibility that I have to be there, be right there in the House of Commons, then I'd have been off, I wouldn't stay in Britain at all. I'd have been off . . .

CLARE: You'd have been . . .

GRANT: I'd be a dirt farmer somewhere in Guyana or Africa. I'd prefer that to living in this situation in Britain.

CLARE: So really, it's the mission, it's the duty that keeps you here?

GRANT: Yeah.

CLARE: Is there anything else? What is there about the life you lead here other than that sense of mission and duty, that gives you satisfaction, or even pleasure?

GRANT: Well, I think having said that I feel a sense of duty, I also have to say that it is quite pleasurable sometimes being in the House of Commons, being at a place where things happen, where events unfold, great events have unfolded over the past five years. We've been very lucky in a sense to have some of the great speeches and to see the downfall of great politicians and to be part of that, even though you're just a minute part of it. I think that has been very important. But I also think that the things that I like about being in the House of Commons, the thing that I like is that it gives the opportunity of meeting people that you would never meet outside of the House of Commons. I've learnt a lot of things. I met somebody, some black people from Tuvalu and from Fiji and other places, people that I would never have an opportunity of meeting. So that I see the place as an important place in terms of contact and in terms of the ability of an MP to go to different parts of the world and meet different people and to carry on my theories because I have my own theories of how life should be lived and to test those theories out with people all around the globe. I try to go to various countries to meet not only the politicians but to meet with the ordinary people to see whether in fact a person who is a native of Guyana is the same as a person who is a native of Zimbabwe. To see whether there is a real link there and that at some future time we might be able to link up all these people of like mind in order for us to have a decent world to live in. And, so that's important, you know, and the House of Commons allows you to make those sorts of contacts.

CLARE: But are you something of a loner there, because it's something of a club where, clearly, people are committed to many things? It must be difficult for you because an awful lot of what goes on there must come across in a sense of another world.

CLARE: Sure. I'm naturally a very sort of gregarious person and I think this is something the people don't understand. I mean, when I see myself as a representative of people in Tottenham generally and of black people in particular and I always like to do things collectively and I think this is part of my make-up and a part of how I was brought up, that we did things as a group, you know, as a family and that type of thing, as a people. I am very much involved in that sort of thing and the House of Commons isn't the sort of place for that to happen, because the House of Commons is made up a number of individuals who are always trying to outdo each other, stab each other in the back.

CLARE: Competitive place.

GRANT: That's right, competitiveness in order to get patronage and to gain a thing. I'm not into that so that I miss out all of that, so I don't go into the bars and the places where all the gossip goes ahead and so on. I just stay in my room. I have a lot of meetings, I have people coming to see me in the House of Commons, so I'm not lonely in that sense. But I don't mix a lot I think with a lot of the other MPs, apart from a select group of people within the Campaign Group of Labour MPs who are socialists like myself and who have a certain perspective on politics.

CLARE: Do you see yourself as a role model? Are you conscious of the fact that you might be saying to young West Indians and Africans and so on, 'Look, it is possible to do what I am doing'?

GRANT: I'm a bit troubled by this. I've never felt myself as a role model. I have always seen myself as doing things in a certain way to try and get the best out of a situation, more and more I have begun to realise that people see me as a role model, whereas it's almost as if I've got nothing to do with it. So therefore, that has had to temper my behaviour in certain situations. I mean, I'd like to be a bit more radical and a lot more outspoken and make a lot more fuss in the House of Commons. I remember I was thinking of being thrown out once by the speaker and I'd have been the first person to be thrown out on television and so on but people said, 'No, no, no, no, no, no, you can't, you can't do that,' and they explained why it is that I can't be the first person. Because, you know, I'd have been the first black person to be thrown out on television and so on and people would feel that that would be like a stain on black people, so therefore I've had to draw back my natural inclinations in a whole number of areas in order to sort of have some kind of role model. But I'm not happy in this position as a role model because what I think role models are might not equate with what people generally think. But I accept that in the position I am in, I have to behave in a reasonable manner so that young people could perhaps look up to me and so on.

CLARE: Seeing you as a role model means that somehow you've no private life, that anything you do is somehow going to set a standard or is indicating how other people should live. You're saying to me, 'That's not something I really wanted but it's been foisted on me.'

GRANT: It's been foisted on me and I've got to live with it, unless I am able to disappear into Africa somewhere, in the bush . . .

CLARE: I remember when I interviewed Arthur Ashe, he talked very tellingly about the conflict for a black man in the United States. That he could either behave like Mohammed Ali, 'If that's the way you want a black man to behave, I'll show you, I will be your firebrand, I will say the unsayable, I will act out your fantasies of what a black man is.' Or in Ashe's case, you have to be a super gentleman. You have to be, in a sense, more controlled than the controlled. I wonder was there something equivalent here, in Britain? Do you sense that, if you were to be really yourself, if you were to be really fiery, people would say that gives the wrong image of a black man in Britain. On the other hand, if you behave in a more controlled way, some of the people, some of your own people will say, you've sold out, you've become a white man, a white man's black man.

GRANT: Well, I think if this is what Arthur Ashe says is the position in the States, it's not quite the same here, thank God. Because I think here that you're able to act more out of the ordinary, say, and it'll be accepted, than perhaps a number of other countries. I think on the continent it's vastly different.

CLARE: Really?

GRANT: You can still have a measure of independence and go your own way and say a few things as long as you don't go too far. I think that there is a certain amount of tolerance in British society still that allows you basically form your own path. But it's becoming more and more difficult to maintain that balance and to have that fine divide.

CLARE: More and more difficult?

GRANT: It's becoming more and more difficult because I think the press in particular now, they move into one's private life and so on, so much that it's becoming very, very difficult to be yourself. I think that what the press and the media want and particularly tabloid press are basically, you know, carbon copies of people that they decide how they should behave. And I think that as far as I'm concerned there's no way that I'm going to act like that but I have to take that in mind and that is sort of cautionary, that sort of restricts my movements in some way but it's not as bad as having to sell out.

CLARE: Is it fair to ask yourself this, do you see yourself continuing in politics in Britain for the foreseeable future or do you have a life plan that involves a change of direction at some stage?

GRANT: I have a sort of a plan but I know that things change into the opposite so I know it's a waste of time having any sort of real serious plan but generally I would like perhaps to do another term and then just retire somewhere and do something else, getting involved in helping the movement in another way. I doubt whether that will happen. It would depend on whether there are other people coming up who'll be MPs but if by the next election there are only a handful of black MPs again, I mean, you can't just resign or leave it like that because people will still be depending on you. So it would depend on whether other people come forward. I'm particularly keen to get young people interested in politics and coming up because you know, we want to hand on to other people so that we can keep up the pressure. That would prevent me from giving it up if there is nobody else to take it over.

CLARE: You've talked about your Afro-Caribbean inheritance, and of course, your Guyanese life and experience, but you've also reminded me, as if I needed reminding, that it's a colonial experience that you had in those first nineteen years and we've dwelt to some extent on some of the negative aspects of that, the racism and the way in which power was distributed and so on. When you look at your life, what would you see, or would you see a positive inheritance of the colonial experience for you? What would you be able to say to the British, if you felt like it, that they might, in their guilt-ridden moments, feel better about, that you feel you owe to this society, or you're grateful, if one is grateful about these things, but anyway, you appreciate that experience and set it against some of the more negative ones? What would you identify in your own character and experience?

GRANT: Well, I think that the education and freedom that one has, I think that is perhaps peculiar to the English-speaking world, the Brits and the Americans and so on. I don't think that you get it, certainly you don't get it, you don't appear to get it amongst many blacks in the other languages. I think that perhaps British colonisation was different from the others.

CLARE: Different in that . . .

GRANT: Well, I think that they allowed a lot more development of the people themselves, politically and otherwise and in some of the other colonising countries. I mean if you talk to the French, you see the restrictions that they have had and the restrictions that still exist today on them. If you look at the Portuguese, if you speak to Portuguese blacks, if you speak to Spanish blacks, they all tell you that in Britain you know, we have a lot more liberties than they have and this goes back, I think, all the way to colonisation. I think that maybe if we were to be colonised at all, maybe the Brits were the best of the bunch. That's as much as I'm prepared to go. The other thing that I think that Britain is very good at is the whole business of organisation. Because of African people's experiences in terms of enslavement and colonisation, I think that there is a sort of restlessness, a sort of lack of application to certain things that we have. We have very bright people, you know. It's like the West Indies cricket team of a few years ago. They had brilliant individuals but they could never work together as a team and I think that what the British are good at is that organisation and that application and I think that that has been very good for British blacks. If we can add that British sense of organisation and so on to the natural flair and natural talents of people of African origin then I think you've got a very unstoppable combination.

CLARE: What is left of the Jesuit's religious education? You said you're not a religious person. What do you see death representing, the end of everything?

GRANT: I think that this is the little bit that the Jesuits have left in me. I still can't accept that, you know, that one day I won't wake up and I won't exist any more. I know this is what the Marxists say, 'Oh, well, you're born and you die and that's the end of it,' but the Jesuits say there's an afterlife and so on. But I don't know and obviously we can't prove it, but I think that there is that doubt in me and I just can't believe that, you know, that when death comes, that'll be the end for me. I just somehow think that I'll exist in another form or something else and I think that that's the bit of the Jesuit that's still left in me.

CLARE: I read somewhere that you have diabetes.

GRANT: Yes.

CLARE: Does it from time to time cause you real troubles.

CLARE: Yeah, yeah, yes, very serious, yes, very serious. I've got a very virulent form of diabetes, affects my eyes.

CLARE: So you're insulin dependent?

GRANT: Yeah.

CLARE: Has that affected your attitude to life? When did that happen to you, when did you have it diagnosed?

GRANT: I was diagnosed in about 1975 or something like that.

CLARE: So you were in your thirties.

GRANT: But I think that I've always had it because I can remember as a young kid I used to always be thirsty and everything but nobody knew anything about it and you know, the health checks and so on weren't existent then. I think I've always had it and it's got worse and worse. It does have an effect on me. Some people say that if your sugar is low you get very angry quickly and that type of thing. I don't know whether it's true or not. But I know it affects me just on a daily basis and just keeping up the struggle because diabetes is a very emotional ailment and politics is a very emotional subject, so I'm in the wrong profession for a diabetic. So that when I get angry or if I get upset my sugar level goes up. So it does have an effect on me, yes.

CLARE: And do you still get angry, do you still churn up?

GRANT: Sometimes I get very angry when I see injustice. This is another thing I got from the Jesuits, I'm totally for the underdog, right. I'm always in that position. I always find myself in that position and sometimes, when I see injustice happening against people, I just get so angry I just, you know, burst into tears or something. But I can't do much about it but I get very, very burnt up inside. I get very emotional.

CLARE: What do you do to ease it a little?

GRANT: What I try to do is to do something about it, even if it's just asking a question in parliament or raising it in some way. Somehow that kind of eases my conscience, makes me feel that I've done something at least, and I haven't just ignored it, seen something on television and ignored it. So I have to take some action. Depending on the situation obviously, that determines the action that I might take but certainly, I have to do something, I just can't sit and watch something on television and just leave it.

CLARE: Because I sense you're angry, your anger is quite visceral, that you actually have physical associations with it. You actually held your chest there when you were describing it. So you will feel physically churned up.

GRANT: Yeah, my heart, my heart starts hurting and stuff.

CLARE: Sharon or somebody would say here, 'Cool down, Bernie, it's not worth it.'

GRANT: That's true.

CLARE: Yes?

GRANT: 'No, no, no,' I'd say, but now I'm learning to control it a bit more. It's not a violent anger but it's an anger where you feel frustrated that this is happening and there's not much you can do about it. That's the kind of anger.

CLARE: Is it a family trait? Your family, are they easily moved?

GRANT: I don't think so.

CLARE: That sort of thing, of injustice, is that something very bound up with you?

GRANT: I think it's bound up with me. I think it's bound up with me. I think I got it from my mother because she has this very strong sense as well.

CLARE: Is she still alive?

GRANT: No, she died a few years ago. About three years ago, unfortunately, it was a tragic loss. She was the head of the family and, you know, it's never been the same since.

CLARE: You miss her?

GRANT: Oh, absolutely, yes, yes.

CLARE: What did she do for you?

GRANT: You go to her no matter how bad things are out there, if you got to her and you talked to her she would just sort of say, 'Oh yes,' and she would accept you for what you are, you know, straightforward, regardless of what you say and what you do. She would just be there and she was always rooting for me and she was always getting clippings and this and that and the other, keeping me in touch and then she would ring me up and say, 'Look, I don't think that you should have done this,' or, you know. She gave me a lot of advice.

CLARE: And she spoke her mind clearly?

GRANT: Oh, yes.

CLARE: She'd say what she thought.

GRANT: Yeah.

CLARE: And your father, he's still alive?

GRANT: Yes, yes he's still alive and I've got a great relationship, a reasonably good relationship with him. We don't argue and stuff like that but he's different, you know. I think he's much more materialistic perhaps. I'm a bit of a dreamer, I think I've always been a dreamer as a youth. And he's not, he's not like that. He's much more hard headed and so on. But he's nice and we all get on well together and so on. And, of course, he knows a lot about the African history and about the struggles in places like Guyana and the colonies, you know, during colonial times and so his kind of knowledge is invaluable in that kind of historic context.

CLARE: But he's more phlegmatic about it?

GRANT: Yeah, he doesn't get involved in all these, like movements and so on. He keeps saying, 'You shouldn't do this and you shouldn't do that because you'll upset people and they'll do this to you and you know, they'll kill you,' and all this type of thing. So he tries to pull me back, whereas my mother would say, 'Go on and do what it is you want to do. Be careful but go ahead and do what you want.'

CLARE: Do you ever worry about your physical safety?

GRANT: Sometimes, not too much, not too much. People worry more for me than I worry for myself and as a result of that, people are saying that you've got to have people with you at all times and make sure because I've had a lot of death threats.

CLARE: Have you?

GRANT: People have sent bullets and stuff in the post and that type of thing. Whenever there is a big flare-up in the papers we always get deluged with cuttings from the press, you know, particularly the tabloid press. We get all sorts of different things, of what people will do to me and that type of thing. And I remember once, when we were in Haringey and this happened, we had two people opening all the mail. After about two hours they couldn't cope with it any more and these were people who were just like workers, you know. It was so vitriolic and the things that they were saying were so nasty that we had to change people every two hours to open the kind of mail that we got. I've got a big room at home, it's all full of stuff, things that people send in to me. So any time I feel as though I want to give up and so on, I just go and have a look at some of this stuff and it fires me again.

CLARE: Really?

GRANT: (Laughs.) Yes, so that I can carry on again because there's no way I'm going to let those people win over me.

CLARE: That's what it does to you?

GRANT: That's right.

CLARE: It fires that feeling?

GRANT: That's right.

CLARE: It doesn't say, 'Oh to hell, this is too much?'

GRANT: No, no, no, it makes me more determined.

CLARE: It's a repugnant kind of vision that you get periodically of what people can be really like. What do you offset that with?

GRANT: We, I go to pensioners, right, who are not the most radical group of people in my constituency, and I go to meet them, you know, and they ask me to come and talk to them and so on and I go and I feel really shaky about talking to them and they say, 'Oh, Bernie, it's just great what you have been doing,' and, you know, I just love it when people respond like that. And people do it quite a lot, you know, not only in my area. Sometimes I go up north, up to Scotland and so on and people are saying, you know, 'You're doing a grand job, keep it up,' and that type of thing and it's just those little things, you know, that really keep you going. It's by no means all black people, about 50/50 I would say of people who write to you or who meet you somewhere and just give you a nod and a smile. To me, that's good enough, it shows that some people appreciate what you're doing, anyway.

CLARE: When we talked about your diabetes, you mentioned the fact that it's quite a virulent form and it has affected your eyes. You've had a retinopathy. When I asked you about death, perhaps what I really should have asked you about was if you worry about getting old, or getting ill, or getting sick, or being disabled? You're such an active man and you clearly like to go out and do, you're a doer and I wondered the extent to which that worries you?

GRANT: No, not really, I think that one of the reasons for that is that as a part of our struggle for rights generally, particularly when we were in Haringey, we worked for disabled people and we worked with elderly people. We worked with young people, we worked with lesbians and so on so that I understand how those people feel. Because I've worked and fought for the rights of those people, if I became disabled and so on, I don't think it would be a problem. I constantly think what happens if I go blind or something, because that's one of the things that happens to diabetics, particularly from the Caribbean. And I just say, 'Oh, well, I'll just have to function and I know Jock, and I know this person who is actually functioning,' and because I had to fight with them to get some aids or adaptations for them and so on, so I understand it. So I don't think it's a problem. It would come fairly naturally to me. I would just have to operate differently but I think that I'd be able to cope pretty well and I'm not worried about that at all.

CLARE: Do you have any profound regrets?

GRANT: Any profound regrets, apart from the fact that I couldn't make the West Indies cricket team? I don't think that I've got any real regrets. I'm constantly pinching myself to see that I'm in this position. Because I'm thinking, you know, you're just a fellow from Guyana and the colonies. When I was ten or eleven or twelve, going to college, I would never have thought that I'd be speaking to you in the Radio Four studio in the midst of London. I think I've been incredibly lucky so I don't have any regrets at all. I just feel that somehow things might change and I wouldn't be able to do what I'm doing for whatever reason, something might happen. But I certainly don't have any regrets. I think I've been tremendously fortunate to be able to do what I'm doing and to be able to serve people, because I like working for people, I like working with people. I like to have people around me a lot, I don't like to be on my own. So if anybody wanted to harm me, all they have to do is lock me away somewhere on my own and I'm sure I'd run mad very quickly.

CLARE: Bernie Grant, thank you very much indeed.

GRANT: Thanks.

Bernard Knight

It is my experience that many people, particularly journalists, appear convinced that those professionals whose work takes them to the frontiers of life and death – cardiac surgeons, Arctic explorers, racing drivers, forensic pathologists – must be extraordinarily reflective, sagacious and introspective individuals. Over many years I have from time to time been asked by television companies and weekly magazines to interview this surgeon or that mountain climber and the underlying assumption is always the same. He (it is almost invariably a male) would be absolutely fascinating if I could but persuade him to talk revealingly about the thoughts and emotions he experiences in the course of his life-challenging work. In vain do I caution the contrary – that many heart surgeons and racing-car drivers are amongst the least introspective and most phlegmatic of people, that they will describe what they do in a laconic, unemotional and prosaic fashion and they will eschew the kind of speculative and interpretative analysis that the producer or editor most desires to obtain.

Since Freud, there has been a reluctance to accept that unemotional people may indeed be just unemotional. Instead, the mental mechanism of denial has been introduced to explain why a brain surgeon, whose daily work often involves life and death decisions – to attempt to tie this bleeding aneurysm, to remove that malignant tumour – contrives to make it sound like changing a wheel. But denial in this instance is meant the tendency to repudiate any painful emotional experience – distress, disgust, fear, anxiety – associated with the professional activity in question and to maintain in the face of events, behaviour or situations that would ordinarily produce profound emotional reactions an absolutely stoical and imperturbable psychological stance.

Professor Knight certainly leaves his listeners in no doubt concerning his emotional reaction or lack of reaction to the more disturbing and distressing aspects of his work. A man whose daily job it is to examine the wrecked, ruined bodies of people murdered, raped, tortured and dismembered describes it as just that, a job – 'I get up at nine o'clock and I do the day's work and I go home and do something else'; 'You finish, you wash your hands and you go away and see what's on the telly.' He is adamant that it is a secure compartment, separate from the rest of his ordinary, everyday life. He loses no sleep, never gets depressed and hardly gives a thought to the incongruous and awesome aspects of his work.

The only chink in the armour, if armour it is, concerns not his waking hours but his sleep. Professor Knight tells of a recurrent dream, a dream which he understands is dreamt by other forensic pathologists. It involves him doing a post-mortem on a member of his family – his wife or son – and they're still alive! Yet he had opened them up and has to close them by four o'clock and it is five minute to four and there is this 'panic situation' lest he not 'finish' it.

Ever since Freud, and indeed before, people have laid great store by the meaning of dreams. In Freud's massive work, *The Interpretation of Dreams*, he quotes with approval the saying, 'Tell me some of your dreams and I will tell you about your inner self.' At the heart of the analytical exploration of dreams is the belief that it is not possible to think of any action in a dream for which the original motive has not in some way or other, whether as a wish or desire or impulse, passed through the waking mind. For Freud a dream can be amongst many things the fulfilment of a wish or fear.

Professor Knight's dream belongs to the category known as anxiety dreams. There is mounting panic throughout it. The manifest content of the dream is anxiety-arousing – cutting up a live body in a setting, the post-mortem, in which the person ordinarily would be dead. The *latent* content, Freudians would argue, contains the disguised wish. Professor Knight dislikes human life, even that closest to him. He takes pleasure in his work, involving as it does not living people but dead ones. The desire to turn life into death, however, is distorted in the dream – what Professor Knight appears to be undertaking is an operation but Professor Knight, and those other pathologists with similar dreams, do not operate on living, anaethesised patients but carry out dissections on dead ones. Is it the fact that the body is a living one that arouses panic? It is unclear whether he is operating on or killing his subject! Is the anxiety that mounts an anxiety that the patient will wake up before the deadline, before Professor Knight has killed him?

There are those of course who believe that dreams are froth, or in the words of a nineteenth-century sceptic merely the 'ten fingers of a man who knows nothing of music, wandering over the keys of a keyboard'. Dreams have been compared to the cacophony of noise – voices, snatches of music, atmosphere – heard when you turn the dial in a random fashion on a radio. So does the dream experienced by Professor Knight and many of his pathology colleagues tell us anything about their inner lives? Well there is the fact that the dream clearly relates to his work as a pathologist. It is not simply noise. Nor is it random. He has dreamt it repeatedly. It is not unique to him but is shared by people who work in his field. As to its content and the wish-fulfilment analysis, is there anything else about Professor Knight which might in any way support the notion that buried within this affable, unemotional, matter-of-fact man are violent fantasies, murderous desires, sadistic impulses?

He insists that he himself has no desire to murder, rape or abuse people and he does not understand what it is that leads others to do such things. He is at pains to emphasise how separate his work as a pathologist is from the rest of his life, including his attitudes and beliefs. Professor Knight makes no bones about the fact that he holds humanity in general in considerable contempt. As he puts it with uncharacteristic passion and venom – 'humanity stinks'. The effect of seeing the fruits of man's inhumanity to man – particularly the impact and consequences of the mass abuse of human rights and the humiliation, degradation, torture and killing of innocent civilians in countries such as Rwanda where Professor Knight has been called to apply his specialised skills on behalf of organisations such as Amnesty International – has only served further to emphasise his disgust with human kind. He insists that he would hold such views whether or not he was a forensic pathologist, which only raises the disturbing possibility that it is partly because he holds such views that he is drawn to and able to function as a forensic pathologist. Like many passionate haters of humanity he idealises animals. At one moment he concedes the innocence of children by blithely comparing them to dogs. This turns out to be a high compliment when delivered by Professor Knight, for in his view animals are innocent, loving and lovable whereas the human race 'is a malignancy on the face of the earth.' The forensic specialist who can coolly set about dissecting and analysing the remains of some violated woman retrieved from behind the wall of a modest house in Gloucester admits, 'I couldn't be a vet, never be a vet. It'd break my heart to be a vet. I couldn't stand to see them suffer.'

But of course whatever dream analysis may reveal about the latent content of Professor Knight's fantasies we must be wary of attributing reality to such unconscious wishes, if that indeed is what they are. To dream murderous dreams does not make Professor Knight a monster any more than dispassionately cutting up dead bodies while cracking jokes with mortuary attendants suggests psychological instability! Freud himself was aware of the erroneous logic which equates what people may unconsciously desire with truth and what they consciously express as desire with deception. Plato's dictum that the virtuous man is content to *dream* what a wicked man really *does*, quoted at the end of Freud's book, acquits dreams and underpins the important distinction between psychical reality, what happens in dreams, and material reality, what happens in actual conscious life. We all do have murderous impulses and most of us, fortunately, repress them. The most that can said of Professor Knight is that his work may well activate such impulses to a greater extent than more prosaic work but he is able to contain and suppress them so that they only surface in his dreams.

Professor Knight does acknowledge that there are internal tensions even if he is somewhat coy about identifying them as his own. The small band of international forensic pathologists, he reveals, are characters with a quirky sense of humour. Humour is 'a safety valve' which enables pathologists and mortuary attendants to cope with the work they do. It is, in Knight's words, 'a defiant counterbalance' to the job. But of course such a 'manic defence' against the horror can break down. Professor Knight reveals that forensic pathologists do appear particularly prone to suicide. But being the man he is – 'coping is my password' – he is confident that he can and will survive.

His pessimistic conclusions concerning the human race are those of a man with no religious faith, no view of man as the centre and pinnacle of God's creative plan. In this context, one of the oddest letters I have received during the years I have been involved with radio interviewing was one which arrived last year and rebuked me for neglecting the issue of religion! In fact, hardly an interview passes without some discussion concerning belief, the purpose of life, the challenge of mortality, the nature of creation. Indeed, one critic took me to task for being overly concerned with an agenda which he felt had been set for me by the Jesuits who educated me back in my secondary school days! He has a point. In this collection, for example, a number of the contributors, most notably Professor Blakemore, Sir Colin Davis, Marjorie Proops and Professor Winston, discuss their religious beliefs while in the case of my interview with Professor Bernard Knight it was the subject of religious belief that proved to be unexpectedly controversial. Indeed, few interviews have caused such a flurry of animated, passionate correspondence. Whereas I had expected that there might be some reaction to his detached, phlegmatic attitude towards the bleak, macabre and morbid aspects of his own work as a forensic pathologist or to his unequivocal denunciation of human beings as a dreadful species, these provoked modest comment. It was his unqualified dismissal of religious belief as 'a form of mental aberration' that led to shock and horror on the part of many listeners – although a substantial minority confessed to being absolutely delighted that a man of such eminence and experience of the dark side of life had the courage to say so bluntly and explicitly what they and others believe.

Once again, it is Professor Knight's straightforward, no-nonsense approach to the issue of life and death that is so striking. He does not know what all the fuss is about. We are born, we live a few years, we die. Being dead does not unduly worry him. He equates it with being asleep. It is the process of dying that disturbs him. He is impressively pragmatic. The rest of us can sleep more easily in our beds knowing that there are people such as Professor Knight prepared to do the kind of work that must be done and he does so well. On the basis of my impression of him, he is psychologically well prepared to do it too. He copes.

CLARE: Bernard Knight is one of the most eminent scientists in a field which frequently attracts lurid headlines and intense public curiosity. He is Professor of Forensic Pathology and the Director of the Wales Institute of Forensic Medicine. As a consultant pathologist to the Home Office since 1965 he has worked on such high profile murder investigations as the macabre killing of Vatican banker, Roberto Calvi, who was found hanging under London's Blackfriar's Bridge, and more recently the identification of the victims buried at 25 Cromwell Street in Gloucester.

Bernard Henry Knight was born on May 3rd, 1931 in Cardiff, the only son of a ship broker. He trained as a doctor at the University of Wales, qualifying in 1954. He served as a captain in the Royal Army Medical Corps and in 1967 qualified as a barrister.

As befitting someone who gives writing as his recreation in *Who's Who*, Professor Knight is a prolific author. He has had published over twenty books of non-fiction and text books as well as eight crime novels under the pen name of Bernard Pincton. He has received many British and international awards and honours and in 1993 was appointed Commander of the British Empire.

Professor Knight, you must be the first person in the psychiatrist's chair whose professional work not only does not call for, but seems to preclude, any speculation about human psychology, and so I wonder whether such things as motives, yours included, are of any particular interest to you?

KNIGHT: Oh, yes, I think so. I'm interested in the motives of the people who provide my customers, so to speak. As long as it doesn't interfere with objectivity. Certainly I'm interested in people's motives. You can't but help doing that in a criminal practice, so to speak.

CLARE: The more general picture of a forensic pathologist, rooted in the objective realities of the corpse in front of him, does need to be modified a little?

KNIGHT: Yes, I mean that's the official face of it. My report and statements have to be totally objective but that doesn't stop my mind wandering hither and thither about why this happened, and how it happened and is it going to happen again.

CLARE: Are you seen by others as a particularly detached, objective observer of the human condition?

KNIGHT: I don't know, I don't think so, really. I think it's not such an impersonal, sterile sort of job as people imagine, or is portrayed on the television and in books. It's a pretty chummy sort of job with the police and our collegues and I wouldn't say light-hearted but as with all macabre jobs you have to have a bit of light-heartedness to leaven the occasions. So, off-stage so to speak, it is quite a jolly business I suppose.

CLARE: What was it that attracted you to forensic pathology?

KNIGHT: A single lecture by Professor Keith Simpson when I was a medical student.

CLARE: A single lecture?

KNIGHT: Yes, we had these scientific society things which all students get in about the second year; I think, and I went to that lecture and came out saying, 'I am going to be a forensic pathologist,' and I didn't really deviate from that.

CLARE: And what was it, do you think, looking back, what was it about the lecture? Simpson was a leading forensic pathologist at the time?

KNIGHT: Yes, he was an excellent lecturer. He put things across in such a good way and the whole business gripped me and I wanted to be a pathologist because before being a medical student I was a medical laboratory technician in a path department. So inevitably I was going to be a pathologist. But a forensic pathologist is a sub-branch of general pathology so that steered me in that direction.

CLARE: The only time I think I met Keith Simpson he made it clear to me that the reason he had chosen pathology was that, as he put it, the body did what you could predict it would do. It followed certain rules of decomposition and decay, temperature change and cellular degeneration, whereas living people, and he was quite irritated, I remember at the time, living people didn't really do what you predicted, they got stuffy colds and they reacted in different kinds of ways and life events interfered and personality and so on. So it seemed to me, he rather liked a certain scientific purity about pathology, which, I must confess, I've also rather admired and envied when it's compared to my own field.

KNIGHT: Yeah, I think it's true to a certain extent. I think the older generation of forensic pathologists was a bit too dogmatic about this sort of approach, but certainly most pathologists of any sort tend to want a sort of objective cut and dried profession rather than the more maverick activities of patients. Medicine would be fine if there were no patients, for some doctors.

CLARE: That's right, yes. And I think that may explain why the lay person is rather intrigued by forensic pathology. Let me explain what I mean. The lay perception of medicine is heavily affected by the notion of it as a clinical, a therapeutic science involved with living people, involved with a battle against disease. Death, for example, is a failure of medicine as seen in that particular model. The forensic pathologist is an odd doctor within such a view of medicine. He, it's usually a he, is really, king of the morgue, of the mortuary, of the post-mortem room. It's death rather than life that is his business and that intrigues. The ordinary person is intrigued to know, well, how does someone like this man, Knight, how does he come into medicine which is preoccupied with keeping people alive? Is it death rather than life that intrigues him?

KNIGHT: Not really. I think we're not so far out down that pathway as a forensic scientist. A forensic scientist is about measuring things and it's a very objective matter. The forensic pathologist is mid-way between the two I think. I mean there's a bit of art in it as well as science and, as I say, I think we're the end product, or the end of the medical line where we, it, the buck stops, so to speak, in the mortuary. There's nowhere else to go after that except the crematorium. And I think this attracts a certain type of doctor, the one who doesn't want to be a clinician and there are many who don't want patient contact. I wouldn't say that's true of me. I did a bit of general practice once and – I'm not sure I liked it but they liked me, I think.

CLARE: Yes, what did you make of it, what did you make of clinical contact?

KNIGHT: Well, I did some clinical medicine in the army as a regular medical officer in Malaya and as well as being a pathologist, we had general duties and I did some general practice, and in a way I liked it. But the general practice I did up in one of the Welsh Valleys was ninety-nine per cent social work, you know, giving certificates to people. I think general practice has changed since the 1950s when I did that, but really, there was no medicine in it. I saw one lady who was really ill and I sent her to hospital and she died of a pulmonary embolism. I thought, 'Well that's a jolly fine thing I've done. I've seen one patient with something serious and I've killed her!' So perhaps that's why I backed out of general practice!

CLARE: Your medical school was?

KNIGHT: Cardiff.

CLARE: You went in following a period as a laboratory technician.

KNIGHT: Yes, I started as a farmer before that. I've done a sort of series of professions.

CLARE: And during medical school, when you were exposed to the clinical side of medicine, paediatrics and obstetrics and clinical medicine itself, did that in any sense affect your decision to be a pathologist?

KNIGHT: No, no not all.

CLARE: It was absolutely fixed.

KNIGHT: I liked clinical medicine. I liked people. I'd have been quite happy, I think, to be a clinician. It's just that, you know, I got stimulated into this pathological avenue. Because of being a technician, that was the obvious route to take, but if someone had said, 'Well you can't be a pathologist, you've got to be a clinician,' I wouldn't have been all that distressed about it.

CLARE: And the appeal for you of pathology?

KNIGHT: Well, although I did four years of histopathology, it doesn't appeal to me much, the thought of sitting down looking down a microscope all day at biopsies, it's appalling. I'd much rather do what I do, getting out and about and doing different things and again, perhaps the law. I mean I did the law later on, ten years after medicine. And the legalistic aspects of it are much more interesting than just sheer morphological descriptions that many pathologists do. It's a matter of choice. I mean they like doing it. I don't like doing it.

CLARE: You did indeed qualify as a barrister about thirteen years after you qualified as a doctor. It was 1967?

KNIGHT: Yes, 1967, that's right.

CLARE: What kind of things would you be doing that would involve the law and medicine and that would interest you?

KNIGHT: Well, I like court work. I like going through material, written material, and producing a report out of it, picking the bones out of it and then giving evidence in court. A lot of doctors hate court but I quite like it. I like it as long as I've got my facts right. I hate going to court if I'm at all unsure. But if you've that chalk line beyond which you're not prepared to go in chancing your arm, so to speak, then it is fine, I enjoy it and going there. I had thought of becoming a coroner at one time which is really why I did the Bar because London coroners have to be doubly qualified and the whole legal process interested me. It meshes so well with the type of medicine I do, that the two things welded together very well.

CLARE: But your court presentations, as you say, rest very much on the facts that you marshal.

KNIGHT: Yes.

CLARE: The scientific data, and they, in turn, are derived, initially at any rate, first of all from the crude post-mortem and then the subtle examination of systems and organs and cells and so on.

KNIGHT: It's not exclusively that of course. There's a lot of civil work about seat belts and industrial accidents and it's not all just bodies in mortuaries.

CLARE: No. But talking about bodies in mortuaries, when would you have seen your first dead body? Do you know?

KNIGHT: Oh, I was a technician before I did medicine.

CLARE: Do you remember it?

KNIGHT: Yes. I used to have to go into the mortuary to take messages in or go and get specimens or something and I can still remember that there was a door with one of these circular portholes in it, a swing door and this ghastly sort of fluorescent lighting and these rows of pale, white feet. I remember that now. It's still etched on my memory. But then you just get used to it. I don't even notice now.

CLARE: You don't. And is there any of that sense of Simpson's view? He, I think, took a certain delight, satisfaction in the fact that there are laws that are followed. It is not as arbitrary, as, say, the behavioural sciences which are much more speculative.

KNIGHT: Oh, most certainly, yes, yes. There's much less biological variation in what you find in a dead body than, as you say, in a living patient. Though there is a lot of variation and we have to be very, very, very, very wary of overstepping the mark. In my big text book on the first page I've got an aphorism, 'seldom say always, seldom say never,' which is a pretty good rule of thumb, I think, because some of my colleagues, certainly in the past, were much too dogmatic about methods.

CLARE: So you would be reasonably cautious?

KNIGHT: Oh, yes, caution is the name of the game in this. Unless you can prove something, don't say it.

CLARE: Yes, but of course, you are often under heavy pressure from lawyers to say it because on your evidence a case will swing.

KNIGHT: Yes, but you have to resist the pressure and stoutly. The police are pretty good but sometimes they'll, I won't say lean on you but they'll certainly try and get the best result out of you they can, but you just have to say nothing, say no. And certainly lawyers, they can fight tooth and nail if they want you to say something you don't want to say. You jolly well don't say it. And that's where a lot of doctors come unstuck. They get edged to the precipice. I sit in court sometimes and watch a doctor who's not used to court procedures being edged towards this pit and I can see it happening and I sort of cringe saying, 'Oh, God, they're going to get him now,' and there he goes, over the edge.

CLARE: Did you realise that you, if you like, were temperamentally suited to the legal aspects of medicine. It is, after all, an interesting mix. On the one hand there's the detachment of the pathologist and on the other hand there's the skills of the lawyer and they are not quite the same. They overlap, obviously. I wondered when you realised that you actually enjoyed this kind of cut and thrust?

KNIGHT: Well, I realised I enjoyed it. I'm not particularly introspective about it all. People tend to attribute, er, introspection to us and think, 'Do you enjoy this, do you?' I never really think about it, really, you know. It's a job, you know, I get up at nine o'clock and I do the day's work and I go home and do something else. I wouldn't sit there beating my breast and tearing my hair about my life's mission or whatever. You just do it.

CLARE: All right. But are you intrigued by the interest in what you do? For example, there is a whole genre of crime writing which is bound up, accurately or inaccurately, with the doings, the thinkings, the work of the forensic pathologist.

KNIGHT: Yes, and mostly inaccurately too.

CLARE: Do you think so?

KNIGHT: This is one of my standard lectures and my senior lecturer, Steve Leadbeater, is also very interested in crime fiction, an expert on it. We've got standard lectures of debunking the well-known crime writers.

CLARE: Like who? Ruth Rendell?

KNIGHT: Ruth Rendell's not so bad, but I suppose the worst is Agatha Christie, absolute drivel. Marvellous entertainment, what's it matter anyway, you know, is it entertainment or is it authenticity? But to get it so badly wrong as she does. I mean there are good writers like P.D. James and Ed McBain and people like that.

CLARE: And do you read it?

KNIGHT: Oh yes, avidly.

CLARE: You do?

KNIGHT: Yeah. That's why I started writing crime fiction because I thought, some of this stuff is so awful I can do better myself. Way back in the sixties I started writing some. And then I went straight and started writing historical stuff and biography.

CLARE: Do you still write fiction, crime fiction?

KNIGHT: Yes, but not books. I write for radio drama and television and stuff like that.

CLARE: And the name, Bernard Pincton?

KNIGHT: I've dropped that now. In the days when doctors used to sit with their back to the television camera, I just adopted a name of a pub I used to live in, an old ex pub, Pincton. But now it doesn't matter. I just call myself Knight.

CLARE: What about the temptation, given what you must feel confronted by vagaries of the human condition, the things that people do to each other, the extraordinary behaviours that people get up to, what about the temptation to be profoundly sceptical, cynical even, about the human condition, about humanity?

KNIGHT: Oh, yes, I think humanity stinks. I'm a pathological animal lover. I'm not so keen on *Homo sapiens*. But not because of that. What upsets me much more than criminal activities and horror is the abuse of human rights, which I've been involved in quite a bit. I've done a couple of missions for Amnesty, to Uganda and Kuwait and done a lot of work in Britain for victims of human rights abuse and I think that's much nastier than the criminal work. Criminality is often impulsive but the abuse of human rights is so cold blooded and premeditated that I think it's awful.

CLARE: And you'd be working to verify and confirm some of the things that are done?

KNIGHT: Yes, yes. I went as a doctor with an Amnesty team to Kuwait just three weeks after the Gulf War ceased. Then down to Kenya to look at Ugandan victims of the Obote regime. Some of the things I saw were awful, much worse than I'd seen in the criminal sphere.

CLARE: What sort of effect does it have on you? For example, would it interfere with your sleep? Would you sometimes find it difficult to cope?

KNIGHT: No, this is the standard question. I lecture all over the place and the first lecture is: How do you commit the perfect murder? and the second one is: Does this affect you? And I don't think it affects me. I don't know. I'm not objective enough to know but I certainly don't lose any sleep over it. Though I get these strange dreams and it's strange these dreams, I thought they were unique to me, but other pathologists get the same one. I spoke to a pathologist, a lady pathologist from Malaysia recently, and she said, 'Oh, I get those sort of dreams.' Usually you're doing a post-mortem examination on someone in your family, son or wife or something, and they're still alive but you're doing a post-mortem and you've opened them and you've got to sew them up by four o'clock and it's five to four and you know you're not going to do it and there's this panic situation of, 'Am I going to finish it in time?' And I thought this was just some aberration of mine but it's quite common amongst my colleagues apparently.

CLARE: And how long have you had it? As far back as you can remember?

KNIGHT: Yeah, donkeys years. I mean I've been doing this job for forty years nearly.

CLARE: Would you be more likely to dream this at times of particular crisis or stress?

KNIGHT: No, it seems random, quite random.

CLARE: How regularly would it happen?

KNIGHT: Oh, I don't know, every few months I suppose. But I'm fine when I'm awake and I don't lose sleep over it. It's just these strange dreams, you know, stress dreams I suppose.

CLARE: You've an only son, isn't that right?

KNIGHT: Yes.

CLARE: So it would be your wife or your son?

KNIGHT: Yes, I mean, in your dreams you can't really pin down once you wake up but there's this general feeling that you can remember some of them. As I say, the extraordinary thing is that other pathologists get the same ones, the same type of dream.

CLARE: There is the fact that what you are doing, to you, is very prosaic. You are, I know, at pains to deromanticise it or demystify it. It's a job, you do it. Nonetheless, I have to press you in a way. I remember my very first post-mortem as a student, watching the pathologist. You get used to it after a while I think you'll agree, so when you see it for the first time you're like the lay person, fresh to it. There is this, this extraordinary violation of a major taboo about dead bodies. Dead bodies, in a sense, are preserved, they're protected. And here is this pathologist systematically, very impressively, going step by step, following a ritual. Almost a religious ritual of the taking out and examining and slicing and cutting and so on of organs of the body. And the question I suppose the ordinary person asks is, does the pathologist, do you ever find yourself struck by this, even by the incongruity of it?

KNIGHT: Oh, yes, yeah. I sometimes can stand back and say this is a funny sort of job, you know, and why wasn't I a bus driver or something and this is a hell of way to earn a living. But I don't mind and it doesn't mean I don't like doing it. When you get a decomposed body or you're working in a ditch, it's not so much perhaps in the autopsy room but scenes of crime, because we always go out to any scene of suspicious crime and you're slogging through a wood in the pouring rain, up to your knees in mud to see some dismembered corpse or something or other and you think 'Well, good God, you know, why wasn't I an accountant,' but that's only because of the temporary physical instability as you go through a muddy field. I don't really mind it and I never have minded it, not from the beginning.

CLARE: But the only suggestion that the Knight frame or the frames of your professional colleagues come under strain is this interesting dream and so I wonder, would there be times, for example, when you might go home to your wife, after a particularly distressing experience, called out by the police to some really rather nasty, horrendous child crime or something, would you be able just to compartmentalise that, put it out of your mind or is it something you have to talk about?

KNIGHT: Oh, no, I don't talk about it. I make a point in not talking, usually.

CLARE: Never?

KNIGHT: My wife doesn't want to know. She's pretty revolted by the job I do. I think she can't understand how on earth I do it.

CLARE: Really? She'd ask some of these questions? Well, she probably wouldn't now, but she would have, would she?

KNIGHT: Yes, I mean people ask 'how on earth can you bear to do that job?' but I can honestly say it doesn't affect me, awake anyway, in the slightest. I mean, you finish, you wash you hands and you go away and see what's on the telly, you know. Do whatever you have to do, what everybody, what anyone else does.

CLARE: As you were going through as a student you would have been involved in surgery, you would have done as you are doing now but with living bodies. Did that not appeal to you, the actual surgical techniques?

KNIGHT: Not really, no. Surgery is a very refined form of carpentry in a way. I'm not saying that in a derogatory way of my colleagues but, you know, it doesn't appeal to me, really.

CLARE: Whereas what you're doing?

KNIGHT: Does, yes, there's much more to it, you know. I mean, there's a much wider spectrum of activity if you like. I mean, you get out and about more than being stuck in an operating theatre.

CLARE: Your background isn't a medical one?

KNIGHT: No, I'm a frustrated farmer. As I say, I left school after O-levels and went to work on a farm to do a BScAg. I got dragged back to school then because I couldn't get into university, I was too young. I went to work as a lab technician and it was almost accidentally that I got a place in medical school.

CLARE: Because you left school after your O-levels?

KNIGHT: Temporarily, yes. My mother's family were all farmers going back hundreds of years in Glamorgan and I've still got the hankering after the land, you know.

CLARE: You were an only son.

KNIGHT: Yes, my father was an only son, my wife's an only daughter, my son's an only son. There's a dynasty of only children.

CLARE: Yeah, why, do you know?

KNIGHT: I don't know really. There's only room for one of us in the world I think at a time!

CLARE: Were you, if you like, the characteristic only child? Were you very introspective? Were you a very independent sort of person, self reliant?

KNIGHT: I was independent, I think, yes, very independent. Well I think so, I don't know, just an ordinary kid, really.

CLARE: You grew up where?

KNIGHT: In Cardiff during the war. I lived in the air-raid shelter for a couple of years and collected shrapnel like all the other kids after the air-raids.

CLARE: Your father did what?

KNIGHT: He was a ship broker originally but in the First World War he had to go to France. He was in Ypres and then by the time he came back, they didn't keep careers open in those days, so we rubbed along the bottom for a bit and then the Second World War got him back into ship broking. But there was nothing to do with medicine. There's no one in my family for generations who had a slightest connection with medicine.

CLARE: So when you left after the O-levels you went into agriculture?

KNIGHT: I worked as a farm labourer.

CLARE: Yes, now when you say you were hauled back, who did the hauling back?

KNIGHT: Oh, a school teacher friend of the family, because I'd got pretty good O-levels and they reckoned I shouldn't be working on a farm. Much to my disgust I got pulled back after six months or so, I think.

CLARE: And you did well?

KNIGHT: Yeah, I got a major scholarship but the only reason I went to medical school was another chap in the class sent for a free prospectus to a medical school and I thought anything free is good so I'll send for one of those. So I sent for it, filled a form in and thought no more of it, really. But the first year I was too young. They interviewed me but I was only seventeen so I went to work in a lab then.

CLARE: Today, people would be appalled. You'd be expected to fill out an UCCA form and declare all sorts of passionate involvement in medicine.

KNIGHT: Oh, yeah, not in those days. It was just the back page of a free prospectus in those days.

CLARE: And when you went into medical school, did a great deal of it bore you?

KNIGHT: No, nothing bores me, I find everything interesting.

CLARE: Really?

KNIGHT: Yeah, amateur radio, woodworking, anything you like, I mean, everything is interesting to me. No, it didn't bore me at all.

CLARE: No. What did your parents make of your interest in pathology?

KNIGHT: I don't think they really understood, to be honest. I mean, they were very supportive.

CLARE: Were they ambitious for you?

KNIGHT: I don't think so, really. I'm not sure they even knew what I was doing most of the time. I went off in the morning and came back at night. They were all very approbative or whatever the word is, of me doing good things but I'm not really sure they understood the full importance of it except I ended up as a doctor.

CLARE: What was your father like?

KNIGHT: Oh, an amiable sort of chap, you know, never read a book in his life. A gardener and do-it-youselfer sort of thing. I used to carry the nails for him to make greenhouses. It was just an ordinary sort of childhood.

CLARE: Yeah, and your mother?

KNIGHT: She's still alive, ninety-four, a nice amiable lady.

CLARE: Were they religious?

KNIGHT: Oh, yes, they were both church organists. I had to be in the church choir when I was a kid, I had no choice. My father was a choirmaster.

CLARE: And did it rub off on you?

KNIGHT: Well, it rubbed off completely, yes, being a devout atheist!

CLARE: Tell me more. When you say a devout atheist, that's a fairly strong commitment.

KNIGHT: Yeah well, I will probably get into trouble but I think religious belief is a form of mental aberration, as far as I'm concerned. And it's just extraordinary that intelligent, educated people should believe in some strange supernatural being in an after life. So I just cannot fathom it.

CLARE: What would you say to the person who says, 'Well, what's the point of it all, then?'

KNIGHT: Don't think there is any. We're molecular phenomena, like, you know.

CLARE: But the other night I heard playwright Tom Stoppard say that he felt that to believe that we've evolved from slime into this extraordinary complicated organism is almost as difficult. In fact, he found it more difficult to believe that than to believe there was a God. That in a sense, people believe in some kind of religion because they just cannot make sense of it in any other way.

KNIGHT: No, I don't go along that route at all. I'm very interested in astronomy, in cosmology and all the rest of it, as is my son. I don't see any reason, given enough time, and there's been what, fifteen billion years or something since the creation of the universe, plenty of time for lots of molecules to get together and do the right thing, you know. They say if you give enough monkeys enough typewriters they'll end up with Shakespeare, given enough time.

CLARE: Yours is really the science of causation, in a sense, each time taking a step back asking what's caused this, what's lead to this, what's led to this, what's the point of that? So the ultimate question of causation in turn leads to the question what is the purpose of life?

KNIGHT: I don't think there is one. It's just an accident, really, a sort of chemical accident. It's beyond our comprehension to understand the machinery of it but once you've got hydrogen atoms you can get all the rest if you wait long enough. Only trouble is, who made the first hydrogen atoms or whatever it was?

CLARE: What lead you, the son of two church organists, to become a devout atheist?

KNIGHT: Well, just thinking logically, it didn't made sense, that there's not the slightest proof. I suppose it's because I live with proof, you have to have proof otherwise it's not worth bothering and where is the shred of proof of any of this religious malarkey? There isn't any.

CLARE: And what about another reason that people believe, which is that it sees them through bad times. Have you yourself been through a time when you would ask that question, what's the point of it all, with a greater sense of despair?

KNIGHT: Yeah, I'm sure it must be very comforting to believe. I wish I did in some ways.

CLARE: Do you?

KNIGHT: People who do genuinely believe, I just can't believe that they really believe, if you know what I mean, because it seems so outrageous, but it must be very nice.

CLARE: For example, what do you set against the horrible things you see? I'll tell you why I'm asking you this, because some of the people I see find it very difficult sometimes to sustain a faith in living when they see the awful things that people do, when they turn on the news, when they see some of the things that you've been, as a forensic pathologist, involved in. Here you are and sometimes your work takes you really to the very edge of the abyss of what humanity can get up to. What is it that you set beside that that says, 'Yes, it's worth going on, it's worth living?'

KNIGHT: Well, I never think like that, you see. I just don't think that way. You know, there's a life to be lived, you get so many years and at the end of it you stop. And that's it. Apart from committing suicide, you're stuck with it.

CLARE: Do you ever have doubts?

KNIGHT: About what?

CLARE: About the worth of it all?

KNIGHT: No, not all. Perhaps I'm sort of insensitive or something but these sort of things never occur to me, I just plod on every day.

CLARE: Plod on. You make it sound a tiny bit remorseless.

KNIGHT: Well, no. Well, getting up in the morning's pretty hard but I mean, once the first hour's passed, I'm quite happy then. No, I just take things as they come, you can't alter them.

CLARE: But, there's a large area, then, of human activity, and not just religion, that must rather perplex you. There is the extent to which so many people spend so much time reflecting on, agonising over questions that, as far as you can see, have no answer.

KNIGHT: Yes, well, there's no answer and there's not much point in spending brain power on it. There's so much else to do, you know. As I say, I think the human race is pretty rotten. You know, the more I see of it the more rotten it becomes. I think we're a malignancy on the face of the earth, the things we've done to the environment and the animal kingdom. I'm a passionate animal lover, I can't pass a dog in the street without speaking to it or touching it if possible.

CLARE: But, again, it could be said it's just another collection of cells that have evolved.

KNIGHT: Yeah, but it's a nice collection, it's a nice innocent, usually innocent and unselfish. You know you go home and the dog comes up to you and wags his tail, he's glad to see you. No subterfuge. I couldn't be a vet, never be a vet. It'd break my heart to be a vet, I couldn't, you know, stand to see them suffer.

CLARE: And it's to do with an innocence that you see, the very fact that an animal can't make the choice to be bad, I suppose?

KNIGHT: Yeah, I think that's part of it and I just love dogs, I mean, the way they look at you and, you know, everything about them.

CLARE: Do you have one?

KNIGHT: Yes, yes.

CLARE: Would you feel that way about animals in general?

KNIGHT: Yes, I suppose it would be a bit difficult to be friendly to an alligator or something.

CLARE: You prefer animals to children.

KNIGHT: I suppose it is an awful thing to say but, yes, in a way. Not that I dislike children, I mean I'm very fond of kids, but these days you're not allowed to approach a child, and I think that's a disgusting development in the last couple of decades. You daren't say hello to a child in the street or in the most innocent way, you'd get locked up or someone would throw stones at you. I think that's awful.

CLARE: Suspect you of molestation?

KNIGHT: Yes, you daren't look at a child, almost, these days.

CLARE: Would your feeling about animals extend to small children or do you feel that the contamination begins early in the human condition?

KNIGHT: Probably starts in schools when you get collections of children who contaminate each other. Before that they're pretty innocent. But, yes, I sort of, class little children as with dogs, so to speak. But they don't stay that way as dogs do, you know.

CLARE: And when you talk about humanity as a malignant species, the logical conclusion of that would be that it would be better if ours was a species that really, in the end, became extinct.

KNIGHT: I think it will but the trouble is it will have done so much damage by then most other things will be extinct with it. When you look at things like Rwanda and, as I say, I've done these Amnesty visits to various places and seen the things that people do to other people, far worse than some of the things I see in the criminal sphere.

CLARE: And yet you're moved to work for the people who are abused and tortured and intimidated and humiliated. You're moved to do things. This view of the human condition doesn't lead you to say, 'To hell with it all, I'll go and till my garden?'

KNIGHT: No, I don't go out of my way to do it. I don't rush around looking for work but whenever anyone asks me to do it I'm very happy to do it.

CLARE: But why would you bother?

KNIGHT: Well, again, I don't like to see injustice which is again part of the job, I suppose. Injustice crops up in my work both ways, the defence and the prosecution get it wrong sometimes. I'm not interested in the verdicts in cases but I get very hot under the collar when I see scientific or medical facts either deliberately got wrong or just got wrong out of apathy or ignorance and that causes some injustice.

CLARE: Right, but to an extent that's somewhat cerebral, somewhat intellectual. But the objects of the injustice are human beings.

KNIGHT: Yeah.

CLARE: And so there's some element of you that identifies with some human beings anyway, that doesn't take the view that since we're a miserable lot we might as well be left to our own devices. You actually intervene.

KNIGHT: Yes, I think that attitude is a sort of an overview, you know, a sort of umbrella attitude with the whole human race but when it comes down to individuals, or some small group, then I'm as soft a sucker as the next one to try and help them.

CLARE: But you don't feel that we can be redeemed?

KNIGHT: Only by some great mass revolution. When I say revolution I mean as happened in the nonconformism in the nineteenth century, that sort of messianic type of change amongst a very large number of people, and I can't see it happening. It's going the other way, polarising into totally different and antagonistic religions.

CLARE: Some of my listeners will say, but, you know, doesn't Professor Knight realise that whatever about the aberrations that religions have got themselves involved in, some of the central core beliefs of something like Christianity, love your neighbour as yourself, do good to those that hate you, if acted upon, might help us save ourselves, save our planet?

KNIGHT: Yes, I think that there is a coincidence in that people who are, for instance, Christians, real Christians, are probably the nice people who would want to get things put right but tagging it on to Christianity is invalid as far as I'm concerned, but still the people who have these religious feelings are probably nice, nice people who want to do good in the general sense.

CLARE: What about your own humanity? When you talk about the human species, you're talking, really, about us, about you and me. I know that you form your conclusions about the human condition from some of the worst manifestations of what men and women get up to, but does that reflect on you? Do you find yourself thinking, this is what we could all do in certain circumstances? I could do this, if circumstances were different? Or do you feel, no most of this is genetic, it's inbuilt and some people go this way and other people do not?

KNIGHT: I've got no desire to murder or rape or abuse people at all. And I don't know why other people do it but I have to admit that it is their upbringing and their circumstances and perhaps to some extent genetic make-up. I'm not claiming to be, you know, a saint or anything but I've just got no desire to go and do naughty things.

CLARE: The issue of death itself then, your death, does that conjure up any anxieties, fears, or do you again take a rather prosaic view of it?

KNIGHT: I don't mind about being dead, it's the process of dying that worries me. How am I going to die? Being dead is just like being fast asleep. Dead is dead. How I'm going to get to that situation sometimes worries me, especially as you get older and it's nearer.

CLARE: Have you ever been seriously ill?

KNIGHT: No, thank goodness.

CLARE: You've been physically pretty fit?

KNIGHT: Yeah, yeah.

CLARE: And have you ever had anyone close to you die?

KNIGHT: Well, my father, yes, but then he was eighty-five. It's not a sort of unexpected sort of death.

CLARE: No. He died reasonably well?

KNIGHT: Well, he wasn't very well for a couple of years before but I don't think he actually suffered in the sense of real suffering. But it would be nice to live to ninety and have a coronary one day, you know, that would be ideal, but you can't guarantee that.

CLARE: Your interest in crime fiction, is that to correct the misunderstandings and the misinformation of the Agatha Christies, or is it because you find that the actual process whereby crime is committed and then detected, challenging, intellectually challenging?

KNIGHT: I don't think it's either. I like writing. When I was a medical student I was editor of the student magazine. I just liked writing and this was a good peg to hang writing on.

CLARE: Though fiction is interesting, you are not just writing a medical paper or describing a case or techniques or technology or whatever. There's something creative going on in the sense of something coming out of nothing.

KNIGHT: Yes, but I've always liked writing. I mean, writing essays as a kid in school and, as I say, being editor of the journal, it wasn't a scientific journal, it was, you know, the scurrilous rag medical students have. So it was just an excuse to write. You remember, perhaps, the BBC series, *The Expert*, some years ago with Marius Goring. I did the last series of that and that was pure forensic pathology with a fictional twist. So the books have all been of that type.

CLARE: How much do you draw for your fiction on your fact?

KNIGHT: It's all fact.

CLARE: It's all fact?

KNIGHT: I mean it's not recognisable fact but it's a bit of this and a bit of that put together in a mix but all the bits have really happened somewhere or other along the line.

CLARE: Do you ever get depressed?

KNIGHT: No.

CLARE: Never?

KNIGHT: No, only, as I say, at eight o'clock in the morning when I have to get up, but no, I don't. I can only say I don't. I'm quite happy with everything that goes on. I'm stressed very often and don't know which way to turn, running like hell to stand still as far as the work goes.

CLARE: In the sense of things crowding in on you?

KNIGHT: Yes.

CLARE: And, I'm still intrigued that there's this curious fact about the Knights that you were a single son, your wife is a single daughter, you've got a single son and you've expressed some interesting views on the human condition. Are they in any sense related to each other?

KNIGHT: No, not at all.

CLARE: Would you have liked a larger family, for example?

KNIGHT: No, one was enough.

CLARE: Tell me more, why was one enough?

KNIGHT: No, no, no, not really, that's not true really. I enjoyed my son, I love him very much and he's a great character but I don't particularly want to repeat the process, you know.

CLARE: Why not?

KNIGHT: Once you've done it once – well there's lots of other things to do, you don't want to keep having kids, the main trouble with the world is so many people in it.

CLARE: In one sense, you've no great desire because people are a bit of a nuisance. Because again, perhaps there is that link with that lecture of Professor Simpson, death seems more agreeable than life, life is messy and it's contaminating and it's unpredictable in a way. It is a bit of an affront because it spoils things and consumes things and it causes other bits of life trouble.

KNIGHT: Yeah, well that might be true but I don't think it really impinges upon what I do. I mean, you go into the autopsy room and there's half a dozen bodies and they're all dead, and that's it. It's a fact, you can't go backwards so it's no good agonising about it. This is the day's work and we do it.

CLARE: But your dream was interesting because it's about bodies that appear to be both dead and alive.

KNIGHT: Yeah, yeah, that's exactly it. What's even more interesting is I'm not the only one to get them in my profession.

CLARE: Do you, do you think that there's some common thread, apart from the dream, that links forensic pathologists? I wonder whether you feel there is any particular characteristic you'd identify in the forensic pathologist? It's a small group of people isn't it? You would know most of them?

KNIGHT: Oh, very small.

CLARE: The senior forensic pathologists in this country, you would know most of them?

KNIGHT: In the world almost.

CLARE: In the world, yes.

KNIGHT: I think a lot of them are what you might call 'characters', you know, in inverted commas, and they all, or most of them, have got a quirky sense of humour.

CLARE: Black, macabre?

KNIGHT: Not necessarily, they're just jovial sort of people. Well jovial is perhaps the wrong word but matey sort of people, convivial sort of people. There are not many sort of schizoid, gloomy characters. My contemporaries are all jolly lads and a couple of lasses. People ask me how on earth can I be a forensic pathologist and I think it's a process of natural selection. Those who don't want to be it, don't be it, or they give up, and quite a lot of people give up and there's a high suicide rate. It's such a small specialty, the numbers aren't great but five, I think, of my colleagues have committed suicide, and I think that was one way of getting out of the job, perhaps, but others just leave it and go and do something else.

CLARE: So, in a way, the kind of personality you have is protective because, as you said to me, you don't get depressed and therefore I didn't even bother asking you the next question, whether you ever find yourself thinking life just wasn't worth living. But clearly, some of your colleagues did think that.

KNIGHT: Yes, and perhaps then they weren't suited to the job, they shouldn't be in the job, and instead of leaving they took another way out, perhaps. I mean, that's one explanation I think.

CLARE: Because it does call for a remarkable detachment. I don't know whether you acknowledge that or not but I keep pushing you on this because I know that if there's one branch of medicine I could not do it's that. I couldn't do it and I know why I couldn't do it. I think I'd have more vivid dreams than just the one you have, and I'd certainly have that one. But to an extent, you are protected because of the nature of your personality, which is very practical. You don't spend too much time speculating.

KNIGHT: No, this is it. Far more people ask me all these questions but that's the only time I ever think about it. I never think about it at other times. I don't go round, you know, inspecting my navel and wondering about life. There isn't time. I'm so blessed busy and there's so many other things to do extramurally, you know. There isn't time to tear my hair and beat my chest about what I do.

CLARE: Yes, even though I feel the need to remind listeners that you will see scenes that if they were to be portrayed in the living room or in the cinema, well, in fact, they wouldn't be because the censor would just remove them straight away. In a sense, you should be corrupted by what you see, it should in some way disturb, distort, your psychic health. You're often exposed to the victims of terrible sexual crimes, frightful violent crimes, often systematic sadism. Of course a lot of your work doesn't involve any of those things, it involves, as you say, much more routine matters. Nonetheless, you are exposed to those. So, I suppose people would ask, 'Now, why isn't Bernard Knight turned off or disturbed by all of this?' It is so distressing.

KNIGHT Well, I think I do the job because I'm the sort of chap who can do it. Literally, I've done what, twenty-five, thirty thousand autopsies. I've seen every horrible scene ten times over. There's nothing I haven't seen. And yet I can go to a horrible scene and when it's finished, ten minutes later, I can think of something totally different – you know, where am I going to plant my delphiniums when I get back. It's not an act. I just don't think about it. You turn, you switch on to another topic.

CLARE: Would you be affected by something you might hear on radio, or see on television or in the cinema? In other words, fictional violence?

KNIGHT: Well, I never go the cinema. But on television I think there's too much gratuitous violence. I'm saying this almost as an author rather than a pathologist now. It contributes nothing to the plot and is thrown in there gratuitously.

CLARE: Would it disturb you?

KNIGHT: It doesn't disturb me. It might incense me, as it were, rather than disturb. I just think it shouldn't be there. I couldn't care less about the violence. That's kiddies' stuff, you know, compared to the things I've seen.

CLARE: Well, precisely, yes.

KNIGHT: But I think it shouldn't be there in public view.

CLARE: What, therefore, would you say has contributed to your ability to be a forensic pathologist? I don't mean now your technical ability and your skills, I mean your personality. Is this something you would see in your genetic make-up, your parents, or is this something quite unique, in a sense, to you?

KNIGHT: I think I'm quite different from my parents. There's nothing about them which would contribute to a forensic pathologist's make-up. I'm just me. There's just this pattern that my genes have dropped into which makes me not be bothered with nasty sights. And I suppose I've gradually got to it. It didn't happen the first day. I was a lab technician, saw the mortuary gradually, then went to the dissecting rooms as a medical student, four years' in histopathology, so I gradually worked up to it. I can honestly say it never affected me, ever, nor is likely to, I suppose, after forty years.

CLARE: You were never tempted to become a full-time barrister and move away from medicine?

KNIGHT: Yes, I was, but it was financially impossible because at that time I was well into my thirties, had a small child, and I couldn't have done it. But I was tempted at one stage.

CLARE: Because, what was it that tempted you?

KNIGHT: Well, just something new, really, I'm always looking for something new to do. I almost went back into general practice after being a senior lecturer in forensic pathology, but I was rescued at the last moment, at least the local population were rescued, I think!

CLARE: You don't think you'd be too good?

KNIGHT: Oh, I think I would actually, I think I put myself down there. I think when I did my locum the patients wanted me to stay, which said something about it.

CLARE: You work very hard?

KNIGHT: A workaholic I think.

CLARE: Why do you say that?

KNIGHT: Well, I never, hardly ever, stop working unless I actually physically remove myself from either the office or home to a place down in the country. That's the only place I don't work, there's nothing there to work on.

CLARE: So what do you do when you're not working? Do you miss work, do you physically miss it?

KNIGHT: No, it's a damn nuisance to be honest but there's so much of it I have to keep bashing away at it to try and get through it all. But I retire in just over two years' time and it'll be marvellous. I'm not in the slightest way apprehensive about retiring.

CLARE: So you're not dependent on the work in the sense that you're not one of these people who, when not working, have almost withdrawal symptons of irritability and concentration?

KNIGHT: Never had a chance to find out, really.

CLARE: No, but when you go to your house in the country?

KNIGHT: Oh, no, there's, you know, other things, I'm back to being a farmer then, you know, hacking grass and building things and digging holes in the ground.

CLARE: Do you take holidays?

KNIGHT: Not really, no, I've got all these blessed conferences and go abroad to other universities and things, travelling too much.

CLARE: But you don't enjoy it?

KNIGHT: But I can never sit on a beach or anything for more than half an hour anyway.

CLARE: But if you go to a conference in some exotic city, would that interest you, would you then take yourself off or would you come back immediately from the conference when you'd done whatever you had to do?

KNIGHT: Well, I usually do because the courts. It's a job to get away, with the blessed courts. It's an awful lifestyle. I live in my diary, juggling the diary dates round all the time. The courts are so unpredictable. You just can't plan anything. You just try to snatch a few days here and there to go to a meeting or something.

CLARE: How has your wife coped with that kind of life, living with this man who really doesn't talk too much about what he does, and anyway, if he did, she'd be distressed beyond words.

KNIGHT: Oh, she seems to cope very well. She's used to it. She was a lab technician herself, not that that's anything to do with it, really, but she understands the medical lifestyle, I suppose. She seems fairly philosophical about it.

CLARE: Would she ever say of you that your job had affected you, or changed you, hardened you?

KNIGHT: I don't know, again. I haven't asked her. Not so radically as myself I don't think, but she's pretty disgusted with some of the things that go on in the world I think, too, like most of us are, I suppose.

CLARE: Sure. But at the same time, you're in a speciality with a lot of friends.

KNIGHT: Yes.

CLARE: And you're in a profession that, for all its faults, is altruistic. Medicine is about intervening, preventing suffering, helping. I'm putting myself in your shoes in a way and thinking, 'Well, one of the ways I suppose I cope with the dreadful tide of mess is to remind myself, consciously or unconsciously, of those elements of humanity that are admirable, praiseworthy.' The fact that there's someone like you traipsing through a forest late at night to sort out an answer as to how some dismembered body got there, is itself praiseworthy.

KNIGHT: Well, I never think of it like that. I've never given that a thought. It's, as I keep saying, it's prosaically a job which I enjoy.

CLARE: So you can hold a fairly pessimistic view of the human condition because it doesn't affect you, it doesn't then make you feel bad about yourself?

KNIGHT: Oh, no, no.

CLARE: Which is what happens to a lot a people. What depresses them out there begins to depress them about themselves.

KNIGHT: No, I never get depressed. When I'm tramping through that wet forest I'm usually with a gang of detectives who I know well, Bill and Joe, and we have a good chat and it's all very pally and I enjoy it.

CLARE: But even as you speak I think there are so many good things about human beings. You conjured one up almost immediately the good humour . . .

KNIGHT: Companionship.

CLARE: Companionship, which you clearly value.

KNIGHT: Yes.

CLARE: You like that – people faced with some ghastly actual reality, nontheless, being humorous and personable and supportive.

KNIGHT: Yes, I recognise it as a safety valve, I think. I think we do react like this and there's always a sort of joke cracking that goes on. It has to be a safety valve. It's like many sort of mortuary attendants are very noisy people who bang trays about and drop things and shout as a sort of defiant counterbalance to the job they do.

CLARE: Yes, which is bleak.

KNIGHT: Yes, so in a way, perhaps I do the same. But I never think about it objectively. It's just something to do.

CLARE: But as you say, the time when you do think about it is when you're asked by people like me.

KNIGHT: Yes, the only time.

CLARE: The only time?

KNIGHT: I never think about it any other time.

CLARE: And so when I asked you to be interviewed by me, you knew that I'd ask you these questions?

KNIGHT: Yes, they're the standard questions at the end of every lecture. I lecture a lot to various people. I was in Oxford Union the night before last. First question was: 'How do you commit the perfect murder?' the second question was: 'How does the job affect you?'. I know those two questions come up every lecture.

CLARE: The first one of course taps your factual, professional, technical knowledge.

KNIGHT: And taxes my evasive qualities!

CLARE: The second of course reveals more about the questioner, really. The person is trying to understand what it is like for you.

KNIGHT: It's usually a girl, a woman who asks that one. I've identified the questioners, even, over the years.

CLARE: And what do you make of that?

KNIGHT: Well, I just assume that it's such an awful thing I do that she couldn't possibly do it and she's trying to find out what sort of monster I am because I can do it. That's the analysis of it.

CLARE: And what you're saying is, 'I'm not a particular monster.'

KNIGHT: I don't think so, no – kind to dogs and small children.

CLARE: Yes. The Freudian would say there's a lot of repressed aggression in this man. Look at what's coming out in his dream, operating on his living relatives. Talking about your personality for a minute, and it's always difficult, I really would need to talk to your wife or your son, but I'll have to rely on you. In terms of the kind of feedback you get from the people close to you, are you seen to be an irascible man?

KNIGHT: No, I think the opposite. Placid to the point of dullness. I mean, I can't be bothered to lose my temper.

CLARE: Do you ever? Are you one of these people who rarely does but when they do it's ferocious?

KNIGHT: I hardly ever do, as I say. You'd have to ask my wife but I can't remember. I can never generate enough adrenalin. Perhaps my adrenal's a bit slow or something but I can't be bothered. I tend to withdraw.

CLARE: Do you?

KNIGHT: Well, I just go quiet.

CLARE: You don't like arguments?

KNIGHT: No, avoid them like the plague.

CLARE: Were there many in your childhood?

KNIGHT: No.

CLARE: No? Well I have to say one thinks of Welsh people as having certain Celtic bravura.

KNIGHT: Yes.

CLARE: But that wasn't so?

KNIGHT: No, I don't think so.

CLARE: They were like you, in that sense, your parents?

KNIGHT: Yes, well, clip round the ear perhaps now and then for doing something wrong but that's it.

CLARE: But otherwise quiet?

KNIGHT: That was a long time ago. Yes.

CLARE: Dull?

KNIGHT: Yes, I suppose. I suppose I'm pretty dull really.

CLARE: What's your son like, is he like you?

KNIGHT: No, he's the opposite. No, he's red-haired, a red-haired giant with a terrible temper, which goes up and down as fast . . .

CLARE: And what does he make of you? Does he try and goad

you? Are you the sort of person who makes other people try and shake you a bit?

KNIGHT: Oh, no. But he's a typical red-head, you know, red hair and a red beard and a temper to go with it.

CLARE: And would you get passionate about anything?

KNIGHT: Animal cruelty.

CLARE: You would?

KNIGHT: Yes, well, if I saw somebody maltreating an animal I might get pretty shirty.

CLARE: Anything else?

KNIGHT: Don't think so, no. I might do something about it but not in an enraged way. I'd write one of my letters or something like that, or do something practical, but not lose my rag.

CLARE: Apart from your work and your writing, what sort of interests do you have? What do you like doing?

KNIGHT: History, reading about history. I've written a couple of historical novels. I'm interested in the Dark Ages, Celtic history, twelfth-century Roman history.

CLARE: The past?

KNIGHT: Yes. I'm interested in Roman medicine and have given a couple of lectures on that. The past, yes.

CLARE: Do you do a lot of reading?

KNIGHT: Yes, not so much now as I used to. Haven't got time or the eyesight.

CLARE: Are you someone who has an ambition, that there's something you want to do, that you haven't done?

KNIGHT: Well, I've done so many things. I suppose there's lots left, you know, but I can't really pinpoint anything. I'm pretty contented, really. I've had a good life and a well paid job.

CLARE: Do you think of yourself as a Welshman?

KNIGHT: Oh, yes, absolutely, that's what I want carved on my tombstone in Welsh: Here Lies a Welshman.

CLARE: Tell me, what do you see as the marks of a Welshman, apart from being born in Wales.

KNIGHT: I don't know really, a lover of literature and artistic things and a sense of history, a sense of being, of living on the edge of Europe, of being pushed there by everyone else. Your country's done a bit better than ours in surviving but I'm interested in Celtic history and it would be an awful shame if we disappeared.

CLARE: So, would you have other Welsh charactertistics? Do you have a passionate interest in rugby or the language?

KNIGHT: No, I don't know a round ball from an oblong one.

CLARE: You're not interested in sport?

KNIGHT: And I can't sing!

CLARE: How about the Welsh language?

KNIGHT: Yeah, well I'm not fluent. I'd give my right arm to be fluent in Welsh. I've been learning for about thirty years but unless you actually speak in it every day it's hopeless.

CLARE: Yes, but I gather you speak Hungarian?

KNIGHT: Oh, no, just a few words.

CLARE: Really?

KNIGHT: My son is a linguist.

CLARE: In Hungary?

KNIGHT: Yes.

CLARE: He wasn't drawn to medicine.

KNIGHT: No. He went the furthest direction from it I think, probably because of me I should think.

CLARE: Really! Why? Would he have known anything very much about what you did?

KNIGHT: Oh, yes, yes, I think he knows a lot, he knows a lot. He used to come and see what I did but he didn't want to be a doctor. He saw me getting up in the middle of the night and not coming back for a day or so. And he wanted nothing of that. And he's a good linguist. Not that it's done him all that much good in his career, so to speak, but he's a very erudite sort of chap. But he certainly didn't want to do medicine, much to his mother's disgust.

CLARE: She would have liked him to?

KNIGHT: Well, she would have liked him to have a profession – the law or medicine or something.

CLARE: You would have been an easy-going father?

KNIGHT: I think so, yes.

CLARE: You'd have left it to your wife, would you, to . . .

KNIGHT: I think she's the motive force in our family, yes.

CLARE: Really? Would you have been an absentee doctor father?

KNIGHT: Oh, no, no, not really. I pulled my weight when he was a little one. I was the guy who pushed him around in a pram a lot, and dangled him on my knee or whatever fathers do. I think he had a fair whack from his mum and dad. And he's a good boy too. It's just he's got these strange career prospects, like speaking Hungarian!

CLARE: Returning for a moment to this issue of religion and evolution, it's clear that, from what you say, that you don't actually think that the human condition, human beings, the human species, have necessarily improved over the thousands of years of evolution? Almost every evolutionist tends to suggest that there is a progress here, that what distinguishes man from the animals that you, if you like, empathise with, is the ability to choose and reflect, consciousness, and, of course, the ability to do noble and ignoble things. But what I'm rather intrigued by in your summation of all of this is that, as far as you're concerned, it's a dead end species, better dead than alive. The cost of human evolution outstrips the advantages.

KNIGHT: Yes, it might be an extreme view I suppose. I think we're heading that way. Maybe haven't got there so far but we're doing our level best to ruin the world around.

CLARE: How long has that pessimism been a feature of your life?

KNIGHT: I think since nuclear weapons came along, really. I never expected to live this long. I thought I was being vapourised before now. Way back in the sixties, I suppose, when, you know, the nuclear confrontation was really growing.

CLARE: You would have been in your thirties?

KNIGHT: Yes. I went as far as to get some morphine and keep it at home in case we ever needed it in some terrible nuclear catastrophe. Those days have gone, thank goodness. I hope they have anyway.

CLARE: And you stored the morphine at home?

KNIGHT: Yeah, legally. I wanted to die quickly.

CLARE: Did you know anyone else who did that?

KNIGHT: No. It just seemed a sensible thing to do at the time.

CLARE: Did your wife know?

KNIGHT: I don't think so.

CLARE: No?

KNIGHT: But that was the time of Cuba. We damn near came near it at Cuba. I remember the shop I bought it in – in Hackney somewhere.

CLARE: That was the Kennedy/Kruschev show-down over Cuba in 1962. You would have about thirty.

KNIGHT: Yes.

CLARE: Up to then would you have been a fairly easy-going man? Or would you always have had that slight tendency to feel the human condition was going downhill?

KNIGHT: I don't think this was any kind of earth shattering change in my lifestyle. I'm always a practical guy. If there's something that can be done or something you can do, I go and do it. If it's having a bit of morphine in case you have to put your family out of their misery, I'd do it. I didn't. You know, you've done that, you were prepared, you go onto the next thing then.

CLARE: OK. But in fact it was the bleakest vision of all. Now it's eased a little?

KNIGHT: Oh, yes, considerably I think. Unless we get some crazy Third World country that lobs a nuclear weapon in our direction, but I don't think we're in the same danger as we were ten, fifteen years ago.

CLARE: But I don't sense that this has modified your pitiless view of humanity.

KNIGHT: Well, I think we're a dangerous and unpredictable race and therefore you have to make preparations to make the best of it you can. Twenty years ago I was all for digging a nuclear bunker but the ground was a bit hard so I gave up.

CLARE: Did you try?

KNIGHT: Yes. I went down about a foot. I just try and match results to the needs, you know, if there's a need to do something I'll try and do it.

CLARE: It might be said that you might pay for the job that you do, is that not a rather undiluted view of human wickedness?

KNIGHT: No, I don't think it's anything to do with it. I don't think what I do is anything to do with that business.

CLARE: But it doesn't exactly alter it, does it, or stand as a contrast?

KNIGHT: No, but if I'd been a clinician I'd have still had the same attitude, I think, about the human race. I don't think what I do makes any difference. At least I don't consciously feel it does.

CLARE: Well, nonetheless, every time some pretty malevolent occurrence occurs in Britain, you or somebody like you will be called out as you say, at any hour of the day or night, and you will see it in all its full horror. Whereas I, as a clinician, the only death I'll see are some suicides and some of the consequences. I'll see some of the things you'll see but I won't see anything like the same number. But much of what I'll see are people suffering as a result, not so much of what other humans do to them, though sometimes, but also what biology, evolution, does to them. However, I can still hold in my head a picture of human beings which, warts and all, suggests that they are more lovable than hateable whereas your experience is less diluted by the positive.

KNIGHT: I still think my work is in a compartment which is separate from my perception of the rest of human life.

CLARE: But your dream suggests it isn't?

KNIGHT: Yeah, well you're the expert, I wouldn't know about that!

CLARE: I said 'suggests'! All right but let's accept that your work for some reason is compartmentalised, then, of course, I am particularly intrigued as to where your fairly bleak vision of humanity does come from because after all, it's not widely shared. There are of course some people, and I have to say this before I'm deluged by people who say Professor Knight is absolutely right, there are of course people who take that view, but there are others who would find it difficult I suppose to be so single-mindedly bleak, because they would find it very difficult to keep going. So, maybe for the worst of reasons, they idealise certain aspects of the human condition. Nonetheless, you don't, clearly, and I'm intrigued why you don't, because your parents were decent parents, you apparently had a happy childhood and you describe yourself as a sort of rather balanced man.

KNIGHT: Yes. I think maybe you're overdoing the bleakness. I don't go round looking around me and thinking what a bleak world it is, I never think of it. It's only when you actually draw my attention to it that I think this. I've got so much else to think about. These thoughts don't really occupy me much unless someone actually discusses them like you do, which is pretty, pretty rare, really. We've only been around what, three million years, the dinosaurs were around for a couple of hundred million years. We've gone along one alley which might be a blind alley. Couple of million years time there might be highly intelligent ants that are doing things. Why have we got this arrogance to think that we are the be-all and end-all of the universe? We're just three-million-year short-termers, nothing, perhaps, compared to other species. We've got further but that's not to say we might not fizzle out and somebody else go a lot further. Perhaps with six legs, how do we know? Three million years is a fleabite on the history of the world.

CLARE: Yes, and I also sense that you wouldn't care much one way or the other.

KNIGHT: I'm pragmatic, I suppose pragmatism is my main characteristic, it's not going to affect me. I'll be dead in twenty years. I don't care twopence what's going to happen.

CLARE: Pragmatism is one of your cardinal features, yes. You do what can be done and if it cannot be done, you're not going to waste too much time.

KNIGHT: No, I'll go on to something else.

CLARE: Yes. So when we come back to the issue that I suppose confronts you so regularly, death itself, this is not something you speculate much about. You worry of course about the process of dying, how you'll die, but death, as far as you're concerned, is a reality and that's that. You just have to accept it.

KNIGHT: Yes, death is all in the past when I see it. By definition it's all over when I get there and I'm there to pick up the pieces and make the most sense of it that I can on behalf of the community, law enforcement or whatever. I can't alter one whit of what's happened, so why bother, so why worry, not why bother but why worry about it? I don't worry about it. It's happened, it's all retrospective. I'm a retrospective doctor.

CLARE: And feelings? What do you actually feel when you're confronted with it?

KNIGHT: I'm not callous. In the past they used to use terms, well in America, terms like 'the meat wagon' and all this sort of crudities. I think that's awful. I wouldn't have any truck with that at all. And when I'm there, cutting a brain, for instance, I wonder what this brain was thinking twelve hours ago. But it's a sort of dispassionate sort of contemplation. There is nothing I can do about it. The brain stopped working twelve hours ago. I still wonder about it and I'm often very sorry, yes, and I'm upset for the relatives. Relatives have to identify bodies to me sometimes in the most awful circumstances. I must say I try to dodge that sometimes because I find that a bit traumatic. Sometimes I can't and that's the worst part of it. Not the dead body, it's the living relatives who are so distressed. That's the bit that rubs off most difficulty on me.

CLARE: But you cope?

KNIGHT: Oh, yes, coping is my password, I think!

CLARE: Professor Bernard Knight, thank you very much indeed.

KNIGHT: Thank you.

Joanna Lumley

I met Joanna Lumley once before the *In the Psychiatrist's Chair* interview. It was in the late seventies and involved a most peculiar lunch party at a house in Berkeley Square hosted by something called the KIB Foundation. The initials stood for Koestler (Arthur), Inglis (Brian) and someone called Bloomfield who, I was told, had made a lot of money out of margarine. What united the three men was an interest in the paranormal – in the case of the late Arthur Koestler it was a genuinely scientific interest, in Inglis's case a semi-religious interest but in the case of Mr Bloomfield, who attended the lunch party with Brian Inglis, it was an unshakable conviction that not only was there something out there but it regularly took it upon itself to intrude on anything and everything back here.

What I was doing there I have no idea. But sitting beside me was the delectable Joanna Lumley. She now cannot recall why she was there either but I do recall myself sitting dumbfounded as with great seriousness she proceeded to wind up Mr Bloomfield to heights of ecstasy with her astonishing account of the transformation of her then-husband, Jeremy Lloyd, into a Yeti! I still do not know how much of it all was a magnificent piece of acting. What I do know was that it was the hit of the lunch. I have a sneaking feeling that out of the lunch came a decision to put money into funding a chair in extrasensory perception. One was eventually established at Edinburgh called after Koestler. Perhaps it should be named after Joanna Lumley.

As befits a former model, she is stunningly good at projecting herself. It was to be expected, I suppose, that much of our interview would be taken up with the discrepancy which she feels between the way she is seen by millions of people who know her as one of the most famous actresses and faces of our time and how she sees herself. She has been an actress all her working life. She started with many walk-on parts in dreadful sitcoms with scripts which would simply describe her as a pretty girl. She was one of the vacuous blondes in the 1968 Bond movie *On Her Majesty's Secret Service*. She starred for a brief period as the upper-class girlfriend of Ken Barlow in *Coronation Street*. She was in her early thirties when she became famous as Purdey in *The New Avengers*. The way you are treated, it has been said and she has said it herself, tends to be the way you think you are. Now, treated as an exceedingly successful and public star – she has been described as a heroine of popular mainstream culture – she faces the familiar dilemma. This time the conflict is between the character of Patsy, the drink-befuddled, fag-fisted, empty-headed, foul-mouthed grotesque she portrays in *Absolutely Fabulous* and the real Joanna Lumley, who is durable, intelligent, glamorous and, she is at pains to insist unconvincingly it has to be said, ordinary, even dull and psychologically uncomplicated.

She does what many stars do, and that is insist that behind the dazzle and away from the lights she is just another woman, one of the many 'who scrub floors or put arms down lavatories and paint things'. I believe her when she describes herself thus. That is to say, I believe that she is intelligent enough to know that she must keep reminding herself that tinsel is tinsel. But it is only half the story. As she herself makes plain, from very early on she has been a performer in love with performance and capable of being seduced by the wowed audience. As a child she delighted in showing off, making others laugh and keeping herself amused, being the extrovert clown revelling in drawing attention to herself. Indeed, she herself dreamt of being the very sort of person she now rather resents the public for believing her to be. On the other hand, she finds it sad that so many people expect her to be very rich, very accomplished, very powerful, 'the sort of Hollywood dream', a female Orson Welles inhabiting huge houses with servants and a dazzling life of parties and beautiful people. On the other hand, the fantasy that fuelled her when she was starting out is close to being just that and wonderfully revealing – 'a woman standing on a Manhattan balcony . . . satin evening gloves and strapless dress . . . about to light a cigarette . . . and behind her the lights of Manhattan in the blue evening sky'.

Joanna Lumley is one of those people who can enthusiastically immerse herself in the action, the glamour, the nonsense that constitute the milieu of the contemporary star while simultaneously maintaining a certain ironic and amused detachment, skilfully debunking the fuss while energetically enjoying it. But maintaining this kind of psychological high-wire trick is relentlessly demanding. Interviewing her was fun – she is humorous, witty and hugely self-mocking – 'shallow as a puddle' is her self-description – but I know she is too bright to believe it. She laughs a lot and indulges in a very English form of modesty. But the interview was hard work too. Conversation does not flow but rather ebbs and surges, a sort of billowing tide with small, gentle waves followed by a massive tidal rush. Behind the silky laugh and subtle flattery is a wariness. She deftly leads me away from anything too painful or too deep. Re-reading the interview I am struck by how willing I was to be led! Left to herself she can come full circle, seemingly contradicting herself in full flow.

Is she narcissistic? It is not an unreasonable question given her career first as a model than an actress, her well-known reputation as one of the brightest people around – in the early eighties she dazzled a cluster of highly intelligent academics who were invited by Jilly Cooper to sit the common entrance examination – and her remarkable looks. The answer starts negatively. No, she insists, you cannot bewitch yourself, cannot look at yourself and say that what you see looks good. I am not so sure that you cannot and say so. Then she admits that what she only ever wanted to look like was Brigitte Bardot and Marilyn Monroe 'because they were the dream purveyors'. She not entirely convincingly demurs when I suggest that such an ambition in her case had a little more realism to it. She has, after all, always been a very attractive woman. Hers is of course a familiar dilemma. A good-looking, intelligent woman is largely defined by others in terms of her physcial appearance. Clearly Joanna Lumley knows she is bright and funny and clever and more than a match for others but she finds herself enmeshed by the web of physical allure and sexual attractiveness. That which publicly defines her privately constricts her.

Joanna Lumley's recurrent dream involves the Thames flooding while she tries desperately to warn people sitting unconcerned in riverside meadows. She discusses its possible significance in the context of a constant, nagging realisation that everything we do, every West End role or TV advertisement, every relationship and enterprise eventually comes to an end. All things must pass. The dream is of happiness interrupted, life ending. The interruption is predictable but catastrophic. But she is privy to the knowledge and others remain indifferent. The dream suggests a person who knows well the pain of trauma and indeed her own life has had its fair share of rupture. Aged twenty-two she became pregnant and she brought up her son, Jamie, as a single mother. It was a struggle. She was never out of the red until the television series *Sapphire and Steel*. She married then separated from scriptwriter Jeremy Lloyd, had a lengthy relationship with actor Michael Kitchen, and now lives with conductor Stephen Barlow. For all the turmoil and change she insists she is not complicated, not neurotic, not very interesting. I am unconvinced.

Joanna Lumley preferred not to talk about those nearest to her. It is an understandable request. Only the subject of an interview consents to talking uninhibitedly. Relatives have a right to privacy. So I do not know how her parents or her elder sister have coped with the fame and the publicity that Joanna's success has produced. It does of course limit the interview, particularly given her view that her family has been the greatest influence on her development. There are constant hints, particularly towards the end of the interview, that I am getting a carefully controlled package with not too much in the way of personal revelation. There is the robust insistence that all in all the show goes on. There is the revealing hint of a 'swishing steel curtain' and an explicit reference to the relevant fact that the things she would say to me 'as a psychiatrist' are quite different from the things she is saying to me as part of a radio interview being broadcast to an audience. We have, she reminds that audience, an enormous responsibility 'to the people we know'. She is absolutely right. It does limit what is done in *In the*

Psychiatrist's Chair and it answers those journalists who repeatedly suggest that because I am a psychiatrist this gives me licence to ask anything I wish.

And so the interview ends as it begins, with reflections on what Joanna Lumley refers to as the two sides of the coin – fame and anonymity. Joanna Lumley is not one of those people who privately lament the glamour and the celebrity status while relentlessly milking it in public. She enjoys and resents it simultaneously. It is the story of her life – the pursuit of fame and public adulation *and* the desire to be the simple, uncomplicated Joanna who can slip into the local Co-op for a packet of biscuits without being besieged by a pack of fans expecting her to swear like Patsy. She likes it at the top and hates it. She is one of those people sitting happily in the meadow and she is roaring at herself that it is all going to end. Meanwhile she gives herself and lots of other people enormous enjoyment and seems at the mid-stage of her life to have attained a level of peace and stability sufficient to satisfy her and not enough to bore.

CLARE: Joanna Lumley is the top television comedy actress of the year. Before her current success as Patsy in *Absolutely Fabulous* on BBC 1 she was best-known for her role as Purdey in *The New Advengers* and also as the author of several books, including an autobiography *Stare Back and Smile* and *Forces Sweethearts*, out this year in paperback. She is a former columnist of *The Times* and a champion of many good causes. She was born in Kashmir on the May 1st, 1946 the younger daughter of an army officer. Convent-educated, she went on to become a fashion and photographic model during the 1960s. When she was twenty-two she had a son, Jamie, who she brought up on her own.

She is often referred to not only as a great and enduring beauty but also as a very nice person. Indeed, according to the findings of a recent gallup poll, she is the woman most men would want to kiss in this country. However, she is happily married to her second husband, Stephen Barlow, the orchestra conductor.

Joanna Lumley, is there, do you think, a gap between the way you are often depicted and the way you really think of yourself?

LUMLEY: I think quite often as an actress, you get a sort of strange sliding thing about the person you're playing on screen, particularly on television, and your real-life person. So that's one sort of strange division which happens. The other division, which I think must be the same with all of us, is between the person you appear to be to other people and the person you are inside your head. So now I've got two barriers in front of me, and how that might appear to other people in ordinary life, and then that ordinary-life peson acting and becoming Patsy or Purdey or whoever it is, usually taken up by the media or the press, who sometimes get slightly muddled between that on-screen character and your off-screen character. People tend to think that you make up your own lines or you really do drink five bottles of Beaujolais at lunchtime.

CLARE: Do you ever get muddled?

LUMLEY: No. No, I don't get muddled any more than you feel muddled when you've got no clothes on or when you're fully dressed for the show. I mean you always know when you're stark naked or when you're fully clothed, i.e. stark naked is what you are in your brain and fully clothed is you out there in front of two thousand people or ten million people except that you know it doesn't feel like that.

CLARE: I ask that because from quite early on you had this desire to perform in public.

LUMLEY: Show off?

CLARE: To show off, perhaps, yes.

LUMLEY: Yeah, oh yeah. That's entertaining. Yes, absolutely, but that was, that was really just to make people laugh, to keep myself amused, to do things because I like doing silly voices and things like that and showing off, just showing off and having a good time. It was better than just not showing off. It filled up what I perceived to be awkward pauses, which in fact were fragrant silences which I wrecked, but still . . .

CLARE: How early did you realise that you had a certain talent for showing off?

LUMLEY: Oh, I never felt that I had a talent, I just knew I was a show off. I think you know, then later on you learn words like extrovert and introvert and I guessed I must have been an extrovert because I like fooling around and telling funny stories or clowning around, actually, clowning around. It didn't feel as though I was trying to draw attention to myself, but of course I must have done. It didn't feel like that. It just felt like being completely normal and natural. If I had something to say I would say it at once out loud, you know.

CLARE: To what do you attribute that particular personality trait? Is it something that you feel came out of your genetic background, your family background, or is it something that came out of, say, your boarding school environment?

LUMLEY: Oh no, no, it happened long before I went to boarding school, long before. I suspect we're just born like it. I think the way you're treated could, maybe, damage a little creature but as I was treated kind of the best, we had kind of VIP silver-star, five-star upbringing, just the best you could get and so we've just flourished. My sister and I just flourished the way that we were brought up to be and I just turned into this sort of show off, you know what I mean. A bit obnoxious, probably.

CLARE: Yes, I'm interested in this.

LUMLEY: Bumptious I think is the word that came to me at boarding school, that they all called me, bumptious.

CLARE: Confident?

LUMLEY: Smart alec, lippy.

CLARE: Partly due to my own profession's preoccupation with pathology, we're used to thinking of people who make their names in the face of childhood deprivation, set-backs and so on. But there seems to me to be a group of people, and one finds them in the arts, who are performers precisely because early on they were much prized, much valued and they got an immediate feedback when they performed in public as children. They were the doting children of admiring parents and that generated a desire, or at least a naturalness about just performing in public. Was that the kind of Lumley background?

LUMLEY: Yes, I must just quickly say this, performing in public I still find absolutely terrifying so that's different from showing off.

CLARE: Showing off in public I should have said.

LUMLEY: Showing off is when you're just being your ordinary person.

CLARE: There is a link, isn't there?

LUMLEY: This might be building it up a bit bigger than it was. It wasn't as though they said, 'Oh come on, Jo will do this and do this.' That never happened.

CLARE: But showing off assumes an audience. That people are showing off . . .

LUMLEY: Yes, but an audience could be one?

CLARE: Oh indeed, yes.

LUMLEY: Yes, it can be one, preferably one. I mean when I'm performing . . .

CLARE: But who was the audience in the Lumley home?

LUMLEY: Well, my sister was great, she was great and always laughed at me. I mean she was just great.

CLARE: She was younger?

LUMLEY: No, she is two years older than me. Maybe I'm making too much of this thing of showing off because a lot of us showed off in those days and the people who could do the best accents or could do the best back bends or swing from the highest tree. I mean this is all a kind of exuberance, I think, rather than a showing off but I found it easy to put my hand up and answer a question and not be consumed with shyness. What I mean actually is that I wasn't shy, so I don't mean I necessarily was anything, I just wasn't shy.

CLARE: You had a confidence about yourself?

LUMLEY: Yes.

CLARE: In public situations?

LUMLEY: Only up to a certain stage.

CLARE: But how did that get altered into the performer, or the model?

LUMLEY: Oh, the model was nothing. I don't mean it was nothing but it was no intention of mine to become a model. It wasn't a goal of mine. I couldn't see what you could be as a model except to be photographed. You can't do anything as a model except be photographed. You can't do anything as a model. You can kind of drape your limbs more successfully. It's an extremely hard life actually. But you can't redeem yourself by saying something smart or getting out of it or doing something flip or fly because that's not your job. Your job is to be statue-still for hours on end in the most uncomfortable conditions and climates. So modelling was out.

CLARE: Acting?

LUMLEY: Acting was because I was put in school plays, you know. Also I had a great dread, which I suspect I share with most of the world, of actually having to go to work and therefore if you have to grow up and do something, it seemed better to do something that was agreeable rather than these awful things like offices. I think I've discovered that I'm sort of numerically dyslexic in that I can only remember telephone numbers if I say them out loud and then write them down from hearing the echo in my head. I can't see numbers straight, so that has put me in a very bad way with computers and maths and all these things like this. It's no good . . .

CLARE: Does it affect reading?

LUMLEY: No, not at all.

CLARE: And scripts?

LUMLEY: No, no, no, no. Photographic, photographic, but not with numbers, not with numbers. Is that odd? Semi-odd?

CLARE: Semi-odd!

LUMLEY: My excuse anyway.

CLARE: It's not accompanied by anything else. You don't have difficulty with names or identifying and naming objects. It's just an isolated factor.

LUMLEY: I think so.

CLARE: This issue that you mention about showing off, school plays, and the distinction you draw between showing off and performing, you said, 'I didn't have any anxiety about putting my hand up in class,' but you then mentioned that there was an anxiety associated with performing.

LUMLEY: Yup.

CLARE: Now that will strike people as something of a puzzle. They would have assumed that the reason you were so good in school plays was that you had such confidence and you didn't seem to be fearful.

LUMLEY: Well, this is the truth, that if I could rely on myself I would be all right but of course, when you're doing a play you're relying on somebody else's words and you are also responsible to other people to whom you must speak and things you've got to do in the right order.

CLARE: So it was the responsibility?

LUMLEY: Yes, of getting it right for other people, for making it all right, for not letting them down, not letting the audience down. Most actors' great dread is drying because you're going to let people down and the play's going to grind to a halt and everybody's going to forget that they were watching a piece of fiction and become impatient in their seats and so on and you'll have spoilt it. You will have spoilt it for everybody.

CLARE: Because reading what you had to say about yourself in your autobiography and one or two other things I saw attributed to you, I was struck by the recurrent theme that you're somewhat frightened of responsibility, fearful of it in some way. You emphasise it, you mention it from time to time.

LUMLEY: Well, I think quite the opposite. I think I kind of gather up responsibilities and grapple them unto me with hoops of steel. I don't know what responsibilities you mean. If you mean getting a proper job?

CLARE: Yes, you said something about acting enabling you to stay something of a child, avoiding the responsibilities of being an adult. That was one that stuck in my mind.

LUMLEY: Mmm.

CLARE: Then just now you talked about the responsibility you feel in a play to others. It's an interesting emphasis.

LUMLEY: But I do feel that responsibility and therefore I don't forget my lines, then I do do it properly and I don't let people down and I don't not turn up to the theatre or turn up late. So, I've always taken and shouldered those responsibilities. What I don't want to be is part of an enormous chain of selling cars.

CLARE: Does it fuel a fear, that responsibility? I mean, does it get to the point sometimes where it's too much?

LUMLEY: Black out, pistol to the temples? Oh no, no. The idea of having to work in an office would do that. It would drive you insane.

CLARE: No, no, the stage fright or a fear of going on?

LUMLEY: No, no, not this one. Oh, stage fright, stage fright if it comes to get you, which it has, it has in my life once or twice, he is the worst and the most criminal flatmate because he lives with you until he goes and there's nothing you can do about that. But that is a kind of panic. We call it stage fright because we're actors but I suspect it might be a kind of panic that visits all sorts of people at different times in their lives.

CLARE: Yes, it looks as if it is that way.

LUMLEY: They call it a nervous breakdown. It's probably just a sort of real insecurity attack which you can get from anything, I think, but I think actors call that stage fright and it comes out of the blue.

CLARE: Did it in your case?

LUMLEY: Oh yes, completely out of the blue.

CLARE: You weren't under strain for any other reason?

LUMLEY: Well, yes, but you can't gauge which bit of the metal is weakest when the thing goes wrong. You know, everything seems to be going along and you seem to be managing. And we've all got stresses and strains. We don't crack up under them, but maybe sometimes something has been gnawing away at you and that's the bit that goes ping and you're never sure what it is, which bit of it.

CLARE: In your case can you remember what it might have been?

LUMLEY: I was anxious about my cousin who was very ill and it seemed that she was going to die and she was terribly close to me and that was awful and I was anxious about her. I was anxious because I was in a play but I wasn't getting very much money which was neither here nor there, really, if I was firing on all cylinders. I became fearful in the way that you suddenly can become fearful. I can't explain it. You can feel it coming upon you like a terrible illness, like a cold. I don't actually get ill but I know the symptoms. We can certainly spot it in other people. We go, 'Oh I don't like the way so and so was, they were yammering. Did you see them? Something's going to go wrong.' Snap. And maybe other people can see it happening in you before it happens to yourself. Also, you push it away, you push it away, it can't be true. And also, you always feel that it's your fault, a lot of times when you're ill or distressed or anything. I mean, if somebody drives their shopping trolley over my heel in Sainsburys I say, 'Sorry!' (Laughs.) We come from the bunch of people who say sorry, you know.

CLARE: Yes. What sort of people do you come from? What was your father like, for example? He was a military man.

LUMLEY: Yes. My parents are both alive, thank God, and they're the best people in the world. He was in the army but he wasn't a military man. People immediately imagine people with colossal moustaches slapping at their boots with a great riding crop. Completely the opposite.

CLARE: Yes, stentorian commands and so on . . .

LUMLEY: Yes.

CLARE: He wasn't like that?

LUMLEY: To us as children they were intensely kind and funny and easy. We were the most important things in their lives.

CLARE: Was going to boarding school difficult for you? You had to do that quite young.

LUMLEY: I was eight. Well, I was homesick but we'd only just come back from the Far East from Malaya and I was also homesick for Malaya as well. I was homesick for them. They'd gone to Scotland and I couldn't think where Scotland was, I didn't know on my map where Scotland was. And I was also homesick for heat and the smell of Malaya and (sighs) and I managed to get over it, although funnily enough I was thinking about homesickness the other day and, and remembering that there are some sort of secret things, secret pains which we all have to endure and it's very odd because when you're going through them, I can remember thinking, I will get over this, but this is it now. I can remember going to new schools and thinking, I don't know what this is like yet but soon I will know it and then I will not have forgotten this, but this feeling will become irrelevant, this sense of not knowing where a door leads to or what the nickname for the science mistress is, you know. I knew I'd know it eventually but nevertheless, newness is very frightening.

CLARE: Still, for you?

LUMLEY: No, not now.

CLARE: No?

LUMLEY: Newness is great. But I think that newness might be what makes people angry about other people. You know, if it's different, you kind of hate them or hate it. I'm sure that's why people are so paranoid about death because it's the ultimate newness, it's the only thing we've got no information about. And so people do back flips not to face up to being dead, you know.

CLARE: You think about it quite a bit?

LUMLEY: Regularly, every day. Not with any sort of mournful attitude but with interest.

CLARE: Can you remember your first encounter with death?

LUMLEY: Not really. It would have been with an animal I should think and I can't really remember. I think what you're trying to say is when I can remember my first encounter with death when I realised that that was death, i.e. my death?

CLARE: Yes.

LUMLEY: You know, the stopping of life. I think it takes forever. I think probably one doesn't even believe it now.

CLARE: It emerged just now in the context of separation. I was talking about leaving home, going to a new school, your parents up in Scotland, you at school in Kent.

LUMLEY: They'd only gone for a fortnight's holiday but, do you know, it's the train pulling out syndrome when we all cry, that's the truth of it. The train pulls out and you cry, then you're on your journey and it's exciting and you eat sandwiches and look out of the window and it's different. But I think there will always be the time that the train pulling out or the ship pulling out and even now, when I watch films, there's something about a huge vessel irrevocably leaving that is just, 'Oooh.' Now you can say, 'Oh, but that's because you spent your life on ships toing and froing and leaving,' but I wasn't leaving anybody behind, I was travelling with my family. I was completely happy. But that's why *Brief Encounter* is a great film, pulling away, taking somebody away for ever in a train, inexorable.

CLARE: Like death.

LUMLEY: Like death. So we've got a series of mini deaths through our lives, inexorable partings from people, leaving school even though it's time to leave school. It's a strange wrench to know that you're not going to be the prefect or the girl in the sixth form who everybody knows.

CLARE: We've all our own ways of coping with this issue of separation, every separation, every separation a little death, moving towards our own death, we build things around us. Some people seek their supports in other people, some in a career, some in a vocation or find the support to see them through these things inside themselves. You come across, and this is why I'm back again to the gap between how you seem and how you are, you come across as quite a resilient, independent person and, I wonder, are you?

LUMLEY: I think I am. I think I am. I do try to be because I think it's nice to be independent. I also think that we were built separately and not like Siamese twins because we're meant to be independent and not to drag too heavily on anybody. 'If all men count with you but none too much,' as Kipling said.

CLARE: Would anybody have said you're quite distant, you're hard to get to know?

LUMLEY: I don't know why they would say that because I don't think I am. I think I am as shallow as a puddle, you see. I think all I am is just sitting here in front of you. There's nothing else there and in fact, I'm as deep as my eyeballs and no further. (Laughter.) But people have said, one or two people have said 'cold', and I think my voice has got something to do with it. I've got the kind of accent, I suppose, that people could find off-putting. I didn't think of changing my voice any more than I would expect anybody else to change their voice. I don't find other people's voices unpleasant or ridiculous. But people accuse you of having a voice. That doesn't actually lead anywhere. I'm tall and a lot of photographs taken of me as a model had a haughty expression because that's what they expected. You know instead of grinning insanely as one does now, you had to suck in your cheekbones which weren't very much as you were eighteen or nineteen and rather pudgy, so you looked haughty and so people said you were cold which was not true. I am a furnace, Professor, of friendliness, and I'd give my coat to the first person who asked me, and they know that too.

CLARE: A furnace suggests that you can boil and bubble as well. Can you? You seem in control, not the sort of person who necessarily explodes. Yet you used the word furnace and I wonder are there times when you do explode?

LUMLEY: I have lost my temper once or twice. I don't like losing my temper because I do lose it, I try to avoid anything that could get me into a temper. And I do counsel myself as I drive or with things that could possibly get one into any kind of confrontation. I loathe heated arguments.

CLARE: Why?

LUMLEY: Because I'm not combative. I don't like fighting with people. And I think that if I really lost my temper I'd be so hugely unpleasant and say things I would bitterly regret, maybe crush the person I was going to fight. Rise up and, having appeared to be David, I would be Goliath's grandfather and crump them all to bits and then be left with these little corpses on my hands.

CLARE: So most of the time you would keep all of that under tight control lest every now and again it might erupt.

LUMLEY: Well, if not tight control, simply drive away from it, do you know what I mean? Simply motor round. You can usually see when things are going to come up and people are going to be bloody. And sometimes people write me, very occasionally, beastly letters of unbearable cruelty.

CLARE: Really!

LUMLEY: Just occasionally, quite often triggered off by their own unhappiness. I have to walk about with those, you know, walk to and fro a bit and stop myself shaking because they're sometimes frightful, but completely outweighed by the letters of friendliness and kindness I get. Somehow, madly wrong letters really get to me, the injustice of that letter. I might add it's not really, not usually about me they're about, you know, about perhaps one of the charities I support or something like that and they are people who themselves may be slightly off-beam. And I know that I've got to get over the rage I feel or the sense of injustice and calm down and write some sort of reasoned response rather than what I actually thought first of all. Sometimes you can't write at all because most of those people don't bother to write their own names and addresses.

CLARE: In your personal relationships would that have been a feature? That you, by and large, keep a good deal of control but there would be occasions when you would erupt?

LUMLEY: I suppose so. I don't think so more than anybody else. I don't know. I can't bear rowing. You know, people say a good row clears the air. It does the exact opposite. It leaves stains all over the place as far as I can see. Ghastly things that you can hear the echo of those awful words you said, or they said.

CLARE: But I'm intrigued because I'm not sure where would you have been exposed to that that made you come to that conclusion?

LUMLEY: Oh rows, oh shouting matches at school, dramas in rehearsals of theatre things, people who one knows having rows at parties. I've come across rows all the time. In one's life people have rows in the street.

CLARE: But not at home?

LUMLEY: Not at home.

CLARE: So in a sense it's your unfamiliarity with it in your close personal relationships that made you so dislike it when you came across it in school?

LUMLEY: Well, is it wrong? Is it strange to dislike rows? Is it odd?

CLARE: No. I'm not saying it's right or wrong, I'm just saying that it's a feature. You find people who could be sitting here and they'd be saying to me, 'Oh, we rowed all the time. Oh, a terrific explosive family we came from, we were always fighting and shouting. I'm sure that's one of the reasons I'm this or that or the other.' It's the familiarity people have with family disagreements.

LUMLEY: Well then, I'm unfamiliar with them, I'm unfamiliar with rows.

CLARE: You're not familiar with them?

LUMLEY: . . . and also, any smell of one, any sight of one, I'm off, I'm out, I'm away.

CLARE: And yet the ordinary man in the street thinks that a lot of drama productions, rehearsals, acting is full of drama and confrontation.

LUMLEY: Yes, but it's not personal rows. There can be great heated discussions about how the play should be, but that's actually a different thing. I imagine that's like any production meeting, making a new car, or presenting some new margarine. People can to and fro and stamp around and get very excited about that. It's personal rows I hate. It's personal. It's people saying personally ghastly things to each other. I can understand that to some people it means nothing and it never did mean anything. But in my world it does mean something when you tell somebody you hate them.

CLARE: Right.

LUMLEY: I don't want to get drawn into them saying it to me or me saying it to them on a sort of spur of the moment rage.

CLARE: You described yourself as uncomplicated. What was it again, 'a furnace of friendliness'?

LUMLEY: (Laughs.) Yes. Huge mouth, huge teeth, rushing up to people with babies and dogs, helping old women. I like it, that's why.

CLARE: What is it you don't like about yourself?

LUMLEY: Vanity. The vanity that made me accept this sweet invitation of yours. It's only vanity to sit here, to imagine that anybody other than your most intimate friends and family, who know you in any case, could be interested in this. Why am I coming to talk? Partly curiosity because I've never spoken to a psychiatrist before – but sheer vanity. This is vanity, allowing myself to be photographed is vanity. I know it's part of the plays I do, that you have to do it. It's written into your contract. I try not to read the press about me because it's no good. If they say good things you go, 'Thank goodness for that.' If they say bad things you storm and phone up somebody who is in the show and say, 'Is this fair?' And they say, 'No, but have you read what they said about me?' So that's just silly.

CLARE: Do you wish you weren't?

LUMLEY: Yes, look, I combed my hair and put on lipstick to come and see you because we were going to have a photograph taken. So what is that but vanity? If I was true, and I have been true to myself, and at home I usually go out looking like the wrath of God, and then the press unfortunately send down photographers and say, 'She looks really, really dreadful,' and so I tend now to try to look nicer in case the press are waiting with their photographs and will make people upset in the newspapers by saying, 'Joanna Lumley is moldering away in front of your eyes. Tragic figure stamping about in Clapham.' So I try to make their lives a little nicer by putting on lipstick.

CLARE: And, of course, there is the dilemma that basically you become public property.

LUMLEY: Oh, yeah.

CLARE: You have to be the way someone else wants you to be.

LUMLEY: Yes, that's part of acting though. It's something you go, 'Can I gamble with this? Can I gamble with this? Will it let me off the hook?' And the answer is no. And what you do forfeit, and I think if I'd known I probably would never have gone into acting, much as I love it, is the loss of your own private self which is inestimable.

CLARE: But you could stop.

LUMLEY: No, not now. How can you? I can stop but the face walks about still. So then you become the has-been. I can remember Katie, the woman who did Oxo cube commercials. She was in the 1960s. I can see her face in front of me now, it's 1994. So my face won't die away. So even though I might have stopped working, people will still recognise you and then people are always hugely sympathetic which is much worse. And sometimes even if you are only in a play in the West End, they go, 'Oh dear, so you're not on television any more. What, just in the West End, dear, oh dear.' Of course, that's the peak of an actor's career to be in the West End but this is now perceived as some tragic loss, you know, complete failure. And God help people, many of my best friends, the most talented actors in the world are out of work now, and to listen to the public going, 'Oh what, resting are you?,' you know. You'd never dream of asking a man who's just been sacked from a

Scunthorpe colliery if he was resting, would you? But actors are always a joke. So part of the joke is that you also lose your private life but you don't know this before you get into it because when you first start you never think you're going to be successful. You just think it'll be good fun. Then when the terrible spotlight of success turns on you, which is, of course, immensely rewarding in many ways, you realise that it's sealed off all the exits and you're in this sort of Colditz thing with only one way out and that's through the floodwater which is rushing towards you and every step is going to be very heavy and you're going to need crampons and you're going to be swept back every now and then and be back in the terrible floodlit pool. But I've got sticky fingers and I can climb round the roof. I'll get out, I'll get out. You can get out, but it's getting harder.

CLARE: How do you get out?

LUMLEY: Well, you go to countries where they don't have television.

CLARE: So they don't know you.

LUMLEY: Yes, that's good. You go to countries where they don't have British tourists, you know, like tourist spots, like hot places like the Seychelles. Although the Sychellois wouldn't know you, the people who go to the Seychelles all come from here and so they would know you. And so you get away from people who can recognise you and then you can be you again and stand, if you want, and look into a museum thing at some ancient artifact, you can stand there for four hours if you want to and not have people looking at you as if you're in a museum and taking photographs of you.

CLARE: And, of course, you're right when you said it at the beginning, there are obvious reasons. People out there are saying, 'Oh, there they go again,' you know, 'going on about the price of power and fame and so on,' and you're rightly saying 'Well, hang on, there are certain advantages, obviously, there are certain satisfactions.'

LUMLEY: Of course there are. There are wonderful advantages.

CLARE: But, but just sticking with this, you said you wouldn't do it if you had known.

LUMLEY: No, because nobody in their right minds would. This is the frightening thing, Professor, that young ones who you talk to today and you go, 'And what do you want to be?' Do you know what they want to be. Famous. They don't want to write or be a great thing, they just, they don't want to be a singer or a bank manager. They just want to be famous. All they want to be is on television. And they perceive being on television, no matter what you do on television, if you're recognisable on television, that is where their Mecca is. That puts you in a bit of a spot, you know, to be in that Mecca position because they see me now as in prime position. What more could life hold for me than being on television?

CLARE: Being famous?

LUMLEY: Yes.

CLARE: That's why at the outset I asked you about the effect of that on you. Now you've described some of the external effects, the fact that you can't relax if there are people around and you can't stand and look into a window for four hours.

LUMLEY: Well, you can and you do.

CLARE: Or you can but it's difficult. Well, what kind of psychological effects does it have on you?

LUMLEY: I'll tell you what I love about it. People don't do this to movie stars and certainly not to people in the theatre, but because you're in their living rooms on that little box they feel they know you and so people talk to you in a completely different way. They feel familiar with you and speak to you at once, as somebody they know and I love that. That is lovely. So you can short-cut quite a lot of the preliminaries of getting to know ordinary people.

CLARE: Is it different that you've been Patsy as against Purdey? Does that lead people to treat you differently, two quite different characters really?

LUMLEY: Yes, oh, completely different.

CLARE: You are more approachable as Patsy?

LUMLEY: Patsy is more approachable.

CLARE: But let me push you on this. I understand what you're saying about the more social, public effects of this but I'm intrigued to know what this does, if it does anything to you psychologically?

LUMLEY: Well, I'll tell you what I think it is. I think it's rather unseemly. I was brought up in a convent which is excellent. It was not a Catholic one, it was Anglo-Catholic, which is quite high church, but the most charming nuns, clever. Worldly is the wrong word because they were quite opposite from worldly. We were all very young in those days and stayed quite young until we were seventeen or eighteen and left school. I think that the nuns had been wonderful and I write to them every Christmas and sometimes go and see them and they are the most affectionate and forgiving and admiring people. Nevertheless I feel that what I'm doing is pretty unseemly. It's not really acting, I don't mean that. But it is all the stuff that comes in its wake. Being splurged across the papers is not really the way to be if you are a modest woman, which I hope I am. But of course, Patsy isn't a modest woman so Patsy has somehow leeched on to me because I'm recognisably her and somehow, any articles about inebriates or smoking eighty cigarettes a day or behaving badly, somehow I'm there as a photograph. It might be a photograph of Patsy but in some ways they've sort of blended the edges a bit and I've turned into Joanna Lumley. I read an article yesterday which was sent to me which said, 'I love Joanna Lumley, she smokes eighty cigarettes a day' and I went, 'No, that's Patsy,' who is much loved and admired. So they kind of like and admire this person but it really isn't me and I feel that in some ways it's rather odd. I've walked straight into it, I mean, I can't whine and groan about it but sometimes, late at night in bed, reading a book, I think, thank goodness I'm sitting here alone in my bed reading this lovely book.

CLARE: It is a curious thing, that part is so different, then, to you.

LUMLEY: Why?

CLARE: Because . . .

LUMLEY: That's what actors are.

CLARE: Well, is there anything of you in a character like Patsy?

LUMLEY: Well, Anthony Hopkins was asked what he did for Hannibal Lecter and he said he combed his hair back.

CLARE: And changed his voice.

LUMLEY: I know that's a glib answer but that's what he did because he acts it. He just became Hannibal for when the cameras were turning. He didn't have to be it at home. He just did it. That's what acting is, with any luck. That's what acting is. And I really am not, I'm really not Patsy. But it seemed that she'd appeared in my head, or rather in Jennifer's head, embryonically fully formed. All she needed was like a kind of Barbie doll that you pump air into and there she was. And so it's not difficult to be her.

CLARE: I suppose what I'm getting at is as you would expect me to, that is to wonder if there's any tension in you about this niceness, this modesty that you describe? Is there inside you anywhere a kind of embryonic Patsy dying to express itself?

LUMLEY: Oh, of course there is.

CLARE: And that you've found it?

LUMLEY: Of course there is, and in any of our lives which are worthwhile I think we probably cannon between the life of Toulouse Lautrec, you know, hopelessly living amongst the prostitutes and scribbling away in his pockets and getting completely blind on Pernod and you go, 'That's the way an artist lives.' Drawing and writing are so much more in front of my head than acting that I can only admire the mad excesses which managed to make people live. Michelangelo strapped upside down doing the Sistine Chapel and writing poetry, saying, 'Will God ever forgive me for these pathetic daubings?' These are kind of titanic struggles going on with people and I think it would be mad to think that we all simply go about our daily lives and just are. We all, part of us, all want to be like Beryl Cook, that wonderful artist who draws fat women with suspender belts on doing ridiculous things in bread shops with sort of fur coats which open and nothing on underneath, because there's something sort of bizarre and we're all like that. All of us have these bungee-jump-sized dreams which extend in every direction. Could I do that, would I do that? We admire people.

CLARE: But acting lets you do that on occasions?

LUMLEY: Acting lets you do that. Acting lets you do that. You read parts carefully and you go, 'Oh no, not that person again, I've been that one or that's dull. That doesn't go anywhere. That's not even a small elastic band left by the postman, let alone a bungee jump off a bridge.' And so you sort of choose things, and you go, 'Oooh, that's an area to go to.' I did a play by a fine playwright called Bernard Copse which was about a decaying actress who sort of contemplated and even attempted suicide. Now, I'm not a decaying actress and I haven't contemplated suicide, but that was a wonderful road to go down. And lots of it is imagination which we were brought up on. All we read and had read to us as children and read and read and read. Read everything that was to do with the imagination and mind. Making up games, not sitting and watching. Making it up, making it up. We may have seen one film a year, you know, and no televison sets. And so it all came out of our heads or what we read in books. And that seemed to me a very fertile ground for growing great trees of imagination. And now I can imagine my way into anything. I could be anybody, if you just let me. If the part is well written enough or if there's enough meat to be going on, to go virtually in any direction I hope that a human being could go. Which is how Diana Rigg, the most normal and enchanting person to meet, can strangle her children and cough up blood every night on stage, you know. It isn't her but she can go there, she can be there. And of course it's a huge therapy which is why actors come off stage walking on air. All ills cured ready to party till three.

CLARE: But there is something slightly different about television.

LUMLEY: Oh, I know.

CLARE: Precisely that familiarity you mentioned.

LUMLEY: Well, you see, what happens if you go into the theatre or into the cinema, what you have to do, is to sit quietly in your seat until it's over. In the film you can't switch it off and the people are miles bigger than you. In the theatre all you can do is tiptoe out. On television we can be stopped, we can be talked over, we can be taped and made to go in slow motion, we can be made to look completely ridiculous, which of course, in a way we are, but in a way that has never been possible before. We can be made to run backwards. They can run through something which has taken six months' rehearsal. They can put it on fast forward, get to the juicy bits. Do you see what I mean? We are their puppets. They can control us and our destinies. They can switch us off. They can throw us away. You can't do that in a theatre. You can't throw away a movie. You can throw us away. It's quite interesting. So they have more affection for us and more contempt.

CLARE: Which is a little like what you feel about the process. Because you are affectionate but there's a certain degree of contempt.

LUMLEY: I'm only contemptuous of slavish admiration.

CLARE: Are you?

LUMLEY: Mindless, mindless hatred. I hate group opinions and television seems to rely on group opinions. In a theatre if you played a theatre every day of your life you'd never get what I get for one audience of *Absolutely Fabulous*. It couldn't. Every theatre, every night, couldn't play it.

CLARE: Do you need people?

LUMLEY: People?

CLARE: Mm.

LUMLEY: *Natürlich*, Professor.

CLARE: Well, some people can be quite independent, very self-reliant.

LUMLEY: But even if they're self-reliant they're reading books, they're listening to music, they're getting other people's thoughts and ideas.

CLARE: Yes, I meant . . .

LUMLEY: They are listening to the wireless.

CLARE: I meant people more directly.

LUMLEY: Acting people?

CLARE: Yes.

LUMLEY: I love people, I love being with people.

CLARE: You do?

LUMLEY: And that's why I think what I don't like is the change that may come upon them from the fact that I've been on television, because television is only a medium to put forward a play. That's all it is. It itself is nothing at all and yet somehow it's become a new god and to be on it, even to read the weather forecast out on it, makes you in some way a star. And I find that terribly sad.

CLARE: What do people expect you to be?

LUMLEY: Very, very rich, very accomplished, very lazy, very powerful. The dream, the sort of Hollywood dream, the sort of Orson Welles dream of what *Citizen Kane* people were. Huge houses, servants to do things. But this is all whipped up, I've got to say, to the press, who don't want to write about dull people like me who scrub floors or put arms down lavatories or paint things ourselves. That's not really interesting so they put you into a bit of a kind of fab position, you know.

CLARE: So what were the fantasies that fuelled you? They weren't power apparently, or money.

LUMLEY: This is the thing that started it. A photograph, probably advertising cigarettes which I saw when I was in Malaya when I was six or seven, and it was a woman standing on a Manhattan balcony or skyline. Anyway, she was up very high. She had on satin evening gloves and strapless dress and she was about to light a cigarette and some dashing beau in a white coat, a white tux, proffered a flame and behind her the lights of Manhattan in the blue evening sky. Seduction. That was it. I wanted to be that woman and I wanted to smoke cigarettes. Now of course you realise you're not going to do it and if you're up there puffing away you're not going to see yourself puffing away at your cigarette in the blue Manhattan sky and the man's going to be a bore. He might just be a bore. So, the thing to do is to try to get into movies where you can create this extraordinary dream sequence for other people, be part of the dream. That's why I don't want to give up acting, or writing or painting. So it's all part of the telling of the story of the dream and the only thing that keeps us all going is this dream. Oh, the dream. We're lured on the dream holiday, your dream holiday, your dream romance. On Valentine's Day what will your dream Valentine say to you? It's never like that, of course, but we can dream. 'Oh, Rhett Butler' we say, 'Jimmy Dean', it doesn't matter who we pin it on, this is the dream and I love to be part of that dream, that passes it on, passes it on. It's not us. We're not the dream. We put the masks on.

CLARE: But of course, you reminded me that one of the aspects of cinema and television is that you can see yourself, that you can be the person that turns the fast forward, slows it down.

LUMLEY: Oh yes, but you can't charm yourself, you can't bewitch yourself

CLARE: Alas.

LUMLEY: You can't bewitch yourself. You can't do it for yourself. You can only do it for other people. You can't look at yourself and think, 'God, that looks fab,' not a bit of it.

CLARE: Well, some people do, believe you me.

LUMLEY: No, no, no, no they don't, no, Professor.

CLARE: It's called narcissism.

LUMLEY: No they don't. They can't really, truly. Well, maybe then they are more pleased with themselves originally. I find it irritating to see myself because I only ever wanted to look like Bridgitte Bardot or Marilyn Monroe or something so as soon as you see yourself you go, 'Damn, I just look like me again, how awful.'

CLARE: But, hang on, the fact that you wanted to look like them must have some . . .

LUMLEY: Because they were the dream purveyors.

CLARE: Yes, but it must also, it must also relate to the fact that to an extent you, unlike many, many people, you could look like them, or at least, you could think that way because you are a strikingly beautiful woman. That's the fact.

LUMLEY: Professor! Get a grip!

CLARE: That may be a terrible thing to say in the context of the conversation we're having!

LUMLEY: It's not. It's extremely polite and I didn't mean to shout with laughter but it really is . . .

CLARE: But isn't it a burden?

LUMLEY: No, because it's . . .

CLARE: I assumed it would be.

LUMLEY: Strictly speaking not true.

CLARE: Well, we might argue, all right.

LUMLEY: No, we can argue all night. What I mean is that I know what you mean and I can, if combed and presented properly, look damnably good, particularly from a distance, in whatever it is. But in real life I think I'm really only me.

CLARE: But in real life Marilyn Monroe was only her, and Bridgitte Bardot was only her.

LUMLEY: Oh, exactly, she put it on, she, Marilyn Monroe would switch it on and she could sit around just being, like me, just sort of, but she could really switch on the fire.

CLARE: But what I don't want to lose is the fact and I did it crudely and you were right to rap my knuckles . . .

LUMLEY: I didn't, I didn't rap your knuckles.

CLARE: Well, in a sense.

LUMLEY: I actually went into a swooning sort of attitude.

CLARE: But you've talked about the way people perceive you and we talk about things like faulty perceptions of you as haughty and aloof and being tall and in control. But of course, there's also this issue of your looks and whether that also does something, that the way people see you starts them thinking in terms of the Bardots and the Monroes and there is again an expectation there too. I'm interested in the extent to which we're imprisoned by how we look.

LUMLEY: Well, I encourage it. I dye my hair. I draw lines around my mouth.

CLARE: You encourage it?

LUMLEY: I encourage it. I know this is because I'm half-way from Patsy, on to more Patsy and things like that so I've got to keep my hair long, but . . .

CLARE: Long and blonde.

LUMLEY: Yes, I dye it blonde. Well, Patsy's hair is blonde. It's a, it's a semi vanity but it's not really, because I also hacked it off and had it long and pitch black for another part. I actually use my hair. I quite like using myself to fit in, but nothing can cut away from the fact that I am 5' 8'' tall and that I am an English woman with white skin. It would be insanity to cast me as a South American Indian. It would be vanity because it would be lovely to have a crack at it but it would be wrong. It would be wrong actually, it would be terribly wrong. And now, thank goodness, we've stopped all this terrible ridiculous casting we can actually choose somebody. If somebody is, you know, a

Spanish woman of fifty-eight get one, don't get me to do it because that's just stupid, you know. But having got over all that, the parts that I'm playing which at the moment are Patsy and Kate Swift, who hasn't come out yet so you don't know her, they're both English women of a certain height and a certain age. One is more exaggerated than the other, and so I change my appearance very slightly for each of them. When comes the time that I've got to play the person with the big buck teeth and the red hair and things, I'll go and do it. But I did want to look like Marilyn Monroe and Bridgitte Bardot because they seemed to be the people who were cast in the roles. That's changed. In the old days you could only be in films if you were beautiful. That's changed, thank goodness and now you can actually be anything and be fine. Meryl Streep I think is beautiful but nevertheless she's got an unorthodox face and all sorts of people are now catching the headlines, people like Emma Thompson who's got a wonderfully attractive and strong and interesting face but couldn't really be called a beauty in the old terms of beautiful. So there's hope for us all. We can all go and act now rather than just having to be blessed with the looks.

CLARE: But isn't it a curious thing – how do you tell someone who is beautiful they are beautiful because it seems to involve a whole series of almost rather threatening assumptions?

LUMLEY: I know, and why do I behave like that? Why don't I just sit there calmly and say, 'Thank you, Professor,' and then we could have finished with that, instead of which I go, 'Oh no, ha ha ha, give me some more wine,' which incidentally is one of the things I was just about to say. And I get into a sort of false modesty. And also part of it is confusion, you know. I was jolly spotty when I was young and I had really frightful hair, really, really frizzily awful hair, and spotty, and although I wasn't fat I was not really attractive.

CLARE: Well, when did you become attractive?

LUMLEY: Well, when I was modelling I was still a bit spotty and I had those nightmarish things of trying to sort of cover up a spot or be photographed from that side or trying to suck your cheeks in. And I dyed my hair.

CLARE: What age, now, are we talking about?

LUMLEY: This is eighteen, nineteen, you know, quite grown up but enough time to have quite a chirpy kind of character, nevertheless not confident really in the way one looks, which is very odd then to have gone into modelling.

CLARE: Would you have been confident with boys?

LUMLEY: No, no, no no. Only in a sort of joshing way. I felt that I could perhaps run alongside them or give them a good overarm ball if I was playing cricket with them, partner them badly at tennis. But, no, not as seductress or a kind of *femme fatale* or as anybody successful, even remotely, in the humbler regions of love. Not at all.

CLARE: So when did you become conscious that you weren't spotty and you weren't leggy and that, in fact, you made an impact on other people?

LUMLEY: Well, it really did take a long time. I suppose a few people were kind enough to kiss you or say how nice you look (laughs) and so it starts there, the seed starts there. But even now, when I put on make-up I put it on to correct my face, to correct it. To try to make it more like the face ought to be. You know. And I don't know anybody, and I know most of the most beautiful women in the world, who doesn't do exactly that, because there's a slight burden, part of it's a burden and part of it is just the anxiety that you aren't going to look exactly the way that you feel you ought to be looking. I know this is all very surface, but as part of my life is actually how the camera sees me, it's a very odd and important thing, which is why it's lovely to be able to scratch away that person completely and not have to care, which is why Patsy was such a freedom. It doesn't matter where her lipstick goes or what she looks like. She's revolting, revolting.

CLARE: So there is something about her that attracts you?

LUMLEY: Oh, hugely. Oh, I think, oh, absolutely and I would be the first to say that. I think she would be the best fun. I mean, a bit of a menace because she would probably come and stay if you were remotely kind to her. She'd probably come and stay and never leave and go through your purse.

CLARE: But it's the fact that she doesn't really give a damn?

LUMLEY: She doesn't really give a hang.

CLARE: She doesn't give a hang.

LUMLEY: No, and I think that there's something quite agreeable in these straitened ages where everybody's trying to get slim, or trying not to smoke or not drink and live for ever and not get this disease or that disease and you suddenly think, Patsy couldn't give a hang. She's riddled with everything and raddled as well and she's somehow hanging on to life, although nobody knows how, and seeming to have quite a good time and I think a lot of us go, 'God, that's rather great, that's rather good fun. That's rather more fun than I'm having. Patsy who doesn't go into work and gets a salary, how does she manage that scam?' So I think people look at that and think that's rather good fun.

CLARE: You said you think about death, do you think about ageing?

LUMLEY: Things like not being able to do things is a bore. I know enough people who have the menace of arthritis – not being able to grip the top of the marmalade jar and get it off, you know. The bore about going downstairs when your eyes aren't seeing where the edge of the step is and you stumble and fall. I've started to use reading glasses. I've bought about four pairs which I leave around the house and in different rooms. I never knew I'd get to the stage where my 20/20 vision suddenly wouldn't allow me to read a book when I'd just picked it up.

CLARE: Have you ever been ill, seriously ill?

LUMLEY: No.

CLARE: Have you ever been seriously depressed?

LUMLEY: Seriously? Once, when I was about twenty-five, twenty-four or twenty-five. Went into a real black hole then and I don't know what triggered it off. It was a sort of fear. It's always fear, I'm always coming back to this and I'm becoming a bit of a bore by saying the only thing I'm afraid of really is fear. If I could get rid of the fear of fear, which I'm working on all the time, and actually, sometimes, completely triumphant. To be afraid of something seems to me the only enemy I have. And funnily enough, the only thing I'm afraid of is people.

CLARE: People?

LUMLEY: Mm. Because there's nothing else bad in the world. Being munched to bits by a tiger wouldn't worry me. I've never been burnt to death in a fire or nearly burnt, so I'm sure those are frightening, but actually, the only things one can sit in dread of are people . . . (Pause.)

CLARE: What particularly?

LUMLEY: Oh, I don't know. When you read about dreadful things that people do to each other, dreadful things, you know, incomprehensible wars which go on and on.

CLARE: But in your sense, it would be personal violence would it?

LUMLEY: Yes, personal violence, personal violence. Or having to witness somebody I love being personally hurt and that extends to people who I don't know but who I would love by extension, because, sometimes in a funny way, because they've seen you, you've seen them in a funny way, you know.

CLARE: Are there things you often avoid exposing yourself to newsreels or pictures, because they move you, because they disturb you?

LUMLEY: Mm, nightmare stuff. I don't mind violent films. I think they're boring so I don't go to see them but they, they're only actors acting. News, I'm haunted to this day by a picture made by a very brave cameraman down in South Africa who was following some lynch-mob who were following a young man and the cameraman said before, 'I knew they were going to kill him but I felt I had to go and record it,' and it was as if I'd gone underwater because I was trying to get to the knob to turn the television off, but I didn't and I saw on film a youngish man being hacked to death. And the terrible thing is that it is because I wasn't there I couldn't help. If I was there I think it would have been different, I'd have been part of the fight. I'd have been doing something or shouting something or helping, or doing something, but it's watching I can't bear. That's why I hate watching films about real, real tragedies because there seems to be nothing I can do. It can fire you off to trying to do something but if you're confounded again, you get this impotent rage and it is a rage, it's a real violent rage.

CLARE: Is that one of the elements, do you think, in your fear, of being helpless?

LUMLEY: No, I wouldn't be helpless, I'd be violent.

CLARE: No, no, helpless in this situation?

LUMLEY: Oh, helpless in films, yes absolutely, absolutely.

CLARE: And helpless imagining being attacked, or imagining being burgled or imagining being assaulted.

LUMLEY: Oh, these are awful things. I don't imagine those things. I'm not afraid of being assaulted or burgled. Those aren't the things.

CLARE: No?

LUMLEY: No, it's the terror of (pause) of being unable to stop something happening. I've had several dreams where the Thames was flooding, and I ran on the top of the Embankment wall, screaming to people, 'The Thames is coming over its banks, get back, get back,' and people sitting in meadows. It was as if it was the old Thames, but this was only on the Chelsea Embankment, sitting there turning their faces and they couldn't seem to hear me and I was going, 'Get back, you're going to be killed,' and they didn't understand and they didn't listen and it was my fault because, although I'd told them, I couldn't get them to go back. So that was bad. And those sort of dreams come upon me, my warning dreams, which are all completely meaningless of course.

CLARE: Are they?

LUMLEY: (Pause.) Yes, because I've warned nobody.

CLARE: Do you see death as final?

LUMLEY: No, not a jot.

CLARE: So what happens, do you think?

LUMLEY: What happens with everything else. I mean, it's happening all the time, all around us. It's just a pattern, we're just part of a pattern.

CLARE: But what will happen to you?

LUMLEY: Be part of the pattern. Body goes crimp, crump, crump and turns into whatever it is, turns back into matter again. Mind goes into mind bank, you know, whatever it's called the cosmic soup, is that the word they call it? And I melt down and get picked out for more babies in years to come, who get the same old brains. I mean the truth is, I'm perfectly sure that nothing, including the water, nothing has left this planet since time began, apart from the odd meteorite crashing into it. So this is all the same stuff, we are made of the same stuff as Abraham.

CLARE: How far would you take it? Would you take it to reincarnation? Would you believe that you've been here before?

LUMLEY: I don't think you can help being reincarnated, whether you believe it or not. You're going to be recycled, lets put it like that. In some way, whether you will come back as me, Joanna Lumley into the spirit of a, something or other, I'm not sure about that, but I certainly can remember things that have never happened to me so it's got to come from somewhere.

CLARE: Like what?

LUMLEY: Oh, places I've been to, or familiarity. You know, this *déjà vu* thing, this complete certainty about people or the sudden closeness you feel to people who you don't know. The sudden familiarity of pieces of music, the absolute attachment I have to certain bits of furniture which you suddenly come across and go, 'OK, I don't care, I don't care if I have to work for the rest of my life, that's mine, that's got my name on it, I'm going to have that.' It's not really even because you like it. It's because you recognise things. We recognise this amongst people. That's how you hunt around, who, who's the man I love?

CLARE: Why do we go wrong then?

LUMLEY: We can't help it. The whole point of it is to go wrong. It can't just go right 'cos the whole game would be up then, the whole jig would be up. The whole point is setting it up so you go wrong so you can go right. The whole thing is this great sort of thing. As much good as bad, as much right as wrong, as much this as that, as much darkness as light, you know yin and yang. All the balances. If you can just see this binary code thing about everything and not get into a stew, as much life as death, as much death as life. And then you stop getting into a stew about things.

CLARE: Do you?

LUMLEY: Yeah.

CLARE: But you get into a stew about things, it doesn't stop you?

LUMLEY: Yes, but that's part of it, because part of my life has to be in a stew because the other half is so transparently happy. So, to counterbalance a fab happy life, you've got to have in-a-stew life otherwise it would be a pesky bore.

CLARE: It is a happy life?

LUMLEY: It's paradise. I think it's paradise. I don't think I will ever see anything lovelier than the things you can find here and the feelings you get here on this earth, and the potential . . .

CLARE: Then is the fear, the conscious recognition . . .

LUMLEY: It's of damage and destruction.

CLARE: And it'll end?

LUMLEY: No, no, no, no, that's fine. No, no, no. My life is fine because it just blends into the next thing. It's a damage and destruction . . .

CLARE: But wait now, wait now, wait now.

LUMLEY: It's destruction, Professor.

CLARE: I know, but you're very persuasive, I suddenly went with you there and then I realised, 'Well, hang on a minute.' I understand what you mean in the great cosmic sense that we all in the end come to dust, and to dust we return and our spirits go God knows where and your theory is as good as anybody else's. But at the same time, it does mean that Joanna Lumley, and we referred to this earlier when we talked about death, otherwise why would death have any sting at all, Joanna Lumley will cease. It used to be said that one of the great consolations for people living miserable lives is the knowledge that they would die, whereas now you might say one of the real threats to people who are living reasonably satisfying lives is that they will die. It's one of the paradoxes of being happy. People are nervous about being happy because they know that it'll stop.

LUMLEY: But look, Professor, we're only called these names while we're here and we've only learned in these bodies while we're here. You've just got a man's body and you look like that and I'm stuck like this and this is what our parts are and this is who we are. I know Shakespeare said, 'All the world's a stage' – this wasn't such light, frivolous banter chit-chat that he was saying. All we are is being these people for the moment. It's not a great me, me, me, me, me thing, because just as I leave a theatre at the end of a three-month, six-month run, and you look around the old dressing-room and you go, 'God, oh, I forgot to take that card down, there we are, done that, put the tights down there, costume hanging there, bye, bye, costume. Look around here, well I won't be in here for a bit,' and out you walk. And the part's gone. The notices, the notices are all there, got the old photographs . . .

CLARE: Yes, but you feel something?

LUMLEY: Oh yes! This is the train going out.

CLARE: That's right.

LUMLEY: Irrevocable. Off you go. Bye bye. Tear runs down the face. But that's all, and life goes on.

CLARE: Mm, it does.

LUMLEY: And on Monday morning the sweeper comes in and she puts out the clothes for the Chippendales.

CLARE: Right, but the point I'm making to you is this. When you talked about your fear, one interpretation of that fear, of the tide coming and you warning people, is that you were warning people it would end.

LUMLEY: Yes.

CLARE: Was I right?

LUMLEY: Completely happy and quite right.

CLARE: Yes. And of course, what you're warning is that there's inside you, as there is inside me, particularly at moments when things are going well, a bat's squeak, an echo of the fact that the train will go out, the sea will come in, the ship will steam out.

LUMLEY: And what will happen will be that people will die in dreadful pain, I think that's what I can't stand. So films like *The Killing Fields* affected me dreadfully, you know.

CLARE: Do you worry about dying in great pain, do you worry about pain?

LUMLEY: No.

CLARE: You don't?

LUMLEY: Not if it's my own. I worry about other people's pain, not my own.

CLARE: Why do you worry so much about other people, do you know?

LUMLEY: I don't know. Do you know what I do sometimes, preferably if the train's going slowly through places like Clapham Junction? I look at people's houses and I'm terribly anxious about how they manage to live.

CLARE: About what's going on there.

LUMLEY: What are they up to, and my brain gets fuller and fuller of what is the world up to, being up to. How can it, how is it managing? I don't know how it's managing. I'm managing mine. I mean this is certifiable language so I do hope that you understand what I'm talking about. What I'm trying to say is that sometimes I seem to know everything but without the exact details and I flick past and it's like a kind of kids' game and I look at the houses and I go, 'De . . . de . . . de . . . gas bills, de . . . de . . . de . . . and are children at school?' and I've got to somehow absorb all that. It's only a kind of game, but I don't mean to play it, it happens. I look at people and I go, 'How will you manage, how can you get that shopping home, how are you going to get your baby up those stairs?' You know. Of course they manage.

CLARE: Why do you then describe yourself, given what you're saying, the sorts of things you think, the sorts of feelings you feel, the sort of preoccupations you have, why did you, at the outset, describe yourself in terms of 'What you see is what there is?'

LUMLEY: Well, you can see it beaming out of me.

CLARE: No, you said something, I wish I could remember the phrase.

LUMLEY: Shallow as a puddle.

CLARE: But you're not shallow as a puddle.

LUMLEY: But who knows who's shallow as a puddle.

CLARE: Well, you used the phrase.

LUMLEY: No, well, I know, because I suspect we all are.

CLARE: But you know that's not true, you know that there are people . . .

LUMLEY: Well, I don't know.

CLARE: Would you say that you've met people who you would never describe as shallow as a puddle?

LUMLEY: Well, I know, but sometimes they're not as deep as all that.

CLARE: Yes, I accept that but . . .

LUMLEY: You know, sometimes they're just an old boulder. Do you know what I mean? Of course it's colossal but it's only a boulder, you know. I mean we can't get too reverent about people or too scathing about other people. And I don't feel any different really. And this is why what's going on in my head I put into everybody else's heads, and I wonder if they're thinking like me how they're managing because their heads must be flying around. And that's why I try to warn them and help them and do this because if they've got this, which they probably have, they just don't get the opportunity to speak to you on a green microphone.

CLARE: Well no, that's one of the reasons I like speaking to people like you speaking on the green microphone because you would be surprised the letters that people will write in, and they'll say things like, 'I do exactly the same, sitting in the train, passing through Clapham. These are the same preoccupations.' It's precisely because people don't normally talk this way.

LUMLEY: Well, don't they?

CLARE: Well, not in public they don't, no.

LUMLEY: Do you know, this is the other good thing about television. People do now talk to me in the most strange shorthand way, they jump straight across barriers and they talk to me a little bit in the way that if I was elegant and kind and courteous, I would be talking to you now, which I hope I am, but they spill out things to me in the way that I am spilling out, Professor, stuff to you because they short-change it. And I knew, I knew your face before I knew you, so you're a friend, so I can talk to you.

CLARE: How did you, how do you mean?

LUMLEY: Well, if you're a complete stranger in a train . . .

CLARE: Oh yes, I see.

LUMLEY: I'd be asking you more questions and you'd have to answer them.

CLARE: But you do intrigue yourself?

LUMLEY: *Natürlich*, because we have to. You can't just bore yourself to bits and, also, if you bore yourself to bits you can always go and read a book.

CLARE: You have a technique which is very disarming, which is to imply that when I ask you something that the question applies to everybody – 'Doesn't everybody do this, you know,' but everybody doesn't.

LUMLEY: How do you know?

CLARE: Well, because I've spent twenty-five years talking to people and there'll be people . . .

LUMLEY: Oh, what an awfully impertinent question, of course you have.

CLARE: Not at all, it's a very reasonable question. But people will write to me and say, 'What a crazy woman, that she talks about these things, I never talk about these things.' The blanket statement, 'We're all shallow as puddles!' or 'Doesn't everybody do it?' are a way of deflecting me because I can only answer by saying, 'Yeah, you're right,' and we can move on or I can say, 'Hang on a minute.' Some people would find our conversation, you used a word 'certifiable' but if you're certifiable so am I because I'm engaged in this conversation, but you used it because a bit of you recognised that out there will be some people who will not tune into this, they don't understand these experiences. They say, 'No, I never sit in the train passing through Clapham, I just look down at these houses and thank God I'm not living in them,' or whatever. But they won't go through what you've just described and I'm saying to you there are certain things about you which are really quite unusual. People, in my experience, maybe it's the kind of people I've met, but in my experience people are very reluctant to talk about some of these things. Maybe you're right, maybe they do, but I'm tempted to conclude that some people don't actually have these kinds of experiences about life or they don't think this way about life. Let me give you an example. I would have interviewed on this programme last year, a scientist like Colin Blakemore, a very interesting, very complicated man, but he didn't speak like this. He spoke in a different kind of way about life.

LUMLEY: Well, we're all so very different in the way that we're sort of triggered off by things.

CLARE: But that's why I'm interested to know the extent to which this aspect of yourself interests you to the extent that you wonder what triggers it off in you. Where does it come from? Perhaps I shouldn't be interested in it, but I am.

LUMLEY: I don't know, me too. I tell you what, it just sort of suddenly occurs. It isn't mine.

CLARE: It isn't yours?

LUMLEY: No, it's as if one sort of gathered up piecemeal somebody else's bag in your luggage, that's all, which is why I believe in this sort of old cosmic soup thing. I think sometimes we collect quite large conglomerations of thoughts or perceptions which may have drifted molecule-wise your way because then you suddenly have this huge, this sort of pan-world interest in people. I'm actually so fanatically interested in people and the way they operate and how they operate around the world. I couldn't give sixpence for the next coloured lipstick, or whether I'm thin or fat, these things don't interest me. What does interest me is the way people think and the way they injure each other.

CLARE: But let me just make an observation about our own interview, that what is striking is the extent to which I really have not got a picture from you of the people immediately close to you. That's to say, your parents, or your sister.

LUMLEY: Well, maybe I'm sort of protecting them. They are important.

CLARE: Well, of course they must be.

LUMLEY: But of course I'm awfully reluctant because we're this kind of family where it's not really right to discuss . . .

CLARE: It's like the nuns again and the modesty?

LUMLEY: Sort of, because they are without any shadow of doubt the most profound influence that can be on my life, my mother, my father and my sister, into whose world I grew, they were everything to me.

CLARE: All right, well let me just ask you this, which I think you can answer, because I do appreciate this dilemma, is it very difficult to talk about people who are not here and who are alive and who are influential?

LUMLEY: And who don't like being talked about.

CLARE: And who don't like being talked about. But, if I said to you, thinking of the kind of person you are, how much of it do you derive from them? Do you recognise certain things in yourself that you would see in your mother or in your father?

LUMLEY: Oh, of course, of course.

CLARE: Which of the two would you be more like?

LUMLEY: Well, my mother would be the one who would be the first to rush and help people and immensely practical and . . .

CLARE: A doer?

LUMLEY: Tough, a doer, tough to the point she would go without anything. My father's enormous sense of humour, enormous sense of clowning, and from them both and from my sister, a passion for books and reading. Although they were all three light years ahead of me, my sister light years ahead of me in almost every subject. In reading, in painting, in games, in writing, in everything.

CLARE: These are awfully crude distinctions, do forgive me, but she would have been the brains, she would have been seen as brains. Would you have been seen early on . . .

LUMLEY: As brainy? No – smart, bright, smart, smart, photographic memory.

CLARE: Quick.

LUMLEY: Quick, quick, yup, quick.

CLARE: What did your sister do?

LUMLEY: Well, she was brainy, she writes a bit, she sculpts, she's an artist you know, and she got married. She's inherited from my father the philosophical. They played chess together and things like that. I suspect I was the lightweight of the family, you know.

CLARE: Would you have been seen as sort of scatty?

LUMLEY: No, they adored me.

CLARE: I don't mean that as a criticsim. When you say the lightweight of the family?

LUMLEY: Lightweight, no, well, because if my sister was reading Dickens I'd probably be reading Enid Blyton, do you know what I mean? I'm sort of white trash here, Professor. But the thing is, it's really such good fun and they all just laughed at me and thought it was great and they laughed in that loving, laughing way, you know, that you do to an old clown and it was, it was just great.

CLARE: You were happy with it?

LUMLEY: Completely.

CLARE: You didn't mind being regarded as lightweight?

LUMLEY: Adored . . . well, they didn't regard me as lightweight but I felt as though, you know, because they, there were so sort of great, they just were great. It's very odd to keep on saying this again and again but they were the best starting point that any human being could have in life and I had it, I landed there.

CLARE: And of course, to that extent, that explains the independence.

LUMLEY: Well, it gives you a strength.

CLARE: Resilience, yes.

LUMLEY: If you're a strong little plant you just grow straight up, you don't have to lean on walls or go up twigs or anything, only because you're in this glowing environment with all the best things there.

CLARE: Now, was it difficult when you went out into a world that is far from a glowing environment?

LUMLEY: No, because it was quite a challenge.

CLARE: Is that what you're looking for?

LUMLEY: I love adventures.

CLARE: You look for that?

LUMLEY: Oh, a bit of an adventure, I love it.

CLARE: What about love?

LUMLEY: Yes, that's anywhere. You're civil to people, you're nice to people, you make friends with people, that's no problem. And my parents are there, my sister's there.

CLARE: Would it have left you more vulnerable to the nasty side of life. You know, this thing that if you come out of a happy family, the one snag is you're not streetwise to the nastiness?

LUMLEY: Yes, you're not streetwise, that's exactly the phrase,

Professor, that I would have pounced on if I'd been clever enough. Streetwise, I was not streetwise and so when people have said when I got my first job, 'Will you bring in your cards on Monday,' I actually thought they meant my visiting cards and I hadn't had any printed. I didn't know what cards were. Now this is part of the fault of the nuns and partly the fault of my dear unworldly parents because we didn't know about cards. It wasn't that we were too grand to know about cards. We were just too fey, too out of it all to know about cards. And so those things are a bit of a shock. People being terrifically rude to you or very lippy or very sort of cheeky to you in the street, this was a bit of a shock because if you'd been at a convent, in a boarding school and living in the countryside, you're not exposed to the London thing. None of it was malevolent and people said you're ugly as a pig and you'd kind of go, 'Oh!' and they'd go, 'Oh, come on, you old tart,' and put you in front of the camera, you know, and you'd be fine. It was fine, you just learned a sort of tougher, just a tougher way of toughening up. Nobody was unkind to me. I remember the people on one hand who have ever been unkind to me. I don't mean to take revenge but the fact that I remember them means that they've scored some deep burn.

CLARE: But some of the things you've had to do have been tough, you've brought up your son on your own, that couldn't have been too easy?

LUMLEY: No, but it was joy easy, if you know what I mean.

CLARE: Was it?

LUMLEY: Mm. You've got something to do, brilliant, marvellous, got to have a crack at it. Occasionally you sit down and blub and go, 'Well what do I do?' and then you pull yourself together and get up and go on. But I've got to say it just pales into just like a grey leaf in twilight compared with what people, the tussles people have.

CLARE: But at the time?

LUMLEY: It was great, I had my parents, had my, all my friends, my sister, my boyfriends, all the people around me who all helped, everybody was sweet and nice.

CLARE: Are you someone who is a bit suspicious about self analysis, about examining one's motives?

LUMLEY: No.

CLARE: Why not?

LUMLEY: There's some natural swishing steel curtain, you know the kind that they pull in front of a fire when it's too hot in the old houses, one of those comes swishing in front, between us, when there's a microphone because the things that I would say to you professionally as a psychiatrist are quite different from the things I would say which would be broadcast to the nation because we have the most enormous responsibility to the people we know. In my young life I used to say things because I thought that a) the journalist would be faithful to me because we had spoken as friends and I never knew that they would use it in a different way or make it sound different and I fell badly into several holes because I was courteous and polite and completely honest and truthful and I've learnt to be a bit more guarded. And so, whenever there's anything that means it goes to the wider people, there's some sense of anxiety that that very medium is going to distort the message in some way. So I love being able to speak to people directly rather than through the medium of a journalist.

CLARE: I take your point because people have often asked me about it, and said, you know what's the point of those interviews because there are certain things people won't say. One of my responses is to say, 'Well, even in the closest relationships there are things we don't say.' I accept that there are things we don't say in public that we do say in private but the notion that there's anybody to whom we say everything . . .

LUMLEY: That's mad, and it's too much of a burden. I think we've got different people for saying different things to. And I think that's why it's so lovely, if you're lucky enough to meet different people in life. If ever you have a party for all your friends it's fatal because you know your friends differently. They see you as the working person who's like that or the dutiful niece or daughter or whatever it is, like that, or the doting parent and you aren't the same person to anybody.

You're not supposed to be, none of us is and I think the terrible shock is when you get all your friends together who look at each other with hostility and can't think how they were any of them invited, you know, 'cos they seem so different.

CLARE: Are there things you regret? You said about acting, there was something of a touch of regret about what it had done to you.

LUMLEY: Anonymity, anonymity. Just, just that wonderful thing. You kindly presented me partly as a writer but I mean, that is a major thing and the only way you write is by observing. If you are observed it makes observation practically impossible and the same goes with drawing or anything to do with watching other people. So anonymity is what I miss about acting.

CLARE: But isn't that a paradox?

LUMLEY: Yup, of course it is, because you don't think you're going to be successful, I never thought I'd succeed at anything, I just thought I'd have a good time doing it.

CLARE: To be a success meant that you wouldn't be anonymous. Does it mean . . .

LUMLEY: Yes, but this sounds really odd, I didn't really want to be a success, I just wanted to work.

CLARE: You wanted to do it.

LUMLEY: Yes, I wanted to do it and not to watch it and not to have to dwell on it afterwards or read about it, I just like doing it. I like telling stories and people listening, that's the truth of it. And that's what theatre is. You don't get that on television. You certainly don't get that in movies, you just don't get it. But that's what theatre is, which unfortunately brings along with it its own particular brand of terror and boredom and commitment.

CLARE: But as you well know, there will be people who will say, this cannot be true, I mean, so many people would give their eye-teeth to be Joanna Lumley.

LUMLEY: To be famous?

CLARE: To be famous, yet here she is saying . . .

LUMLEY: I wish I weren't famous – 'The mendacity of the woman,' they're saying. I know, it's very odd isn't it? Anyway, the thing is, you can only know what fame is when you've got it, and I think then you're allowed to say whether you like it or not. It's no use saying, 'Oh, how can she say that?'

CLARE: But as you point out, once you've got it, it's very hard to get rid of it.

LUMLEY: It's the black and white, Professor, it's the binary system.

CLARE: You can fade and that's that.

LUMLEY: You've got to get into it and then you go, 'Oh no, I wish I was out of it.' It's the two-sided thing, everything is like the mask of Janus or the two-sided coin, you know, everything's got the two sides. Don't ever be foolish enough to think that there aren't the two sides. Once you're grasped that point you're fine, you're motoring.

CLARE: What do you want to do that you haven't done?

LUMLEY: Something (pause), well, I mean, everything. I don't think I've actually done anything. I haven't really started yet.

CLARE: Joanna Lumley, thank you very much.

Cecil Parkinson

In his autobiography, *Right at the Centre*, Lord Cecil Parkinson describes the quite remarkable extent to which he is a self-made man. As he puts is, 'For my part I still marvel at the fact that a young man from Carnforth, who set out as a schoolboy to promote socialism should have ended his career working for its destruction; that the son of a railwayman should have committed a Conservative government to the privatisation of the railways; that the son of a "Bevin boy" should have committed a Conservative government to the privatisation of the coal industry; that a former Treasurer of the Labour League of Youth in a small northern town should have become chairman of the Conservative party; that a person who has spent a substantial part of his working life in the City of London, and who had wondered at its exclusive and autocratic nature, should have had the opportunity to open up the Stock Exchange; that someone in the early stage of his life who was a pacifist should have served in a war cabinet.'

It is a formidable litany of altered courses. It might well suggest a man adrift, unconnected to his roots, and perhaps inclined to adapt to the circumstances of his time rather than shaping them. So, on meeting with him, I was keen to establish just what if anything had survived from the young Cecil. He is, I reminded myself, half Irish – a fact not entered in the above catalogue of seeming contradictions. His mother was a refugee from the bigoted anti-Catholic pogroms of Belfast in the 1920s, his father a solid north of England Protestant. However, in his autobiography, he reflected little on his personal life and influences. There are, for example, just a couple of, admittedly revealing, paragraphs about his mother. There is little to explain how a working-class socialist lad from Carnforth should end up with the airs and graces of a patrician Tory in the most radical, right-wing political administration this century. It is a conventional political biography, recording and commenting upon the great political issues of his time.

It is not easy to discern the psychological profile of a man who was for many years the close confidante and heir apparent of that most powerful of political figures, Margaret Thatcher. She was one of four women who appear to have played a cardinal role in the making and remaking of Cecil Parkinson. That she was a strong and formidable woman needs no comment. But so too was the first woman in his life, his mother. She is described, as Mrs Thatcher would be, as a capable woman, a great organiser, the sort of woman people chose to put in charge of this or that committee. It is interesting too to note that it was his mother and not his father who determined that the young Cecil and his sister should obtain the best education going and that Cecil should go to Cambridge.

The woman Cecil Parkinson married is another strong, capable woman, well grounded and firmly directed. Lady Ann Parkinson emerges from the autobiography, from interviews she has given and from the little that her husband has to say about her here, as another firm and decisive woman. Before her marriage Ann Jarvis was running her own travel agency in London and was business manager of the first commercial airline to fly out of Luton. And then there is Sara Keays who has shown in the years since the tragic and painful events of October 1983 immense personal resolve and strength. At the time of the Conservative party conference, it was revealed that he had been having an affair with Ms Keays and she was expecting his child. Lord Parkinson issued a statement admitting that he had offered to marry Ms Keays but adding that he had later changed his mind and was staying with his wife. Sara Keays, however, robustly responded with a statement of her own to *The Times*, designed as she put it 'to put the record straight'. It appeared on the final day of the conference and revealed a number of facts which Parkinson's statement had omitted. He immediately resigned his government post.

Given the circumstances I was bound to explore Parkinson's susceptibility to such women. It provoked one correspondent, a senior research fellow at the Institute of Education, to wonder whether I had under-estimated the 'power' of power, namely the context of politics and the extent to which it both requires and prepares politicians for the exercise of power within the private as well as the public sphere. It is a pertinent point. It may indeed be true that the power which I identify as residing in the various women in Lord Parkinson's life and their influence over his life are of less significance than his power over them. He certainly has charm and he knows it. He himself is sensitive to any suggestion that he was a weak man in the thrall of strong women and is quick to point out to me that Mrs Thatcher, for one, saw him as strong, adding rather cryptically 'perhaps much stronger than a lot of people suspected'.

Lord Parkinson's lament concerning the difficulties he experienced communicating with his father are remarkably similar to that expressed by Professor Blakemore. 'We didn't encourage each other to discuss our lives or our problems', says Lord Parkinson. 'We just didn't have that sort of conversation.' Certainly the image that emerges so regularly from interviews I conduct not merely in this series but in my psychiatric clinic is of men in the grip of an incorrigible emotional reserve, displaying a strong antipathy to the expression of feelings, persistently embodying the stereotype of the controlled, detached, masterful male. There have in recent years been many controversial debates and discussions and arguments concerning the alleged vulnerability of women to depression and other emotional disturbances. Time and time again, in survey after survey, women are found to be over-represented amongst those seeking treatment for anxiety and depression. Less attention has been paid to the fact that in the area of behavioural disorders, such as alcohol and drug abuse, deliquent and other antisocial behaviour, sexual acting-out and violence, men throughout a variety of cultures significantly outnumber women. Women, it has been said, *express* their unhappiness and their stress in words and feelings, men in contrast do not express but *act out* their dissatisfactions.

Those who seek the explanation for these findings in environmental factors are not surprised. Men are continually exposed to role models and environmental cues emphasising the importance of emotional mastery particularly in the public arena. Parkinson's first male role model, his father, is archetypally masculine in the old, patriarchal sense. He is uncommunicative about feelings, private, personal things that really matter but comes to life when the subject is sport or some other public subject. Parkinson senior and junior only manage to have their first real conversation after Cecil Parkinson's mother dies. The worlds of private and public for many men, and indeed many women, are kept very separate and the values placed on them differ markedly. Lord Parkinson is quite honest about all of this. Prior to the public break-up of his relationship with Sara Keays and his political set-back – 'running into the buffers at high speed' as he puts it – he was a workaholic whose family knew little about what he actually did. He lived two worlds, each of which knew little of the other. The extramarital relationship developed because in a very real sense as an active politician, and like many an active politician and indeed other workaholics, he was living two lives, a marital and an extramarital life. It is, as he points out, exceptionally easy to do.

The public aspect of a person's life these days makes inexorable demands on a person's private life. For all the high-minded guff about the emergence of the New Man and of the acknowledgement by the public world of the professions, business, industry, the media and politics of the demands of a personal life, public still takes precedence over private. Business, politics, the professions, still happily schedule conferences, retreats, workshops in personal time because the personal life still takes one of the lowliest positions in the overall hierarchy of social values. The problem is that if the personal side of life has never properly developed and is not clearly valued, and this in the case of many men is the situation, its neglect is inevitable. And then of course comes the irony – a massive disaster, such as Parkinson suffered, can only be survived and mastered with the support of the very people who have been neglected and side-lined in the first place.

It is difficult to know what to make of the statement attributed to Lord Parkinson's friend and fellow MP Robert Rhodes James to the effect that the Parkinson who returned to the cabinet after his period of disgrace had lost his old confidence. But it is interesting to see what Lord Parkinson makes of it. He suggests that it was only then that he began to question. Up to then, so the intriguing implication goes, he just worked and worked and didn't spend too time reflecting on the whys or the wherefores. Some high achievers make a virtue out of the avoidance of introspection. It is as if too much thought might reveal too much of the pointlessness of the daily public process. Many politicians appear at their best when they are at full throttle, unencumbered by much baggage in the shape of the normal emotional doubts, fears and complex feelings that bedevil the rest of us. Not surprisingly, perhaps, there is more than a touch of megalomania in politics – reflected in the scarcely concealed pride with which politicians the world over, as Lord Parkinson does in this instance, regale the bemused listener with chapter and verse detailing just how exhausting, demanding, all-consuming the schedules, practices and procedures of the political process are. In Lord Parkinson's case, the explanation he advances as to why he hit the buffers is close to self-justification. It is difficult to detect in that explanation any acknowledgement that the political system, the late-night sittings, the hectic travel, the endless meetings, the whole rigmarole itself is diseased, is pathological, creates or attracts pathological people and is in urgent need of profound overhaul. He speaks of the system as the male politician he is – proud that he has survived its inane nature rather than concerned that it may well have maimed him, proud that he has coped rather than asking why it is first and foremost a question of coping.

The interview ends, as so many do, with my subject drawing comfort from the fact that he has considerable coping skills. Sadly I did not have the time to tease out quite what he meant. Coping is a complex skill. Lord Parkinson would seem to conceive of it as a skill which one possesses independent of other people. He looks back and sees himself coping with each new demand – marriage, politics, a cabinet post, an extramarital disaster. The interview has come full circle from the opening exploration of all those changes of identity to the introverted man coping with whatever vicissitudes come his way. Lord

Parkinson has indeed coped but has it been a solitary activity? Could it not be said with some justification that his wife and family have played a key role, a familiar role as we know from a variety of similar public political débâcles? His is a very male vision of coping – the lone, sturdy, resilient, laconic man negotiating each new hurdle and all the time seeming to others to be a perfectly balanced, charming and extrovert chap. It is a vision with a special appeal to men. But it is a vision that cries out for qualification given, for example, the uncontestable fact that throughout all his very obvious difficulties Lord Parkinson has been able to count on the support and strength of others, his mother, his wife, Sara Keays and Margaret Thatcher, formidable support indeed.

CLARE: Cecil Edward, or to be absolutely precise, Edward Cecil Parkinson, was born on September 1st, 1931 to working-class parents in the Lancashire town of Carnforth. His father, Sidney, was a local railwayman and his mother, the youngest daughter of an immigrant Irish Roman Catholic family, worked in domestic service. Cecil was educated at Lancaster Royal Grammer School where he excelled both in the classroom and on the sports field. He did his National Service in the airforce, went to Emmanuel College, Cambridge on a grant and graduated in law. He later qualified as a chartered accountant. In 1957 he married Ann Jarvis, the daughter of a wealthy builder.

He was first elected to parliament in 1970. In 1981 Mrs Thatcher made him party chairman, then paymaster general and during the Falklands crisis, a member of the war cabinet.

He left the government over the Sara Keays affair and after the 1987 Conservative victory returned for another spell, as energy and later as transport secretary, and finally resigned when John Major succeeded Margaret Thatcher as prime minister.

Cecil Parkinson became a life peer in 1992.

Lord Parkinson, reading your autobiography, *Right at the Centre,* I was struck by how much you wrote about the politics of the seventies and the eighties, and the personalities and the great political events, and your part in them. I was likewise struck by how little personal information or indeed even analysis was contained there. There were references to your parents, to your sister Norma, to your wife, to your children but there was not a great deal about them in any depth and so I was frankly quite surprised when you agreed to do this interview. I was perplexed and so my question really to you is, why?

PARKINSON: It's a very good question. I've heard your programme. I get quite a number of requests for interviews of one kind or another and I quite often and almost invariably say no but I'd always been intrigued by your programme and in a foolish moment, I said yes and I was thinking about this very question on my way here. Why did I say yes and I honestly don't know, except that I had met you once or twice and enjoyed meeting you and I've always enjoyed your programmes so I think that was it really – I was intrigued as much as anything.

CLARE: Well, I admit I am intrigued by you. Now you are very famous for a variety of reasons but when I read a little about you, the little that you reveal in your book, I was even more intrigued. It seemed to me that you are an unusual man in that you appear on your own account to have almost rebuilt yourself. Let me explain what I mean. I wouldn't have known, looking at you, anything about your background. I wouldn't have in any sense predicted that you had half Irish in you and I've tried this out on a number of people who haven't read *Right at the Centre*. I've asked them. 'What cabinet minister in Mrs Thatcher's heyday had an Irish Roman Catholic mother who left Belfast in the 1920s?' reminding listeners that was a time of considerable political trouble in that part of the world. Not a single person has ever named you. So that's the first thing. You are very different now from what one might have predicted back there on September 1st, 1931 when you were born. You yourself describe a socialist background yet here you are, a former chairman of the Conservative party. You describe yourself as having leanings towards being a clergy-man. Subsequently that seems to have died away. You talk about your pacifist inclinations yet you became a member of a very famous war cabinet. Your father was a railwayman. You were in at the privatisation attempts of the railways. You've been a key figure in the privatisation of the coal industry. You were once an active member of the Labour party. You came from the north of England though as I look at you and listen to you, I would never know that. As a psychiatrist, I'm fascinated. Here is someone – I say this often to my patients who are perplexed by their own identity and wondering what can they do with it – now I might say to them, well there's this man Cecil Parkinson and he virtually rebuilt his. Does it seem like that to you?

PARKINSON: No, it doesn't at all. I just lived my life. I never had any view about what sort of person I ought to be or to become. I just became what I am. It is a fact that people find it surprising. I remember Mrs Thatcher found it surprising.

CLARE: What did she say?

PARKINSON: When I told her that I must be the first member of the Labour party ever to become the chairman of the Conservative party, she was surprised and yet my background's been an open book. I'm proud of it. I never in any way attempted to hide it. I never pretended to be anything that I'm not. People have their own preconceptions about politicians. I think people think we arrive in the world, aged about forty looking rather similar. If you're in the Conservative party and some members of the Labour party, wearing suits that fit and that that's the way we started life and that we all have a uniform background and we all were born with a silver spoon in our mouth. I remember once when I first went into the House, I hadn't even made my maiden speech so I was just sitting listening and it was the very very good series of debates on trade union reform in the 1970 parliament and I was shaking my head when a Labour member was speaking. I wasn't doing it consciously. I was just disagreeing with him and the late Eric Heffer sort of shouted across the floor of the House, 'It's all right for you, but what do you know about having to struggle for anything? You were obviously born with a silver spoon in your mouth.' I saw him the next day by chance outside and I said to him, 'Eric, you know, I'm amazed, I've never spoken to you before but you've got all these preconceptions, perhaps you'd like to know something about me.' And I told him. And he and I became firm friends. I was working in the City at the time and everybody who worked in the city then wore stiff white collars, three-piece suits, it was the uniform. If I'd been a boiler maker I'd have worn overalls but I was working in the City as an accountant and I wore the uniform. Everybody did but it wasn't done to disguise myself or to pretend anything it was just that was the uniform and I wore it like everybody else in my office.

CLARE: But it's not just a uniform. You speak differently.

PARKINSON: Well, again –

CLARE: And presumably you didn't always have this accent?

PARKINSON: Well, again, I've never consciously tried to speak in any way. I've lived in the south now for over forty of my sixty years and if you go to the north of England and you hear an educated northern accent it isn't the 'Ee-by-gum' accent so popular with some comedians. I've never consciously had lessons or set out to eliminate any northern accent. I think it's just that I've lived amongst people who speak like I speak now for more than two thirds of my life.

CLARE: When you came to Emmanuel College, Cambridge, what were you like? Were you the same in terms of your accent and your interests?

PARKINSON: No, I certainly wasn't.

CLARE: What were you like?

PARKINSON: I'm sure I had more of a northern accent than I have now. I can still hear a northern accent in my voice and I have a definite northern inflection. People often say to me they find me very easy to understand and I think that's because I speak in the more deliberate way of a northerner so the pace and the inflection is very much there and certain words. I say 'one' and I say 'poet' like a northerner and I say certain things which come quite naturally to me and I don't want to iron them out and they're there and my wife teases me about it in an affectionate way. When I went to Cambridge I was a little confused politically and personally. I had this ambition to become a clergyman and I'd been a member of the Labour Party for about six years. I'd done my National Service rather reluctantly. I'd become a great admirer of Russia during the war. People's eyebrows shoot up now but quite frankly the Russians played a huge part in defeating Hitler and one should never in any way underestimate their contribution and they made the most enormous sacrifices and millions of people died on a scale that Britian didn't suffer. And one developed a tremendous admiration for their heroism and the idea of joining the forces to be trained to fight against them, which by then they'd been identified as the enemy, seemed to me to be a highly improper thing to do. It wasn't something that I really wanted to be part of. But in the end my headmaster gave me some very good advice and said, 'I can understand how you feel but this will be with you for the rest of your life and it's a very early age at which to make a decision like that.' So I went into the forces but really determined not to cooperate – to be in it but not of it. But during those two years, I changed my attitude to the Labour Party. One was becoming very disillusioned with the fact that England's green and pleasant land didn't become any greener or any pleasanter after six years of Mr Atlee. Bear in mind I was pretty young and I'd had a clergyman who was my form master for five years at school whom I admired tremendously and I think he influenced my view. When I got away from his influence and I gradually started to change, when I was in the forces, I wrote to the Master of Emmanuel, my Cambridge college saying, 'Look, I've changed my mind. I don't want to read divinity or theology' or whatever the Tripos was called and I didn't know what I wanted to read. So I said I'd like to read English. I'd become tired of translating lovely Greek verse into rather pedestrian English and I thought it would be marvellous to study literature without the barrier of language. And so I just chose English. So I arrived in Cambridge with no really clear idea at all of what I wanted to be, having chosen the subject on quite slender grounds and sort of drifting away from the Labour Party as it was in practice but still committed basically to the notions of fairness and social justice which seemed to me to be at the heart of the Labour Party. And so I was a rather confused young man when I went to Cambridge and I had a certain amount of success and I met a lot of people and in the college my running established me as a bit of a college personality. Friends at that time always say they found me very hard to pigeon hole because I was of the Left and my heart was still with the Labour Party although my head was telling me I was wrong. I loved music and singing but I was an athlete and I ran, so I was hearty, but I was really quite a reserved person but once in a while I'd, in the best Cambridge traditions, go berserk and perhaps get a little drunk and do nothing particularly bad but generally have quite an amusing time and have a terrible headache the next day. I would do that once or twice a year but people didn't pigeon hole me at all. Talking to my friends now they didn't know quite what to make of me, really. I had a lot of friends but I wasn't a hearty sportsman and I wasn't an aesthete. I seemed to like to have a foot in both camps.

CLARE: But do people know what to make of you even now?

PARKINSON: Well, I think I've always been quite, funnily enough, reserved about myself. The book which you mentioned, I wanted to call it *A Political Autobiography* because it really isn't an autobiography. It's about my politics. The descriptions of my home town and my life in the north after the war, they were really about how I was developing politically rather than about my family and so on. I think I felt that I've a right to write about myself but I don't think I have a right to – well, I have a right but I didn't have the inclination – to write about my family. I think they deserve their privacy and they enjoy it and so the book should have been *A Political Autobiography*, but the publishers said, 'Well, you know that is the kiss of death, really, and you're much more interesting than that,' but it is really about me as a politician and that's why I don't develop the character of my wife or my children or my parents to any great extent, just in so far as they influenced me politically, really, but I think I like to keep something of myself in reserve.

CLARE: But taking your parents, both of whom are dead . . .

PARKINSON: No, my father is still alive.

CLARE: Your father's still alive?

PARKINSON: Yes. He is eighty-six now. My mother died eighteen months ago.

CLARE: So she lived to a good age too?

PARKINSON: Yes she was about eighty-five when she died.

CLARE: What of each of them is in you? What, for example, was your mother like?

PARKINSON: My mother was a very capable woman. If she'd been born twenty-five years later she would have gone to university and got a very good degree and would have had a good career. She was always, in the little town where we lived, a great organiser. During the war when we had events to raise money to send things to the soldiers on the front, she was always roped in as chairman of the committee or a major part of the organisation. She was a very, very capable woman.

CLARE: She was a doer.

PARKINSON: She was, yes and a very handsome person, too.

CLARE: Was she a practising Catholic?

PARKINSON: No, there's quite an interesting story about that. I'd often wondered why my sister and I were not brought up as Catholics, and I'd never been told but I'd always had the impression that my parents got married in the Catholic church, as you would have expected in a mixed marriage. I had a very, very powerful grandmother who was Granny Parkinson, who was the head of the Mothers' Union and the Women Unionists and a very powerful character and my parents lived with my grandfather and my grandmother when they were first married and they were very young and I'd always assumed that my dominant grandmother just said to my very young mother, 'Look, I don't care what you said to the church, I'm telling you my grandchildren are going to be Protestants.' But I discovered when my mother died and my father and I were talking and I asked him, you know, why weren't we and he said, 'Well, as a matter of fact, my parents would not agree to me marrying a Catholic and your mother's parents were absolutely adamant that she couldn't marry a Protestant and we eloped, and we ran away to Manchester and we got married in Manchester and we came back and said we're married and it caused a hell of a row.' And so I only discovered this at my mother's death and he then said to me, 'I'm not sure you should tell your sister.' Now my sister is fifty-eight and a very well-balanced former headmistress but I don't think as a family we were encouraged to be terribly open. We didn't hide things from each other but we didn't talk a lot. It's one of my great regrets is that until my mother died, I'd never really had a conversation with my father about anything other than our mutual interest in sport or perhaps local personalities. With my mother, too, we were quite a distant family really. I think some of that came from the fact that my mother absolutely insisted that my sister and myself must have every opportunity and my father, and this is not a criticism of him, he felt that young men like me, when they got to fourteen, should go to work. It was at my mother's insistence that my sister and I stayed on at school. It was quite an effort for them. They never had any money. It was an effort to send us off to the Royal Grammar School and then for me to go to Cambridge and so on. They moved us into a world which they didn't know. I found it very difficult to discuss my life as it then was with my parents without making them feel that they were rather parochial and small-time. I'm putting this rather badly but I was moving into the great big world. They never came to Cambridge, for instance, when I was there. Although I would have liked them to they didn't. They just felt I'd moved into a different world and really they didn't want their world to be disturbed by the feeling that perhaps there was a better world which they weren't party to. So although we're all quite good talkers, we didn't talk to each other very much about each other. Very, very rarely. We're quite reticent and if my father was ill or if any of us were ill, we never said we felt ill, et cetera. When my father had a major heart attack I asked him how he felt and he said, 'Oh, I'm all right.' We didn't encourage each other to discuss our lives or our problems. We just didn't have that sort of conversation.

CLARE: Would you see that as a trait in yourself? That you sometimes wished you had been able to say more about how you felt or how you were feeling or what was going on inside your head?

PARKINSON: I think that stays with you. It isn't something that comes naturally and you have to make an effort sometimes. My children sometimes say to me that when they were younger, although I was a very assiduous father, I never missed a school play or a school speech day or anything else that mattered to the girls. We always had all our holidays together and we spent a lot of our time together, they always say that they found that I would go into myself and become quite a remote person although I'm quite outgoing socially. I'm really quite happy with myself. I wouldn't say there are two Parkinsons. When I make an effort I think I can be very sociable, but it is an effort and I'm just as happy not making it.

CLARE: Did your mother have any idea what she wanted you to be, other than to obviously have the opportunities that she didn't have?

PARKINSON: No, she didn't. She just wanted my sister and myself to have the best possible education. After that she just didn't have a concept of what the world could offer. If I'd said to her, 'I'm going to be a member of parliament,' she just would have regarded it as a ludicrous ambition. Parliament seemed so far away and the people in it seemed so grand if you lived in Carnforth. So she just had this blind faith, if you like, that we would be much better off eduated than not educated and that we would find our way in the world. She and my father, as I said, it must have been a tremendous sacrifice for them because they always had very small incomes and yet my sister and I were able to qualify and to go to very good universities and to have careers.

CLARE: Did your mother talk at all about her own childhood, her own family?

PARKINSON: Not a great deal really, no. I met her family. They moved to Barrow-in-Furness and all the boys went into the shipyards there and they all became tradesmen and their sons became engineers and I have a lot of cousins scattered around and we saw each other. We visited each other. I went to Barrow quite often and they came to Carnforth. My mother didn't discuss her family. In fact when I sat down to write I realised just how little I really knew about her life, other than from the time I knew her.

CLARE: Yes. Your mother clearly was an active doer and she had a clear idea at least of what she wanted for you and your sister. Your father, he was English, a Parkinson, what sort of man is he?

PARKINSON: Oh, he's a splendid old man and I only hope I age as gracefully as he has.

CLARE: What was he like as a father?

PARKINSON: Well, we didn't talk to each other a great deal but we shared this love of sport. He was a very fine sportsman when he was a young man and he was very proud of the fact that I won the *victor ludorum* when I was sixteen and I was fourth in the school in junior cross country when I was eleven and there were 300 boys up to age fourteen running. I played rugby quite reasonably, and he got a lot of pleasure out of that side of my life and we talked a lot about sport. I've always been a life-long supporter of Preston North End, they were a wonderful team when I was a boy and they were the nearest team to us, about forty miles away. And he and I used to go to watch Preston and we got on very well then. As long as we stuck to sport we had a lot to talk about. And that's still the case. He's an amazing man because he too had a lot of ability. I once saw his school report and he was quite outstanding but he just didn't have my chances. So we like being with each other but we don't have a great deal to say to each other except about sport and we talk a little now about my mother. And I think I had my first real conversations with him after my mother died. We spent a lot of time together for a couple of days and we talked a lot and we walked around his garden which he loves. But he's a tremendously popular person. He took up golf and he became president of his golf club. He has a mass of friends. My father's never been a threat to anybody and he's always interested in other people. And he loves gardening and he's very natural. He doesn't care whether he's talking to a duke or a dustman, literally. He's just himself wherever he is and as a result he's very popular and has a very straightforward life.

He's never had a complicated life because he's never really had any pretensions and he's been very content with his lot.

CLARE: What does he make of your life?

PARKINSON: Well, he has told me once or twice that he's very proud of the things that I've achieved and I think one of the nicest memories I have of him, and I hope I'll have many more, is of him watching me take my seat in the House of Lords. There's a little ceremony involved when you parade around in these amazing robes, sweltering and with a three-cornered hat under your arm. The BBC filmed the public gallery and there's a very nice picture of my father, sitting with my wife's uncle, Trevor Huddlestone, the archbishop, and these two wonderful-looking old men sitting together. He said to me that it was one of the proudest days of his life. Now he's not given to saying things like that and he genuinely meant it. He told me after my mother died that he would never come to London again so I was really thrilled when he decided he would come for this. But he's not very communicative about these things, but in his own way he lets me know that he's very proud of my life, really.

CLARE: Is there something in all of this that's often said of people from the north of England, that they're a little suspicious of feelings and talking about feelings, a little suspicious, in a sense of introspection? That there's a greater value placed on doing and a bit of a suspicion about too much thinking, about oneself particularly?

PARKINSON: Yes. Yes, I think that's true. I think in recent years I've become much more prone to think about myself a bit. Or to puzzle and to analyse myself.

CLARE: Why?

PARKINSON: Well, I think I had some fairly traumatic experiences from time to time over the last decade. I think that I was much less questioning of myself and of other people until about ten years ago. But I think you're right, I think in the north people get on with it. You know, because actually the range of choices was quite limited. I remember when I moved down to the south I got married and was working in London and we lived in Hertfordshire and, you know, I'd go to a party and you'd hear these people talking about little Johnnie, you know, 'I don't think he's going to make Winchester and I'm afraid he's going to have to make do with Rugby. It's a terrible disappointment.' Well, in the north we didn't have to agonise like that. You either passed the scholarship or you didn't. If you didn't you left school at fourteen and if you did, you went to the local grammar school so one didn't agonise. There was no point in agonising. It either happened or it didn't and so one got on with it. And so I think not having this range of choice which seemed to be open to the much more well-to-do probably made for a less complicated life and therefore made one less introspective. You just didn't have to worry about the choice. It either happened or it didn't. It was very straightforward and equally one felt, in a place like Carnforth, that what was going to happen, whether we went to war or whether we didn't, there was nobody in Carnforth who was going to have any influence on that, so you just didn't worry yourself about the great big world outside. You focused on surviving and more than that, or getting on with life. And so I think that really had a very big influence on me. I did just get on with it.

CLARE: Yes. Until, as you say, ten years ago. I don't want to discuss in any great detail the Sara Keays affair but would it be true to say, though you had obviously an interesting political life up to then, that would seem to me, looking back, reading *Right at the Centre*, that would have been one of the great traumatic moments. And it's more the impact on you than the details of it that I'm quite interested in. You said an interesting thing just a second ago. You said that it was those kind of traumas that made you more reflective, to think more about yourself. In what way did you think more about yourself? What did you ask of yourself?

PARKINSON: Well, I suppose if you look back on my life and you try to sum it up in a few words, I mean, I had enjoyed rather more than my share of success and tasted rather less of my share of failure. I'd been able to go to a very good school, to what I think is still the best university, although I know that's a matter of opinion, and it doesn't really matter, it was a very good university, I was able to go into the City and become a partner, start my own business, go on the candidates list and become a member of parliament, find myself a minister, find myself the chairman of the Party and in the government, in the Cabinet, and after the election, be asked what I would like to do by the prime minister sitting in Number 10 having tea, which would have seemed dream-world stuff if I'd ever thought of or predicted that that would ever happen to me.

CLARE: Were there times that you sometimes pinched yourself? Would you at times be conscious of the contrast of Carnforth and Number 10, of the father the railwayman, the mother the Irish immigrant and, and you, chairman of the Conservative Party?

PARKINSON: Certainly. It just all seemed very improbable and it still does. I still find it difficult to think back to Election Day in 1983 and not pinch myself that I was sitting having tea with Mrs Thatcher in her sitting-room discussing who would be in the Cabinet and what jobs they would have. I mean it all seemed highly unlikely, but the point was it had been a steady progression, if you like, of success in my chosen sphere. Some people might think being a successful politician isn't a move up but in what, in the areas I'd operated in, I'd been successful and then all of a sudden, I apparently ran into the buffers. I think that's not a bad way of putting it, at a very high speed and that's a very traumatic experience. And all of a sudden your life stops and instead of just getting on with what you were doing, you wonder just what am I going to do with the rest of my life? Here I am, I'm fifty-two or fifty-three, in '83, yes, I was fifty-one at the time, I was fifty-two in September, and my life is finished. That's the end. My chosen career is closed to me and, and that's the way it looked, so no wonder one became introspective. And a very good friend of mine, Robert Rhodes James, writing about the people leaving parliament, said to me, and he was a very warm friend and so he said it in a friendly way, that he felt that although I did a good job when I came back into the government, I'd lost my old confidence. I was pretty confident. I never thought of myself as confident but I knew I could handle the jobs I had, but all of a sudden one was questioning. It was the first time in my life really, apart from a short period when I left school and was wondering about the Church, that I'd ever really questioned myself. I just got on with what I was doing. When people said to me, 'Did you want to be prime minister?' it just was, if it had happened I would have been delighted, but I always focused on the job I had and did it as well as I could because I believe in Parkinson's Law, which is that in politics, people like to give you what they think you deserve and deny you what they think you want. And therefore, to have declared ambitions in politics is mad and I just got on with it as I always had and success seemed to follow. Nobody was more surprised than me when I was asked to go to Chequers for lunch and asked to be the chairman of the Conservative Party. But I did it, and we came out with a majority of 142 overall and a lot of money in the bank. I just got on with what I was doing, but I had plenty of time to be introspective after my resignation and that was the first time in my life that I really wondered where I was going instead of following the northern tradition of getting on with it.

CLARE: Did you, at that time, ever feel that you wouldn't be able to cope, that you might come apart?

PARKINSON: I don't think I ever thought that. If I can compare that feeling with anything, it was like being in the dentist's chair. You wish you weren't where you were but you have no choice. I suppose there was a choice, one could have ended one's life, but that was never seriously a choice.

CLARE: Would it have flitted across your mind?

PARKINSON: Oh, I think it crosses everybody's mind occasionally when they are in deep despair but it never really seriously crossed my mind at all. One wondered where one was going and there was quite an extraordinary thing – it's affected me since in my attitude too, for instance, death and people who have lost a relative who've died. I went away for three weeks with my wife and my daughters came and joined us and then we did talk. We talked at enormous length and discussed how we were all going to survive together and the girls and my wife were magnificent and at that point we came home and there were 16,000 letters waiting to be answered. And so the first thing I had to do was to make arrangements to answer them. By the time I'd finished and sorted them out, there were about 200 invitations to speak and letters of support and one of the nicest letters was from a constituency to which I was supposed to speak, their biggest annual event their annual dinner, in Peter Tapsell's constituency. And there was a letter saying, 'We want you to come. We've passed a unanimous vote, please come.' And so, the letters themselves were supportive but answering them got the wheels turning again. You know, I sat and stared at them. Well, I better get on with answering them and by the time I'd finished I'd got my diary starting to fill up and things happening. People in the House were very kind, so life slowly developed a different pattern.

CLARE: In my own clinical work, I'm struck by the fact that it is when a really traumatic crisis occurs that people do talk and it is interesting how quite spontaneously that's come up in our discussion. That background you've got and how your mother, your father were doers, I can understand all of that, and you've put it very clearly. When you've got stark choices there's much less time for the indulgence of contemplation and discussion and weighing up. We come from different professions and I'm aware that mine has its flaws. Perhaps we do occasionally dwell too much on reflection and discussion but it is interesting that you say that in that three weeks you, your wife, your family went away and there was, I can imagine, intense and emotional exchanges and discussions. Would it be fair of me to say that that mightn't have been as much of a feature of your marriage and family before then as you wish in retrospect it had been?

PARKINSON: Well, I didn't realise just how distant I could be and I did become and all my life I have, I am a bit of a workaholic, I freely admit it and I would become totally, totally committed to what I was doing and I would live in that and I would take that home with me. My children now say that I'm so much nicer in a way. We do talk more to each other now and I am more communicative. I've always liked being with them but they said to me I was always preoccupied. And a funny thing, one of my daughters said, 'You know, it was only when I read your book that I realised what you do, what you did.' She said to me, 'I've often, I often wondered, you know, about what your job really was like and what you did and when you were the trade minister or when you were in the war cabinet or whatever, what does a person do, and reading your book, she said, we all know and understand what you did for the first time because you never talked about it, you never said, "Oh, I'm doing this and I've got this problem in Trade." ' The multifibre arrangement the world arrangement, agreement on textiles or the general agreement on trade and tariffs is the sort of thing that they would have very quickly got tired of always talking about. They all now say that I was very wrapped up in what I was doing and I didn't spend a lot of time telling them about it or discussing it with them. But I wasn't taking myself apart, I was just totally absorbed in the job that I had.

CLARE: And that has changed since?

PARKINSON: Well, I think people think that ministers, some people may think, ministers have an easy life but I promise you, most ministerial schedules, certainly Cabinet schedules, would crush the average business man. I see both sides and I see a lot of captains of industry who think they're really hardworking people and there are some. They are very hardworking by their own standards but I think the average Cabinet minister's life would crush them because you don't only have a huge department to run, you have a constituency to look after, you have to spend time speaking in universities, raising money for the party. You have multiple existence and one of them, any one of them, is very, very time-consuming so I think one does get totally, totally wrapped up. I know it's a joke when people say I'm leaving to spend more time with my family but the fact of the matter is that I think families in politics do pay a price because people are totally committed from very early in the morning until extremely late at night.

CLARE: That takes me to this issue of politics and the relationship between the private and the public. One of the aspects of that that's always rather intrigued me, because in any discussion it seems to me to have been neglected, is the possibility, the slightly worrying possibility that an ability to dissemble is part of being a politician and that in a sense, they themselves have a different moral system. Let me quote you. I think it's you who said how you feel inside has no relevance to your public face and elsewhere in your book, you have made a defence of the task you had to travel round Argentina and Chile and shake some bloody hands, steeling yourself with the justification that if we were to restrict ourselves to Western-style democracies there'd be no business. Now, I understand that. I see the world of *realpolitik* and I know what people like you have got to do. What I'm suggesting is, therefore, if people like you have got to do that then rather like certain football skills demand certain footballers, so certain political skills must have to demand certain kinds of psychologies. It would be an advantage, I would have thought, to have a temperament that instinctively keeps a lot to itself, that is something of a cipher to all except the very closest.

PARKINSON: Yes, but I do think you underestimate the commitment that you need to have if you are going to be a success in politics.

CLARE: No . . .

PARKINSON: Let me give you an example, because you mentioned Chile and Argentina. I went at the same time to East Germany, to Romania, to Russia, equally nasty regimes but there I got very little criticism. But when I went to Argentina and Chile I was criticised and funnily enough I saw an article by somebody recently John Simpson I think, recently talking about the fact that I'd been to these dictators but he misunderstood the point. The point was that in both Argentina and Chile there was at that time an emerging civilian governing group. In fact, in each, both Argentina and Chile the military kept total political control but they disbursed economic power. Chile had a privatisation programme that makes ours look like the very beginnings, just makes us look like amateurs. So you had these extraordinary dictators disbursing economic power. The man in Argentina – and the feeling was if he and his economic team produced the success, civilian government would come back to Argentina. So the military would find that they'd created a successful economy by disbursing economic power and it would topple them. And by the way, that's precisely what happened in Chile. Pinochet let some academics run the economy while he maintained total political control and as Chile succeeded, which it has, the people became prosperous and they got rid of him. What we were doing was reinforcing the civilian element who were creating economic success, so we weren't actually pandering. We were playing politics, if you like. We were actually, we hoped, taking part in bringing about the downfall of the military dictators and reinforcing civilian government. And I believed that very passionately when I was there and I made a speech explaining not how General Pinochet was right but how right his economic team were.

So, we set out not to prop up the dictators but actually to support the people whom we hoped would replace them and we had them here and we fêted the civilians, not the generals, they were never invited. One was having to be polite to the dictators but at the same time we weren't there to support them. We were there to support the people who we hoped would replace them.

CLARE: Well, yes, let me put it slightly differently. You describe yourself pre-1983, and I think accurately, that things were happening to you and you moved from one position to another, the chairman of the Party and so on. And the character traits that you had fitted. It was a lot of doing and a good deal of thinking at an intellectual level but not too much introspection, as you've suggested. Let me put something to you because you're obviously the sort of person to ask. I'm struck by the fact that politics, it seems to me, is almost best conducted by people – don't misunderstand me about this because I don't mean it to sound demeaning – but it's best conducted by people who are decisive rather than introspective. I've met many politicians now and they've always struck me, it's only when they've had some kind of trauma or disaster that to be absolutely frank, they become interesting to me.

PARKINSON: Well, I'm interested to hear that but I think it's true of anyone really. You see the chairman of some big company and he doesn't exist as a person when because people say, 'Oh, he's not a person he's the chairman of ICI' – I don't mean that about Denis Henderson by the way – no, he's just the chairman of ICI, he is his job. And then all of a sudden people do a profile and they say, 'Good God, is he really like that?' What people know about us is what you said but it is not necessarily what we are. It's what they're allowed to know but when something happens and they say, 'Well let's have a really close look at this chap,' and then at that point people start saying, 'God, that fellow's a much more interesting character than I ever thought he was.' Actually, he was just as interesting before but nothing had triggered their interest to the extent.

CLARE: But was he? But was he? It wasn't just that other people started to take an interest in you after the disaster. It was you. And it's your children who say of you how much more we learned of you and indeed, how much more interesting you are. And I suspect, though we can't speak for her, that your wife might say something similar. I'm putting something a little more subversive to you. I'm suggesting that often what really intrigues us about public figures, one of the reasons we niggle away to find the clay feet, is that it is the clay feet that humanises them. I'm putting to you that up to 1983 you hadn't any. It was all breaking reasonably well. I'm back to what you put to me. Maybe that's unfair but you might, to an extent, have been indifferent to much of this because it didn't cross your agenda. And in that sense, it's not just that the public didn't bother to look. Even if it had looked it wouldn't necessarily have found very much. And you didn't look. You weren't all that interested in you before.

PARKINSON: I think that's very fair. I think that that is true. You can take it into virtually any life. Take a brilliant young footballer. It's when he gets to about thirty and he breaks his leg or something goes wrong at that point, he suddenly says, 'My God, what's the rest of my life going to be like?' One hasn't had cause to think in those terms. With this background of mine of not being introspective, I suppose one went on. I was still the son of a railwayman. I was still the person who'd been a member of the Labour Party. All the things which you mentioned earlier as interesting about me, they were all there. They were all available to anyone. But I think when something happens to you and goes wrong, people start saying, 'Well, now let's see if his background has anything to do with it or this has anything to do with it.' So, other people start to be swtiched on a little bit. But the facts didn't change. What I'd done in the previous fifty years was there. But all of a sudden it became interesting and people said, 'God, isn't it interesting that the son of a railwayman has finished up as chairman of the Conservative Party?' Well, that was known but the only thing that made it interesting was that I ran into a crisis and a traumatic experience and at that point people start to be interested. One of the things that embarrassed me for two or three years after my resignation was the number of people who used to come up to me and say, 'There but for the grace of God goes I.' And I became, began to understand your profession because I became a sort of figure to whom people confessed their own problems or wanted to share their problems with, and so on. It was an amazing turn-around. People whom one knew, one thought one knew, suddenly confided in me. But of course the difference between them and me is that my problems were public property and theirs were private and known to a small circle of their friends which didn't include me.

CLARE: Let me ask you something else. Had what happened in 1983 happened, I don't know, in 1973, would you have been the politician that you were? You said an interesting thing about when you went back into the cabinet. Robert Rhodes-James made that observation. I'm interested in the observation. Here's this man, Cecil Parkinson, actually more interesting in many ways and complicated as a result, but perhaps not as good a politician as a result. Or to shorten the question even more, is it an advantage for a politician to be a decisive doer, confident, not too introspective, certainly not too tortured about life's grey areas?

PARKINSON: I think it is. That doesn't mean to say you become inhuman or forget your background or the needs of people whose lives might be a little nearer to those of your parents than to yours.

CLARE: Though you might have?

PARKINSON: I don't think I ever did.

CLARE: Coming up to 1980 one of the reasons I wondered whether you ran into the buffers was that indeed you did become detached a little?

PARKINSON: No, no, not at all. I don't know how other people saw one but people have always said to me that I was always very approachable and that I didn't in the House, cut myself off from my friends because I was being promoted and they weren't. I was always accessible and liked being with people. I used to miss being cut off from the House and my friends, and equally I've always been very proud of my background and when I say proud I mean I haven't boasted about it but I'm very proud that I have that background and keen to maintain contact with my home town and the people there. The people who've met me have expected me to be different and they've found I haven't changed. The people I knew at Cambridge have always said that they almost expected change but that I hadn't. So I don't think I became more distant in that way, I just was very busy.

CLARE: As you describe it, coming up to 1983, it's almost as if you had it all really. So some would say, why did you want more? Why did you want another relationship, over and above your family? It wasn't as if you were in a suffering situation because a lot of good things were happening to you.

PARKINSON: I don't know. I really don't know. All I know was that I did, so that's a part of my life that I haven't really attempted to try to explain to myself. I think it's a bit pointless really. It just was the case, as it is the case as I discovered afterwards, with a very large number of people, and that is no reflection on one's own wife or one's family. I think it is just something that happens to a lot of people, especially if they have the opportunity. And politics is a very unaccountable profession in a lot of ways in that your life is so unusual, being at the House of Commons late at night. How many other men crawl into bed at three o'clock or four o'clock in the morning or don't come home at all as they didn't last week when they carried on from two o'clock in the afternoon till one o'clock the next afternoon. So it's a very funny, unpredictable life and as a result one isn't accountable. One has scope and then there are people near one who find one interesting and you find interesting so it's a combination of things. I don't think it's that members of parliament are particularly different from other people. I think it's just that a lot of people, if they're not accountable and temptation or attraction come their way, find themselves tempted or attracted. Perhaps just politicians' lives lend itself more to that. But I don't know is the answer to your question. But all I know is that that happened so presumably, what I had wasn't enough.

CLARE: Are you a person who regrets?

PARKINSON: Yes, I do. I regret the unhappiness, it sounds a little twee, but I do. I regret the unhappiness that I caused other people, and myself, but most of all other people. The disappointment one caused people. Nobody else was in charge of my life so my criticism has to be addressed to myself. I can't blame other people. But I do regret it. I regret that a number of people I care about a great deal were made very unhappy and a number of people who had ambitions and hopes for me and confidence were disappointed. But I can't live on regret and looking backwards so, as I say, reverting to my northern roots, I just got on with it.

CLARE: Your image was hitting the buffers, really coming to a savage, sudden stop. You were careful to point out that you certainly wouldn't express ambition because, as you say, the moment you express it people will set about ensuring it's not fulfilled. Nonetheless, in the small still hours of the night, would you have said to yourself, 'This could be mine. I could, looking round, I could be a successor to Margaret Thatcher.'

PARKINSON: I never said it but it was said. It was said quite a lot. I remember, for instance, the press were pretty unanimous in 1983 that, obviously with the exception of Margaret Thatcher who was the prime minister and won, that the three people who'd had the best elections, were Neil Kinnock, David Owen and myself. And that was a fairly common view. Other people started to say that I was the person Mrs Thatcher preferred and so on. But I can genuinely and truthfully say that I live by my previously declared Parkinson's Law and I just got on with the job that I had. My view was that if you did that well, then there would be another job and if you did it badly, there wouldn't. So, spending time wondering what that next job would be was a waste of time and so I never bothered with it. So I never seriously ever envisaged myself walking through the doors of Number 10 as prime minister. Never, although other people wrote about it and predicted it and funnily enough, still do say things to me of that kind, that that must have been a possibility but it wasn't something that I entertained so I wasn't disappointed that it didn't happen.

CLARE: Do you think it matters what sort of life you led, given the kind of demands we place on politicians, as you say, both in terms of the nature of the task and, indeed, the equipment we give them to fulfill that task, the House of Commons and its strange hours, the multiplicity of demands and so on. You've been well placed to ponder this. Other countries have different value systems. Do you feel, given what it's like to be a minister of state, a secretary of state, what difference does it make, what kind of personal life you have. Do you think there is any connection between the psychology of a man's or a woman's personal life and the psychology of power?

PARKINSON: Well, I find that a very difficult question to answer. There are a lot of very successful politicians who have led totally blameless lives so it's clearly not a prerequisite, not to be blameless, but equally there is a growing number of people in politics in different countries for whom their private life has not been any sort of disadvantage. To give you two examples from the very recent past – President Clinton is now President Clinton in spite of a major campaign to make his private life an issue. Now I'm not qualified to know whether he had an interesting private life or not but all I know is that people really tried to make an issue of it and it certainly didn't damage him. And just recently in Israel has been elected a leader of the very right-wing party, the Likud, having publicly admitted that he's been unfaithful to his third wife who he's only been married to for about a year and he was elected on the first ballot and will, all things being equal, one day become prime minister of Israel. I remember, once, chairing a conference of all the trade ministers from the Pacific Basin in Korea and the Philippines minister came up to me and said, 'Why are you not in the government?' and I said, 'Well, I had to resign.' He said, 'In the Philippines you'd have been a candidate for President.' He was joking. I'm not saying I'm a potential president of the Philippines but it and my own experience suggested that a lot of people didn't regard my private life as a sort of disqualification. When I came back into the government in 1987, I got a standing ovation going into the conference hall to make my speech and Norman Tebbitt, sitting next to me, said, 'It would be very embarrassing if they don't applaud when you sit down, after this welcome.' I think people in a variety of ways were trying to tell me that they felt I had something to offer the government which shouldn't have been blighted, if you like, by my private life. But I didn't see it that way.

CLARE: I'm conscious the listeners of course will say, 'Well, it's two men discussing this issue, that it's a male world, politics, Mrs Thatcher notwithstanding.'

PARKINSON: Well, they may be right, But I would remind you that President Clinton got his votes from an electorate which is more than half women. And if he'd got the whole of the male vote which I'm quite sure he didn't, he would still not be president. Certainly a lot of the most supportive people to me, who wrote to me, were women, in very large numbers, so I think people are not as censorious as the press would have you believe. But as I explained in my book I felt that I could not travel abroad. I was due to go to Japan and America, my first visit abroad, where I'd been touted as the leading figure in the Party and a successful party chairman, to promote trade and so on. That would not have been the case. I would have been surrounded by a huge press corps who would have been interested in my private life and I felt if you can't do the job, you should give it up. That's why I gave it up and I think I was right to do it.

CLARE: But you went back.

PARKINSON: Yes, I went back. I think my overriding motive was that I did not like the fact that the press, certain elements of the press or sections of it, no matter what one was doing, whether one was starting a charity run or doing anything – would refer to 'disgraced former cabinet minister, Cecil Parkinson'. It's a hell of a thing to read yourself, and to have your friends and your family reading and I felt I really couldn't let them get away with that. I didn't think that was the way the public saw me. If it was, I'd better find out and so I decided I must stand for reelection and I was elected next time round with a substantially increased majority and asked to go back into the cabinet and I went back and although Robert said what he said about me not regaining my self-confidence I think I achieved quite a lot in my nearly four years back in government. One of the things I did do was wipe that word from in front of my name or that adjective, 'disgraced'. I hope that doesn't sound as if that was my only motive. I thought I could do a job. Other people thought I could do a job. But it was certainly one of my ambitions to try to remove that and I think I did – not, by the way, just for my own personal satisfaction but also for those who know me and for those I love. It's not very nice for one's family to read that description of their father and so that was a motive. I've summarised what was a very complex set of motives in that one little ambition, but it was one of the things I wanted to do.

CLARE: An interesting incidental aspect of your life is the women who figure in it. Your mother was strong, you talked about a paternal grandmother, very strong. Lady Thatcher is – need I say any more! Sara Keays was a strong woman. Your wife is an impressive and strong woman, I can vouch for her via the contacts I've had in Action on Addiction. You've three daughters. Now, I know God has visited some of this on you but do you ever reflect on that fact that a lot of women, and I've got to be careful how I say this, in Cecil Parkinson's life, are strong women. That you were around when the strongest woman of our century was prime minister.

PARKINSON: Yes, and I think if you ask her, she thinks I was quite strong too. If they were attracted I think the thing that attracted them to me was that I was a strong character as well, perhaps much stronger than a lot of people ever suspected.

CLARE: Do you feel people did suspect you weren't a strong man?

PARKINSON: Well, I think I once made a rather frivolous remark which was misunderstood when I said, 'If there is reincarnation I want to be short and fat and ugly and then people will judge me by what I've done and what I think rather than how I look and dress.' I think there is always a tendency to caricature people, you know, tall, well-dressed – that must be part of the secret of success. Well, I don't think anybody ever gave anybody a cabinet job because of their suits which, by the way, I've always worn off-the-peg suits the whole of my life.

CLARE: It was your looks and your height that made people suspect.

PARKINSON: Well, people comment on it, you know. You are lucky it's women like tall, well-dressed men, all that utter tripe.

CLARE: It's the converse of what many women have to deal with though, isn't it. If an attractive blonde lady with shapely legs finds herself in a position of power, she spends a lot of time explaining the fact that there's a brain there as well.

PARKINSON: Yes.

CLARE: You actually were conscious of the fact that you would have been seen as a sort of matinée idol. I didn't realise the extent to which that probably would have communicated to others a feeling that that's how you had got on.

PARKINSON: Well, that was sort of one of the things that was said. Subsequently, not before 1983, but subsequently. Before 1983 I was sort of the man who started from humble beginnings, won scholarships, been a success in the City, started a business.

CLARE: Did things.

PARKINSON: Got things done and did things. But then, afterwards, all this sort of retrospection. 'Oh, now we see why it is women find him attractive. So that's really what Mrs Thatcher made him chairman of the Party for.' Which was utter tripe.

CLARE: Did she find you attractive?

PARKINSON: I'm sure she didn't. If she did, she never revealed that fact to me.

CLARE: Did you find her attractive?

PARKINSON: I find her a very impressive person and I always have.

CLARE: Attractive?

PARKINSON: I never thought of her in those terms, any more than I'm sure she thought of me in those terms. But that all started later, you know. It was quite interesting. A lot of previous history was rewritten.

CLARE: I never met Lady Thatcher. In the twenty years I was in Britain, our paths never crossed. I sometimes did teeter on the edge of confessing that she did have a certain sexual power and I just wondered, you were close and you're a man with a sexual life and I just wondered whether in fact there was anything in that, that the woman did indeed not just use it, but exuded it?

PARKINSON: No, not as far as I was concerned. I found her a very attractive, well turned out, very impressive person and a colleague. We worked together. One of the things I found with her was that after a time you forgot that she was a woman. You got into the argument, the discussion and so on. She never played on it in cabinet, in my opinion. Some people have said otherwise, but to me, she's a very good friend and a good friend of my family, my wife, my children. We all know her well and like her and she was a really good friend and a very, very impressive person and we all got on very well. We got on very well with Denis. We played golf together and liked each other. But, just as you meet a lot of colleagues with attractive wives and work with attractive women, after a time you know each other well and you have a working relationship and it's based on friendship and work. And that was what my relationship with Margaret Thatcher was based on.

CLARE: The life you now lead, clearly it's a good deal less stressful than your political life because you described yourself previously, perhaps you still are, as a workaholic, by which I deduced that you meant your life really was your work and other things had somehow to be fitted in, which I think is as good a description of an addiction as any, where the practice really becomes the life, whether it's drink or gambling or politics and everything else is fitted in. You used the word 'workaholic' and in a sense you do it deliberately. There is a disease quality to that. There's a suggestion of pathology, and here we are, you and I, discussing this retrospectively. But if we discussed any other disease retrospectively we would be doing it in the context of, 'Is there not something we can do about it? This takes its toll.' I see the spouses and children, not so much the addicts themselves, in workaholic situations. I think that's true of many addictions. Now, has it to be like that? Why have we evolved a system where people are making very important decisions in this stressful, physically exhausting way sometimes at the worst possible time of the day, four in the morning when biological rhythms are at their worst. Their families say, 'It's pathological, doctor, we never see him. He's consumed with this. He doesn't have time for us, he gets involved in drink or an affair or whatever it happens to be.' You're a man who spent a lot of his time trying to change other aspects of the world. Aren't we entitled to say, well, why should we take any of this seriously when the poeple who are so busy trying to change so many of the aspects of the world, resolutely insist on maintaining an absolutely crazy way of running the world. Must it be like this?

PARKINSON: I've met ministers from all over the world in the course of my travels and it does seem to be an absolute feature of government wherever one happens to go. That it is very exhausting. People say that Mr Bush now looks about ten years younger than he did and if you care to look at the pictures of Jimmy Carter when he went into the White House and Jimmy Carter four years later and Jimmy Carter now, you see the same thing. It is a very, very exhausting business as I've said, it's a multiple existence. You have a big department to run. You have a cabinet to take part in. You have to do most of your paper work at night after the day's finished. At the weekend, you have to go off and talk in universities or raise money for the party or do whatever it is, and then you have your own constituency to look after. And it is a very, very exhausting business. But it's also extremely interesting and I think the big killer is boredom. I think being interested, dealing with big problems, the adrenalin flows, you keep going. I used to find that I didn't really have a problem at all until parliament rose and there was a recess and then I would sleep for two or three days and one realised one had pretty well exhausted oneself. But while it is actually happening, government is extremely fascinating. There is never a boring time and so you just keep going.

CLARE: Are you easily bored?

PARKINSON: I'll answer your question in a different way. I would have found life as a back bencher very tiresome. I don't think I would have enjoyed that. I really like to be involved and I really like to be doing something that stretches me and that I think is worthwhile. And so I suppose to that extent you could say I am easily bored but I have a lot of interests. I do enjoy reading. I love the opera and I go regularly. I listen to a lot of music when I'm at home.

CLARE: You do relax?

PARKINSON: I do, yes, and I like to have holidays, but I like to have active sort of holidays where I can run and play golf and read and do a variety of things. I don't like a somnolent lazy holiday. I love skiing, for instance, and I didn't find it until I was thirty-one. I wanted to be a competent skier and I worked very hard at it and I love it still. So I do have a range of interests even on holiday, I like to be active and I would say I don't find just sitting ruminating a wholly satisfactory way of spending time. I like to have time to ruminate. A bit of time but I couldn't spend a fortnight ruminating. I would need to do things.

CLARE: What has happened to that bit of Cecil Parkinson that, for a brief period, thought in terms of being a clergyman? Do you, for example, think much about death?

PARKINSON: I think like most people there was a period in my life, in my twenties, when I thought about little else, actually. That's not quite true but it was a very continuing preoccupation. Recently, extraordinarily enough, I was just thinking about this the other day, I haven't seen a dead person since I saw my grandmother, which is forty or fifty years ago, and it's astonishing to me how the world sort of shields itself from death and dead people.

CLARE: Did you see your mother?

PARKINSON: No, my mother died while I was away and obviously I came back for her funeral but by then she'd been dead for some days, three or four days, and I didn't. My mother was the first of our parents to die so we haven't had a great deal of family contact with death and I haven't given it a great deal of thought in recent years. I must say I haven't.

CLARE: Have you ever been ill?

PARKINSON: Not, touch wood, seriously. I've had the odd flu or something like that.

CLARE: Serious illness?

PARKINSON: No, I haven't for a very long time, thank God. I say that but I don't know why because I'm not a particularly good Christian. I'm not a church-goer although I love church music. I was saying about Christianity, somebody asked me if I was an active Christian and, I know who it was, I was on my way back from Istanbul on an aeroplane and talking to a person who I'd been to a conference with. I was reminded of the Winston Churchill story, when he was asked, when he was a young man trying to become a member of parliament, by a very earnest lady on a selection committee, 'Mr Churchill, are you a pillar of the church,' and he said, 'Ma'am, I'd rather describe myself as a flying buttress, I support the church from the outside.' And I think that's roughly my position. I admire many individual clergymen, and others I don't admire at all. But I don't particularly feel involved. My wife is quite a devout Christian.

CLARE: She is?

PARKINSON: Yes, she is, but I can't say I am.

CLARE: Do you see your daughter by Sara Keays?

PARKINSON: No, I never have.

CLARE: By choice?

PARKINSON: I think the relationship between her mother and myself disintegrated to such an extent that I just didn't think it would contribute anything to her life and I think that I have reason to know that Sara is a very dedicated mother, but I didn't think my presence would add anything to her life.

CLARE: What is interesting as we come to the end is that I'm still struck by the two Parkinsons. You do, even unconsciously, split your life. There is the public and there is the personal. And it is interesting, no more than that, that the pivotal moment of your life was when those two areas collided in a highly unpredictable and dramatic way. As you sift through all of these things that makes Cecil Parkinson, if I said to you what has been the most valuable thing that holds you together, what would you have picked out?

PARKINSON: It may sound very mundane but I think it's my ability to cope. I've been introduced into a whole range of situations which I'd really had nothing but my education to prepare me for and I always had the feeling, whenever I've entered a new phase of my life, be it my marriage or my partnership or any other jobs, can I cope and it's been a pleasant surprise to me that I have been able to. I think that that is really the quality. But I think that you have identified the fact that I'm really much happier talking about events and jobs than I am talking about me. I think that is a legacy, I think a lot of people might be surprised to hear me say that I'm a reticent person. People who know me know I can be rather boisterous occasionally, but actually I've always, to a greater extent than most people think, kept myself to myself.

Marjorie Proops

To judge by the public reaction to the revelation that agony aunts like Claire Rayner and Marjorie Proops have lives as complicated and riddled with problems and conflicts as those of the people who write in to them for advice, wounded healers are what healers are expected to be. Claire Rayner never suffered any adverse affects of talking revealingly about her own unhappy childhood and I doubt that Marjorie Proops's revelations about her marriage and long time extramarital affair have had much impact on her role as one of Britain's most influential agony aunts. She was very agreeable about doing the interview and in the course of it argues that revealing the warts and all about herself only causes other people with problems to feel a kinship. Much of what she discusses with me in this interview had already appeared in her authorised biography published in 1993. It showed a woman oozing contradictions. She is Jewish by birth and still observes some of the religious rituals but had her son, Robert, educated in a Church of England school. She has been a lifelong socialist, friend of such politicians as Jim Callaghan, Michael Foot and Harold Wilson, yet happily sent her son to a public school. She reveals the most intimate details of her sexual and marital life yet remains fiercely secretive about her age. She is a household name for the common sense and sagacity she has brought to bear on the problems of the many thousands of people who have written to her advice column down through the years yet she has, on her admission, seriously mishandled her own problems. She campaigned bravely for better care for battered wives while she herself tolerated a marital relationship in which she was repeatedly emotionally abused and humiliated. None of these contradictions are unique and most people's lives are replete with very similar ones. What makes them interesting in the context of Marjorie Proops is that she has been a woman whose name on the top of her advice column became a byword for sense, directness and decisiveness, of whom indeed it was once said that she had saved more souls than the Salvation Army.

The interview opens with a discussion of her reticence to reveal her age. It is a reticence which, as I have said, is all the more noteworthy in the light of the kinds of things she has discussed in public. The explanation that she gives for her reluctance to divulge it is not entirely convincing and she knew I was unconvinced. She is perfectly entitled to keep her age to herself. But being the journalist she is she cannot be surprised that people are curious and want to know. Later in the interview she describes her profound fear of death and perhaps there is here a connection. She has always been frightened of death ever since she was a child. She attributes this in part to her mother's timidity and she is probably right. She paints a terrible picture of her poor agoraphobic mother – there is a remarkable account of her rushing out of the house calling for her husband, the fear of him leaving her (it was his funeral and the coffin had left the house) overwhelming at least for that moment, her own fear of leaving the house. One of the consequences of being a child of a particularly fearful parent is that the anxiety can be absorbed into the very marrow and core of one's being. Such children often grow up feeling continually anxious without ever quite knowing what it is they are anxious about. Marje Proops was so terrified of death, particularly following the deaths of her husband and her lover, that she couldn't bear to pass a funeral parlour or to find herself caught up in a funeral procession. 'I would,' she declares, 'come out in sweats and physical, awful physical fear.' For people with a profound fear, a profound sense of death, ageing is anathema. To acknowledge age is to have come to terms with death.

Those same fears could well explain, at least in part, her reluctance to leave her marriage despite its unsatisfactory nature. In discussing her disastrous marriage and the love affair she had with an unmarried lawyer on the *Daily Mirror*, she maintains a matter-of-fact approach. Obviously there is a paradox that the woman who publicly advised men and women on their sexual and marital problems was living herself a highly complicated and irregular life. The explanation, if any is needed, may simply lie within the extraordinary psychological ability of splitting public and private life which we all, to a varying extent, possess. It is what many men do when they separate their public and professional lives from the personal, intimate, domestic ones. It is what Lord Parkinson did. Marjorie Proops lived like two distinct people. She describes the humdrum, predictable and dull domestic life she lived with her husband and contrasts it with her exciting, stimulating life as a journalist, meeting tycoons and giants like Hugh Cudlipp and Robert Maxwell. These two lives never seemed to overlap. Her husband, Proopsie, belonged very firmly to the first, her lover Philip to the second.

These days it is likely that the revelation concerning her penchant for dominant, powerful men would cause more of a stir then the fact that she had an affair while married. Indeed, in so far as anything joined her two separate lives together it was her need to be dominated by domineering men. And yet this is no simple tale of a weak woman, financially dependent on an authoritarian bully. Marjorie Proops is no wimp. Her son is on record as saying that she organised her life the way it suited her. She herself admits that she put herself first. Her husband, she reveals, made all the key decisions at home, an area in which she was clearly quite prepared to be dominated, but she was not all that bothered because she had her exciting life outside it. To that extent, Marjorie Proops is indeed a liberated woman, a woman whose life was split in the way the lives of so many men are split. Some of the reactions to her disclosure of infidelity showed a marked gender bias – it was as if what was being revealed was unacceptable because it was being revealed by a woman. And some women were critical. In the *Independent* Margaret Maxwell felt her explanation that she stayed with her husband because she felt frightened she might lose her child was dated. For another distinguished agony aunt, Virginia Ironside, writing in the *Daily Mail*, it didn't wash either and her decision to reveal the extramarital affair so many years after everyone concerned is dead was simply 'tacky'.

It is something of an irony that the woman who did so much to establish the value of telling it as it is and not keeping up pretences for the sake of social niceties should have ended up criticised for talking about her affair and not keeping it to herself. Does it help 'to let things out'? Why do people do it? The conventional wisdom overwhelmingly favours revelation and the past decade has witnessed an extraordinary outpouring on radio, television and in print by people revealing the most intimate details of their sexuality, feelings, experiences, fantasies and desires. When Marjorie Proops opted to do the same as so many of those who had written to her had done and tell her story she promptly collided with the argument that there are some things better left untold. She herself does not justify her autobiographical revelations by claiming that telling her story made her feel better – the most popular explanation advanced these days in defence of public confessions. Indeed, when her autobiography was published she told how writing it was acutely painful and that peeling off layers of your life was a little like peeling layers off an onion.

So why did she tell all? The cynics say that Marjorie Proops is a professional journalist down to her fingertips and she knows a really good story when she sees one. They may be right. She herself admits to an irresistible desire to reveal the truth about herself. Perhaps some of the guilt and depression she has experienced in the past owed something to the duplicity of the life she led and the contrast between what those who wrote to her believed her to be and what she knew about herself. In the interview she is intriguingly contradictory about this very point. At one moment, she denies experiencing any compelling desire to tell people that she was having an affair. Later in the interview, speaking of the counselling relationship she had with her psychotherapist, she says she feels she had to tell 'perhaps based on the desire to cope with the guilt'. Perhaps, and perhaps too there is truth in both these explanations. In writing an autobiography how could she leave out such a central and key relationship? The question surely is not so much why she revealed all about Philip but why she wrote her autobiography? Once she had decided to write it she had to tell of her extramarital relationship. It would have made no sense not to. As for the autobiography, that takes us into the realm of human vanity. Few people with a story to tell can truly resist the urge to tell it, particularly if the story, as in the case of Marjorie Proops, is one of a life lived to the full, passionate as well as productive, romantic as well as sensible. The point missed by so many of the critics is that Marjorie Proops's affair serves to challenge the stereotypical view of her as sane, balanced, hard-headed, everybody's favourite spinster aunt. It challenged her own view of herself as just brain and not beauty, as worthy only of a boorish and bossy husband and not the stuff of which romantic fact as well as fiction is made. 'There were times,' she declares towards the end of the interview, 'when I wanted people to know, I wanted people to know that this very special man loved me because it was something I never thought I'd ever achieve in my life so I did want it to be known.' That sounds real, that sounds authentic. That matches what she has said elsewhere about herself. I do not know how much self-deception is involved in her remark that she never imagined that other journalists would be interested in a 'twenty-year-old adulterous love affair during a sexless marriage', but if they were not to be interested they would not be particularly sharp journalists. The fact is that the affair reveals more about Marjorie Proops than all the stories about the galaxy of socialists with which she had so much in common, her friendship with Hugh Cudlipp and her inordinate admiration for the late Robert Maxwell put together.

CLARE: Often referred to as the doyenne of agony aunts, Marjorie Proops was born Rebecca Marjorie Israel in North London of Jewish parents. Marjorie left school at sixteen, went to art school, was briefly a fashion writer and then became a journalist. In 1954 she joined the *Daily Mirror* as a campaign columnist and celebrity interviewer and has been responsible for the *Dear Marjorie* advice column for twenty-two years. In 1969 she was awarded an OBE for her services to journalism. Marjorie became Mrs Proops in 1935 and has one son, Robert. Her authorised biography, *The Guilt and the Gingerbread* was published in 1993 and revealed that she had simultaneously conducted a sexless marriage and a passionate love affair with a bachelor colleague.

Marjorie Proops, ordinarily in interviews of this kind, people have an expectation, largely I suspect unfulfilled, that all sorts of skeletons will emerge from cupboards but I have to say I've read your biography and it seems to me such skeletons as there are are well out of the cupboard, save for one, which rather intrigued me and that is your age.

PROOPS: I know. It always intrigues people that I don't reveal it, even to you and there's a simple reason actually. A quite ordinary reason, my readers range in age from about ten, or even nine some of them, to their nineties. So I cover a very, very broad age span and I don't want my ten-year-olds, thirteen-year-olds, saying, 'Well, I can't write to that silly old trout,' and I don't want the older ones thinking, 'What the hell would she know at her age. She wouldn't have any sort of contemporary knowledge or feelings or anything.' I mean it's not vanity. You've only to look at me to know I'm not twenty-five. I also think it's irrelevant. When I was a young reporter I was always in dead trouble with the news editor because I used to interview people, I remember years ago interviewing Elizabeth Taylor and I went back to the office and did a story and the news editor said, 'How old is she?' and I said, 'I don't know, didn't ask.' I never thought it mattered.

CLARE: One might say that many other aspects of ourselves can get in the way of the kind of activity you're in and I'm in. That is to say, offering to help other people. For instance that you're Jewish or the fact that you're white or the fact that you're English or whatever it happens to be. But why age? I mean, all of those things could deter different kinds of people from coming forward and writing to Marjorie Proops or seeing me.

PROOPS: Well, that's perfectly true but I think that because of the work that I've done over the years, it must be apparent to the people who write to me that I have no prejudices of any kind, that it doesn't matter to me whether people are black, white, green, yellow, English, whatever.

CLARE: So would it much matter if they knew you were, I don't know, seventy, eighty, ninety.

PROOPS: I don't know, maybe it wouldn't. I mean maybe it

wouldn't. But that is the view I've taken all these years. I think it would matter with the young ones, yes I do.

CLARE: Of course, you raise a very interesting issue. Classical psychoanalysts often argue for an absolute anonymity. They take it to extremes. That's to say, they reveal absolutely nothing about themselves. Indeed, many of them are so well-trained that if you meet them socially you'd be hard put to get an opinion out of them, and indeed an emotion out of them. And there's been much speculation about that. Here you are, and I have to confess I'm in the same position, neither of us exactly unknown and you are known to absolutely millions. What do you feel about that? This issue of people wanting to know about the counsellor, therapist, doctor. Wanting to know a great deal while official training says that some ways the less they know about you the better, the less they will have getting in the way.

PROOPS: Well, I don't know. I think maybe because I started as a journalist, as a reporter and moved into counselling fairly late in my career, I think it's obvious that people knew quite a lot about me anyway from the work I did before. I was involved in all sorts, in politics, for example. I served on two government committees, parliamentary committees, so that you can't be anonymous if you're doing that kind of job. I think that when I started doing the *Dear Marje* work I was fairly well known to the readers of the *Daily Mirror*, in fact, to a lot of people who weren't readers of the *Daily Mirror* because in addition to my journalistic work, I did quite a lot of radio and television, particularly radio at one time so that you're exposed then aren't you, and you can't be a private person. Maybe if I'd been, as you are, a psychiatrist, and therefore trained to be a psychiatrist and therefore reflecting other people rather than exposing myself, it would have been different.

CLARE: Would you have liked to have been a psychiatrist?

PROOPS: Very much. If I'd been educated, there were two things I would have liked to have been, or maybe even three, but two particularly. I would have liked to have been a psychiatrist if I'd had any education and I would also like to have been a politician.

CLARE: Well, reading your biography you could have been the second.

PROOPS: Yes.

CLARE: And yet you didn't take the offer. There was a time when your name alone would have guaranteed you a Labour seat in the sixties.

PROOPS: Yeah.

CLARE: You were approached?

PROOPS: Yeah, twice actually.

CLARE: So what held you back?

PROOPS: Well, I felt strongly that if I was going to go into politics, I would have to give up my work as a journalist. I know that most MPs have two and three jobs, half a dozen maybe, but I have never agreed that that's a good idea or believe that that's a good idea and I don't think that I could have done it. In addition, I had a husband who was a very difficult and very demanding husband. A demanding man, the sort of man who would have resented it very much if I'd been out late in the House of Commons. If I'd had a constituency maybe in the north of England, in the Midlands, a long way away from where I lived and had a son, in fact, I had more than one. I had, my natural son, and two other boys actually, who were part of my family so I had a lot of domestic pressure and I didn't think I could cope with it all.

CLARE: Do you regret that?

PROOPS: Well, I regret that I wasn't able to do it, yes, because I would love to have done it.

CLARE: But you would have loved to have done something else more, being a journalist.

PROOPS: Yes, oh yes.

CLARE: No, and likewise, the same question could be asked about psychiatry, not so much a psychiatrist, because of the medical training but there are these days ways of training to be a counsellor. You had, indeed, a lot of informal training. I read in the book about Eustace Chesser and various things being put your way and you steeping yourself in the literature of therapy and counselling and so on. But I wondered, when I read it whether you'd ever considered a formal training, taking time out and having a formal training as a therapist?

PROOPS: Well, not really because by the time I realised that it would have been wonderful if I had, it was really too late because I was too much involved in doing the job.

CLARE: Let me ask you something about the work you do and the work I do. Do you think that temperamentally you have the patience to see the same people over a period of time? And the reason I ask you that is that one of the real strengths of the work you did was that you were so directive, so no-nonsense, sometimes you must have quivered on the edges as to which way to go but in the end you tended to give clear advice and I, reading that, envied you in a way because that was why they came to you, they wanted a clear answer and you gave them clear advice. Whereas if you were involved with some of these people over a period of time, that might be a good deal less easy to do and I wondered whether you've reflected on whether your temperament found exactly the outlet or the outlet found exactly the temperament?

PROOPS: Well, it's hard to know, isn't it? I have quite a lot of people who write continually, ongoing correspondence, sometimes for years and years. So in a way they're almost like patients. And I have a relationship with them which hardly changes. I remember one reader who, I think she'd been writing to me for twenty years or more, and the original problem, whatever it was, was lost in the mists of time, but in the end she and I became sort of pen pals. In fact I met her eventually, but for years and years she wrote to me and I was a sort of outlet for her and when she was depressed or when she was lonely or whatever she was she simply wrote a letter and it was like a sort of strange pen friendship, but I never felt that I wanted to reject her or neither did I ever feel impatient with her and I've got a lot like that still today.

CLARE: Where did all this come from? When you look back through your life, what do you think the influences or the inheritance was that spurred this interest in other people?

PROOPS: Oh, I know precisely what it was. When I was a child I lived in the pub, in a street called Shepherdess Walk, City

Road, in London, a very rough area of London and the pub which my father ran had two bars on the ground floor. One was the saloon bar, one was the public bar and my sister and I used to be taken through the bar because there was no other exit to go to school. We went to the little comprehensive school down the road and I couldn't understand why the men, they were nearly all men in those days, very, very few women in the pubs in those days, they wore, in the public bar they mostly wore flat caps and the kind of mufflers and shabby clothes and they drank large pots of beer, large glasses of beer and in the other bar there were men with hard hats and neat suits wearing collars and ties, because it was in the City this pub so there were a lot of City gents although I didn't know at that time who they were, but they had small glasses with little drinks and this puzzled me very much indeed. Why were there these two different sets of people? And I used to nag my father and pester my father to explain and one day he got fed up with me and told me that the men in the public bar were hard up, they were, he described them in those days, working class, and the men in the other bar were well off, well paid, could afford the little drinks which were much, much more expensive than the big tankards or glasses of beer. And I thought that that was terrible. I thought this was my very first experience of two classes and I immediately, at the age of about five or six, a very young age, identified with the flat caps from that moment on, I continued to identify with the have-nots rather than the haves, and nothing's changed.

CLARE: Were your parents political?

PROOPS: My father was a Tory. He was interested in politics but he would have loved Thatcher. He would have adored her. And he was a gambler. I mean he was more interested in horse racing than anything else. But I think he would have voted Tory. I'm sure. I mean I don't remember ever discussing his politics.

CLARE: What was he like temperamentally?

PROOPS: Oh, he was lovely. He was lovely. He was a very outgoing man, very affectionate, very fond father, funny.

CLARE: Gregarious.

PROOPS: Oh, yes, very. I mean if you run a pub well you must be gregarious and he was. He was very friendly with everybody and he was the fun member of the family.

CLARE: Do you identify traits in you that you feel you've inherited from him?

PROOPS: Yes.

CLARE: And they would be?

PROOPS: Well, I hope they would be my sense of humour and the sense of the ridiculous. He was a great man for bantering conversation and I've certainly inherited that.

CLARE: And your mother?

PROOPS: My mother was a very nervous, very timid woman. She was so timid that she wouldn't let my sister and I learn to swim in case we drowned and I didn't go to school on a bus on my own until I was sixteen when I first went to art school. She was afraid of absolutely everything. I don't know if she was afraid of my father, I'm not sure about that. I was not aware of what they were like in an intimate relationship but she adored him and he adored her. In fact, I think she had a hard time with him because if you're married to a gambler, as you know, life is very, very insecure and she never knew if she was going to be able to buy the meat at the weekend and she never knew if she could pay the bills. Yet when he died, they'd been married for over forty years, my mother was by that time an agoraphobic.

CLARE: Which was when?

PROOPS: That was in the sixties. The women stayed behind while the funeral cortège went down the road and the men sort of disappeared from the house. My sister and I sat beside my mother flanking her and hanging on to her, to try to console her when she was suddenly aware that the men had moved away and moved out of the house and she got up and shook us off and ran down the garden path and ran down the road, this agoraphobic woman who'd never been out for years on her own, in fact never been out, shouting, 'Alfred, Alfred, take me with you, I can't bear to live without you.' And that, despite the terrible insecurity she must have had in her marriage to my father.

CLARE: Were you conscious of tension, anxiety? Did any of that rub off on you?

PROOPS: Oh, I wasn't aware of it. My mother was very, very protective towards both of us, my sister and me.

CLARE: Did it have a different effect on your sister to you or did you both respond in the same way?

PROOPS: I don't know. My sister and I had a very uneasy relationship and still have to some extent. She's still spikey towards me and I actually blame my mother who I'm quite certain had no idea what she as doing to us when she used to introduce me as the clever one and my sister as the pretty one. Now I could have killed my sister for being the pretty one because that's what I wanted to be and my sister could have killed me for being the clever one and my sister even now, last weekend when we spoke on the telephone, she said, 'How's my clever sister today?'

CLARE: And of course, you've written quite a bit about the effect on you in terms of looks.

PROOPS: Yeah.

CLARE: To the extent that if one didn't know you, on reading it, one would expect when one met you to encounter the beast as distinct from the beauty. It really did leave a mark on you, an enormous one. What was adolescence like?

PROOPS: Well . . .

CLARE: Was it terribly painful?

PROOPS: Terribly painful. Yeah, very painful indeed. And I'm sure the reason I married Proopsie was simply because he asked me and I didn't ever expect anybody, any man to want me, to want to marry me. In those days marriage was the object of every young woman and certainly in Jewish families, middle-class Jews, you know, they expected their daughters to get married and have children and live in Golders Green. I didn't think any of that would ever happen to me. If a boy occasionally talked to me, he'd see my sister and that would be the end of that because she was so pretty. I mean she's still a very, very attractive woman.

CLARE: The expectation of Jewish culture would be that you would get married, rather like, indeed, Irish Catholic culture.

Was there that same notion that if you didn't you were in some sense, on the shelf?

PROOPS: Oh yes, very much so.

CLARE: A stigmatised state. Did you have 'spinster aunts'? Did you have some model of what it might be like if you didn't?

PROOPS: Yes, yes, I did.

CLARE: Such as?

PROOPS: We had a spinster aunt, Lillian, who lived with us, with my mother.

CLARE: Who lived with you?

PROOPS: Actually lived with us and she was very good to us, my aunt. She was the practical one. She did all the cooking and she was a sort of mother figure to both of us. My mother relied on her very much and adored her sister. But I used to have this terror of becoming like my aunt, not wanted by anybody except her sister and her very kind brother-in-law, my father who was very, very good to her, very kind. But my aunt was a figure of charity, in effect. And that's what I dreaded, that I would be like my aunt.

CLARE: When you met your husband, at what stage were you in your own career? What sort of sense did you have that you could make it in terms of your own cleverness?

PROOPS: Well, I'd already started to work and I wasn't doing too badly. I was, you know, earning a few shillings and my first timid footstep was on the lowest rung of the ladder but it was there. And when I met Proopsie, I said to him actually when he asked to me marry him, I asked him two things actually, I said, how did he vote and would he object to my continuing my career, as I called it in those days?

CLARE: But you did ask that?

PROOPS: Oh, yes. And he said yes, and he told me he voted Labour, so I thought, well that's all right, then, and then he said yes, indeed, I'd have his full support and I always did have.

CLARE: Incidentally, your father's political orientation had no influence on you?

PROOPS: No, only in so far as I think it probably stimulated my interest in politics.

CLARE: Would you have argued with him?

PROOPS: Oh, I probably would have done and probably did, I mean I don't remember but I'm pretty sure I did.

CLARE: What was his view of his two daughters?

PROOPS: I was certainly his favourite. My sister was my mother's favourite. I think that my sister fulfilled for my mother what she really wanted in a little girl, in a daughter. Pretty, malleable, good humoured. My father was a very compassionate man and I think maybe there was some element in his affection for me that was compassionate. He was very protective towards me.

CLARE: Did he have any ambitions for you, even if they weren't particularly focused? Did he see you as someone who would go far?

PROOPS: No, I don't think so.

CLARE: You didn't get that sense?

PROOPS: No, I think my mother did.

CLARE: Did she?

PROOPS: Yes, my mother did. My mother was very, very proud of what she regarded as my achievements.

CLARE: But did she have any notion of what you might be, or any wish?

PROOPS: No, I don't think so. You see it was a very alien sort of world to my parents. They knew nothing about newspapers. My father read the racing pages and that was about it.

CLARE: Then how did you get into newspapers?

PROOPS: Well, that was like everything in my life, accidental. I was a fashion artist and a freelance artist and I had an agent, which sounds very grand but actually it was a rather shambling character that used to kind of wander around newspaper offices with a portfolio with a few drawings in. He took some of my drawings and one day he ambled into the *Daily Mirror* office and Hugh Cudlip was there. He was features editor of the *Mirror* and he liked the drawings and he said to this man whose name was Douglas Mount, 'Get her in,' and Douglas Mount ordered me to the *Daily Mirror* which I did, covered in ink and terrified. And there was this man striding about with jutting chin, very aggressive man, Cudlip, and he said, 'Are these your drawings?' and I said they were. He said, 'Walk up and down.'

So I shuffled up and this this little office and he said 'Sit down,' and I sat down. Incidentally, I was wearing an outfit, an awful porridge-coloured outfit, which somebody had given me in lieu of money and it was ten times too big for me and I looked absolutely terrible and also covered in ink and all that, grubby-looking artist. And he said to me, 'Do you think you could represent the *Daily Mirror* at Ascot?' I said yes, hardly knowing what Ascot was, except I remember my father mentioning Ascot. So he said, 'Start Monday.' So I became the *Daily Mirror* fashion artist. He invented the most terrible name, which I was ashamed for years until I began to laugh at it. It was Sylvane, and I thought it sounded like a flower shop. However, he insisted that I was Sylvane and then I left to go to the *Daily Herald* where I really learned a trade, did everything except make the tea and probably did that too and I became a reporter and a feature writer and believe it or not a music critic because the editor had discovered I could read music and that was enough, you know, to be a music critic.

CLARE: I noticed, reading through your life, that you do relate to powerful, complicated men and I wondered how much that was an echo indeed of your father. Hugh Cudlip, Robert Maxwell, but there are others. You do seem to have a fine skill handling these kind of monsters that some people see them as, difficult anyway, multifaceted and quite threatening to many people. Have you reflected on that?

PROOPS: No, not a lot. I certainly have always found that powerful men are attractive. If I meet a man who is wimpish or boring I don't really want to have anything much to do with him unless I have to. But I think that there's something about people in authority, men in authority, who attract me. I need to have some authoritative male figure in my life, if I can, I'm lucky.

CLARE: Now your husband wasn't that, or was he?

PROOPS: Oh, yes, he was very much that.

CLARE: In what way?

PROOPS: He was a bully. He was very dominating and domineering. And because I suppose there must have been and still is an element in me of my mother, the timidity that I must have inherited or learned from my mother, I have always allowed myself to be dominated by these strong men. Maxwell was one of them. I had a very good relationship with Maxwell. I was very fond of him. I still find it very difficult to believe that he was the monster that I knew him to be. Cudlip I adore and always have done.

CLARE: When you say Maxwell, even though you yourself know by virtue of your relationship with your own husband and the kind of things you get written to you, how often these people have these sides to them, you least of all should not be surprised that behind these public appearances are so many quite conflicting private passions and impulses?

PROOPS: I think you can be fairly objective about other people but it's very difficult to be objective about yourself. You can know what your weaknesses and indeed your strengths are but I don't think you can really change them. I know that it's a weakness of mine that I both admire these sort of men and that I have allowed myself over the years to be controlled by them.

CLARE: I also sense a conflict in your relationship with women. On the one hand you do empathise with their defencelessness or weak aspects. On the other hand, often, even within the same response, I noticed that you advocate, 'Stand up for yourself, hit him on the head with the pan while he's asleep. Get out of there, leave him, come back at two in the morning,' and so on. I wondered about that in relation to your mother. I wondered whether in fact you'd found when you were growing up an irritation with your mother's wimpishness.

PROOPS: I'm not aware of it. In fact I think my main emotion, my main feeling about my mother and her timidity was I felt sorry for her. I wanted to protect her from it.

CLARE: Did you ever wish that she would stand up to your father and that she would throw off the timidity.

PROOPS: No, I never did. No, because she loved him so much and they had such a good marriage and he never bullied her. She was never a victim of men like I've been a victim because she had this man, this tender, gentle, loving man, funny man, who made jokes. He was never a bully like the men I've known. He never, ever tried to dominate her. He was very tender with her and very loving with her.

CLARE: You say he was never a bully like the men you've known and you've known these bullies and you've been very candid. You said of the notorious bully, Maxwell, you were fond of him. Sticking with your husband for a moment, domineering and bullying, what was it, do you think, that he did give you?

PROOPS: He provided me with friendship, with the very fact that he was there. Remember that I had this terror of being on my own, of being rejected by men and he was the one who didn't reject me so, there was always this feeling, even when I hated him.

CLARE: Yes, it is like, isn't it, what women who are battered would say?

PROOPS: Yes, yes.

CLARE: Which a lot of people don't understand. They would say, 'Yes, I know, he batters me and abuses me but he's there and in his own curious way he's concerned about me.'

PROOPS: Yes, and I understand that. I write to these women who tell me the most horrendous stories of the abuse that they have to deal with and put up with and they say in the letter, 'Don't tell me to leave him,' and I understand that. I know why it's somehow worse to go then to stay.

CLARE: But you sometimes tell them to leave.

PROOPS: Well I do. I mean, because if a woman's being beaten up and her children are being beaten and maybe her children are being sexually abused, then I feel I have to say, 'Escape if you can,' and I tell them to and I tell them where to go. But I think it's very hard and I think you've got to be very strong or really very, very badly beaten up and frightened to go.

CLARE: So how bullied were you? In one sense you would be seen as quite a strong woman, you seem to stand up for yourself, you know where you stand, you're clear about your feelings. You are a writer in a very tough, very male world. The notion of Proopsie bullying or dominating you might be more difficult than in the case of other women.

PROOPS: I had an escape, didn't I? I could get away every morning at nine o'clock or eight o'clock, or whatever, I could get away from this man and I could stay away until it was time for me to go home in the evening. I also travelled a lot in those days. I went away sometimes for weeks and even months at a time for my job and because he supported me in the job and he had no objection to my working, therefore he knew it was part of the job that I had to travel. I escaped from so much of my life, my married life. Now the women who write to me have no way of escaping. They don't have a job like mine, they don't have independence. Remember I also had financial independence which was very important indeed.

CLARE: Given all of that, why weren't you just silent about your own marriage. You wrote actually in a way that suggested that it was a pretty good one, it was super-duper. It was this that contributed to the view that later you used to justify your writing the book, namely the view of you as someone above problems, with a stable personal life and a successful marriage in a country where marriages were breaking down all over the place. In a sense, if you'd followed what you spoke to me earlier in the interview about, namely this issue of anonymity, the one thing you wouldn't have referred to, you needn't have referred to was your own marriage.

PROOPS: That's true and I think, looking back, I think that what I tried to do was build up a fictitious situation in which I formed a fictitious family life. It didn't exist, which I would like to have believed did exist. I think now, in retrospect, it was like writing a film script and participating in it as a character and all the other people in my life at that time. This was before Philip, my lover, turned up. I wanted to present this picture, not necessarily to the readers of the newspaper or anybody else, but to myself.

CLARE: Did your husband read it?

PROOPS: What, read my column?

CLARE: Yeah.

PROOPS: Oh, yes.

CLARE: Read those descriptions?

PROOPS: Oh, yeah.

CLARE: Did he ever comment on them?

PROOPS: Very rarely.

CLARE: At that stage you weren't sleeping together, you didn't have a physical relationship. It was a marriage largely of convenience.

PROOPS: Oh, yeah. When I say he read it I assume he read it but he had a lot of other interests outside of me, luckily. He was a Freemason which I found extraordinary. I never understood why he would never talk about it because you know it's a secretive sect. He spent a lot of time with his freemasonry and he also had a very interesting job himself. He was an engineer and his work was very absorbing. I think that our relationship was a very strange one. He was playing bridge and very early on when I first knew him he insisted that I learnt to play bridge. I wasn't very interested in it really but I did it to please him the way I have always done things to please men. We used to play a lot of bridge with friends or visiting people and I could never take it seriously. Now, he took it very seriously indeed. To me it was a game. To him it was a contest. It was competition, it was winning and he used to get very angry with me because I found it funny and I used to say, 'For Christ's sake, it's a bloody game.'

CLARE: What's really interesting about the dilemma that you found yourself in during those years and then when the relationship with your lover, Philip developed, was that it wasn't as if you were doing a nine to five job as I don't, a draughtswoman or a PR consultant. You found yourself in a situation advising and responding to people, talking about personal relationships and difficulties, many of which revolved round this very issue of love, intimacy, sharing. I can understand this issue in the earlier years of constructing a fictional life with Proops. Where it gets difficult, where it really gets difficult is when somebody writes to you with a situation virtually identical to your own, a man wrote to you that his wife was having an affair and he said he was trying to preserve the marriage for the sake of the children and you wrote back a pretty Proopsie response, 'You're letting your wife get away with murder. She's a greedy woman who wants to have her cake and eat it and it doesn't matter who else goes hungry.' Now, I'm trying to envisage the psychological state of you writing that letter because it could have been your husband writing in. Your son was there, you certainly convinced yourself that the reason you'd stated with Proops had a lot to do with your son and also the mess of a divorce and so on. Yet here is a statement which suggests that, for you at any rate, doing such a thing makes you a greedy, demanding woman who's having her cake and eating it.

PROOPS: Well, I was, wasn't I?

CLARE: Is that how you felt?

PROOPS: I wasn't aware of feeling it at the time but when I look back on it, yes, I was. But remember I didn't start my column, the *Dear Marje* column until twenty-two years ago. I was married for fifty years, so there were thirty years before I started the *Dear Marje* column and for most of these years I was a columnist writing about politics, about travel, commenting about current affairs, interviewing people and so on. I wasn't giving people advice at that time.

CLARE: No, I accept that. I wondered why you didn't write back and say, not 'You're letting your wife away with murder' but that you might have prefaced it by saying, 'in my experience,' or you might have left that out, you might have said, 'Well marriage is a complicated business and I'd need to know a good deal more about why your wife finds your love and affection insufficient.'

PROOPS: Well, there's a fairly simple explanation to this. All the letters that I publish are anonymous. Sometimes they're a page and a half telling me almost nothing. I can't write back and say, 'Tell me a bit more about your feelings,' and so on. I wish I could. The worst aspect of this job is the one-sidedness of it. Every time a woman writes to me about her horrendous husband I wonder about her and I try to read between the lines and it's impossible. I know nothing about these people.

CLARE: But here you had an interesting insight from your own personal experience.

PROOPS: Oh, yes.

CLARE: But you didn't draw on it?

PROOPS: Because I don't think that my personal experience was probably anything like the experience that this reader would have. I don't even remember this particular letter after the five hundred or so I have every week but I would be very unlikely to draw on my own experiences. What I try to do when I answer the letters is think about the reader and what the reader could do. What the reader is strong enough to do. I'm really very protective towards the readers.

CLARE: I notice in comments about the process you're engaged in that there's often an assumption that people like me, a professional, will be envious or jealous or critical. Now, I'm not, actually, because I know full well that there is a huge pool of unhappiness and misery and morbidity out there and that it's one of those areas where the market demand will always, in my view, exceed the supply so I welcome on board anyone who's prepared to help. I say at the outset and I think anyone who knows me knows that I'm not particularly threatened by alternative therapists, psychotherapists or anything. I am a little doubtful often about effectiveness but I'm a little doubtful of the effectiveness of much of what I do too, so that's shared. No, the anxiety I have is as follows: I notice in many of the comments, not necessarily made by you, in fact I don't think you've ever made this comment, but many people commenting on what you do make a certain assumption. They say the fact that you're there is testament to the fact that people have nobody to turn to, that in this great insensitive world, there's nothing around. And they assume when there's a tragedy that there was nobody there. There was no information. There was nobody to talk to and the agony columnists, they get these thousands of letters. But my experience is that actually at the end of the twentieth century, there's never been so many avenues or so much access. I listed them indeed at some stage before I came to talk to you just out of interest. I was thinking there are helplines, Samaritans, Relate, the Manic Depressive Fellowship, SANE, GPs are far better trained, some of them are very good. There are now psychologists working out in the area, there are acupuncturists, homeopathists, there's all sorts of counselling and various kinds of groups and then there's the orthodox services, groaning under the demand, but in certain parts of the country doing very remarkable work. I also know that when I see people in tragedy one of the first questions I ask them is, who have they sought help from and often people like you are very early on but sometimes they're late on, but there's also this bevy of therapists and counsellors. I'm coming to conclude that the reason there are so many of us around is not only that there are so many problems out there, but that honestly many of those problems are exceedingly difficult to solve. But this issue, this assumption that the demand suggests no response – does it not actually suggest either a response that's inadequate, or that the response is often the best that can be provided and sadly, it's not good enough?

PROOPS: I don't think that. I think that the majority of people, if we're talking about the sort of people who write to agony aunts, most of them say, 'I don't know who to turn to, you are my last resort,' or they end the letter saying, 'I feel much better now I've written to you,' and almost invariably they're letters from people who would not know how to seek all this help, despite the fact that they can read where to get the help. They can ring up the social services department, the women's aid, all sorts of things that they can do but they don't know how to do it and also I think another element is that people are intimidated by authority. People write to me about medical problems, quite a lot, quite a lot about sexual medical problems for example, they suspect that they've got HIV, that they're HIV positive and so on and I have to urge them and beg them to see a doctor. The fact is that I think that they are intimidated by doctors. There's still in this country the sort of forelock-touching attitude to GPs.

CLARE: What do you think you would have said if somebody had written to you saying something like you said to me, that my husband repelled me so I took up with another man, who gave me many splendid and good things. I feel guilt. I suspect my teenage son knows and is very confused. What should I do, Dear Marje? What do you think you would have said?

PROOPS: Well I know what I do say.

CLARE: What would you have said, then, when it was happening to you?

PROOPS: I don't know. I hope I'd have said, 'Carry on getting on whatever you can out of your relationship with this man, providing you are not hurting your partner, your legal partner.'

CLARE: In the biography Robert, your son, suggested that in fact he had been very much hurt by it.

PROOPS: I don't think, no, no. I think again with Robert it's very much a hindsight reaction. It's nonsense to imagine that he knew at the age of five, which he now claims, that he was aware of this, of the marriage. It hadn't even started going wrong when he was five. And he says now that he knew that his father and I were . . .

CLARE: It hadn't been right then, though, had it?

PROOPS: Oh, it had never been right.

CLARE: That's what I say, so when you say, 'It hadn't started to go wrong,' in a sense it had been wrong from the outset.

PROOPS: Yes, but remember Proops was away in the war from when Robert was one until he was five. So his father was a total stranger to him and to me in fact. Proops was a different man when he came back from the army. He was ten times worse.

CLARE: That was a very traumatic time, but your son must have perceived that, even though he was only five or six. I mean the return from the war was one of those moments.

PROOPS: Oh, yes, that was the start of the very bad relationship that he had with his father until his father died.

CLARE: You're very interesting about that in the book. What was he like when he came back from the war?

PROOPS: He was ten times worse than when he went away. He went into the army as an officer, which was unfortunate for him really. If he'd gone through the ranks I think that he would have learned a lot. As it was, because he was a man for whom authority was very important, he went in in charge of other men, superior in rank in other words to other men and then eventually, after four years he became a major which was a fairly high rank I think. I don't really know much about army ranks but I think it's not bad. So he came back even more authoritative and more bossy than he'd been before, and that's saying something. And he was much more demanding of services. He expected things to be done for him because he'd always had a batman doing things for him. He used to sling things on the floor and expect me to pick them up and I was very, very resentful about that. But I think that the thing that actually triggered off the appalling relationship that Robert had with his father was the train journey. I don't know whether it's in that book but shortly after Proops came out of the army he was still in uniform. I mean shortly after he came back from India, I think it was.

CLARE: At the end of the war?

PROOPS: At the end of the war. My parents lived in Walton-on-Thames and we got on a train to go and visit my parents for the first weekend of Proopsie's return and we sat in one of those little carriages with seats on both sides, trundling away down to Walton-on-Thames, and Robert, very excited about it, with seeing this strange man called Daddy, was jumping about this train, leaping from one seat to the other and I kept saying, 'Sit down, you'll hurt yourself. Don't jump about,' and Proops said to me, 'I hope you haven't been bringing him up to be a namby pamby mother's boy while I've been away.' And I didn't respond to that, but felt very angry that he should say that but I didn't want to start arguing with him in front of Robert. And we went to my mother's and Robert became even more excited and we had tea with my mother and she lived in a tall, narrow house, my mother and father, lived in this tall, narrow house with a tall staircase and just when we were about to leave to go home again, Robert tore up the staircase, stood at the top poised, and leapt. No, sorry, I should have said that Proops said on the train, 'Better that he should break a leg than that you should break his spirit.' That was when he was leaping about. And Robert ran up the stairs, poised on the top of the stairs, and leapt to the bottom and broke a leg and he ended up in hospital and I didn't speak to Proops, not even to say, 'Pass the salt,' for weeks and I blamed him for Robert's broken leg. We had to keep returning to Walton to go and visit Robert in hospital. In those days they didn't chuck them out of hospital in three days like they do now with a plaster. But he was there for quite a long time and I feel sure that Robert blamed his father for his broken leg. I blamed his father for his broken leg and I'm sure that if Robert didn't, I probably passed on that message to Robert. And that was the start of this bad relationship and they were terribly, terribly jealous of each other. Proops was jealous of Robert because Robert had been so close to me.

CLARE: And Robert was jealous of Proops?

PROOPS: Of Proops.

CLARE: For coming back?

PROOPS: Yeah.

CLARE: And yet it was clear later perhaps to the older Robert that the relationship between you and Proopsie wasn't a happy one.

PROOPS: Oh, I'm sure it was clear, must have been.

CLARE: Though your son describes you rather like you answered that earlier letter, you know, the greedy woman who got her cake and ate it. He says, 'My mother organised her life the way it suited her.'

PROOPS: Yeah.

CLARE: There is that element of strength and what you might, in someone else's letter, identify as selfishness.

PROOPS: Yeah, well I did didn't I? In fact I think most people do, don't they? They try to. Some are not perhaps ready to admit it but I will certainly admit it. I did organise my life. I did my job, which was absorbing and I loved it. I had all my political associations, my friendships with people like Harold Wilson, Jim Callaghan, Michael Foot, considerable politicians and I was very much involved with them all and involved with a lot of legal reform. I was very interested in homosexual reforms, divorce law reforms, and so on.

CLARE: One parent families and so on.

PROOPS: Yup, yup.

CLARE: The decision that Robert would go to boarding school, was that a difficult one?

PROOPS: Well, it was Proopsie's decision but I agreed with it. I thought that as he was an only son, because the other boy, well he was not adopted but I call him my adopted son.

CLARE: The Nigerian boy?

PROOPS: Nigerian boy, well, he's now nearly sixty.

CLARE: That's right.

PROOPS: My black son.

CLARE: But very good friend of Robert.

PROOPS: Oh, yes, oh, yes, very close. We both thought it was a good idea because he was an only child and Proops was very keen for him to go to boarding school and I didn't object. I also thought that because I was a working mother and working so much away from home, that he'd have a better life at boarding school. Sometimes now he says that he hated it and he wished he hadn't gone to boarding school. Other times he says, 'Well, it wasn't bad.' He ran away when he was a little boy from the first school he went to and he was very unhappy at the first school, but I wasn't aware of it. Maybe I was too absorbed in what I was doing. Actually I think I was a very remiss mother in many ways. I didn't have strong maternal feelings. I adore him and we're closer now than we've ever been, since his father died. Apart from those first five years of his life when he and I were very close together, he slept in his little cot beside my bed in those digs we had and then there was that long period until he got married. Robert, he married when he was about twenty-two and he left home then, of course.

CLARE: But given what we know about an only son, jealousy with the father coming back, the competition in a sense for your attentions, when eventually time would come for him to go to boarding school, it would be painful, wouldn't it?

PROOPS: Oh, yes, it was painful. Yes indeed. And because you never know whether you're making the right decision or not. I often think that parenthood is the one thing that you're never trained for. You trained to be a doctor, to be a psychiatrist, I trained to be a journalist, an artist and to some extent a counsellor, but you never have any training in how to be a parent. How to be a mother. You're in at the deep end until you make mistake after mistake after mistake.

CLARE: But I sense in conflicts about decisions, you would put yourself first.

PROOPS: Well, I don't know about that.

CLARE: When did you not?

PROOPS: (Pause.) I don't think there was any question of it, really, because all the decisions that were made about Robert were jointly made with Proops. Maybe if I'd been a lone parent it would have been a different matter, but I wasn't and remember, too, that Proops was the strong one. Proops was the one who made all the decisions about everything. He designed the homes we lived in. He bought the furniture. He chose the wallpaper, the carpets, everything and every decision where we went on holiday, whatever, they were his decisions and I went along with them.

CLARE: But in a crucial area where many women currently have so much trouble, the decision to go out and work and pursue a career where many otherwise liberated husbands can be so difficult, he wasn't difficult with you on that?

PROOPS: No, he wasn't. And I think the reason was because when he first asked me to marry him, I was a passionate socialist and also passionately interested in doing a creative job. I asked his permission, remember.

CLARE: That's true.

PROOPS: I didn't tell him that this was what I wanted. I said would he mind, would he let me.

CLARE: But on the issue of Robert you were both actually in agreement because you were both pursuing your lives. I wonder if that was something that Robert did pick up, that's why you get this ambivalence in his account now when he looks back.

PROOPS: Yes it might well be, it might well be.

CLARE: When you did respond to these various letters from people, what did you draw on? You point out that psychiatrists and others will draw on theory, perhaps they're encouraged to examine their own personal relationships so they know the extent to which they are drawing on them, if they are. But in your instance, what did you draw on? When people asked you about these conflicts between job and marriage, between lover and husband, between children and personal life, what did you draw on? What kind of framework of theory or personal experience did you draw on, seeing that you were such a contradiction yourself?

PROOPS: I don't know. I honestly do not know the answer to that question.

CLARE: There is out there in what I call the taxi drivers' conventional wisdom, a sense that 'Why should I listen to Marjorie Proops or Anthony Clare because more often than not, their lives are every bit as messy as my own.' Why would they go to Marjorie Proops, Anthony Clare if, when they eventually write their biographies or have them written, they turn out to be as chaotic as them?

PROOPS: I don't know. I can only tell you that after this book appeared there was, as you know, a lot of publicity, I had a tremendous response from readers, all of them, except for a very, very tiny proportion, applauding my decision to tell the truth. They said things like, 'Now I know why you're sympathetic to other people, or why you could help other people because you yourself have had so much pain and suffering.' So I think people now feel I relate to them in a more human way, rather than a detached way that perhaps you might relate to them.

CLARE: Well, perhaps I might except that I suppose increasingly I have to admit that I don't have many of the answers to the kind of problems that come. I'd never be able to write an agony column because of two things; one is I'd keep asking for more information and the more information I got, the more I would acknowledge the complexity of the problem from the outset, unless it was a serious illness that I could, so to speak, treat. But, just coming back to this a little bit, let me ask you did you ever find yourself responding to what you were asked, by drawing on your own personal experience? You've given an example of how you didn't do it.

PROOPS: Oh, yeah, I think I did, I think I did. Indeed, particularly sexually. Because until I met Philip I had a very, very limited sexual experience, none really. I had what amounted to a very brief sexual relationship with Proops, which was appalling, not I think his fault but I simply couldn't cope with sex with him. And then I had no sex at all in my life for years and years and years. So whatever advice, if I'd given advice at that time, which I didn't remember, I wasn't doing that sort of work.

CLARE: You weren't in the business then?

PROOPS: I would have known nothing and so I couldn't have used my own experience in relating to other people's, but after I met Philip I learned what sex was all about and not only technically but emotionally and I learned what love was all about and what response was all about, I was then able to draw on that experience and I did indeed.

CLARE: Did you tell anybody about the relationship?

PROOPS: No.

CLARE: Did you experience the urge from time to time to tell somebody?

PROOPS: No, I didn't.

CLARE: You never felt like writing to somebody?

PROOPS: No, I didn't.

CLARE: There wasn't that sense that occasionally spies have been wanting desperately to say to somebody, 'I'm not what I seem'?

PROOPS: No.

CLARE: Though you weren't what you seemed?

PROOPS: No.

CLARE: You see there's a contradiction, too, in the sense that you say when the decision came to reveal it you were more frightened in a way of what your readers would make of it, because you felt that they thought of you as, you know, having lead a blameless life, whiter than white.

PROOPS: No, I didn't, I wasn't, actually, I wasn't.

CLARE: You weren't?

PROOPS: No, because although I'm sure you'll find this very, very difficult to believe because nobody believes it, I never ever for one minute thought that people would focus on thirteen pages out of a book that is nearly 3,400 pages long.

CLARE: This is what you said at the Foyles luncheon and Barbara Cartland, Barbara Castle I should say (what a Freudian slip), Barbara Castle said it was rubbish.

PROOPS: That's right, she did.

CLARE: But I have to press you on that. You're a hardened, tough, experienced journalist from the centre of British journalism and they're as shrewd and cynical as they come. I do find it difficult to believe because of who is saying it to me. Here is Marjorie Proops, the doyenne, as I say, of agony aunts, a person who is a household name and then out comes a book, *The Guilt and the Gingerbread*, and in it it is revealed that far from the relationship between herself and her husband being an ideal and happy one, it was a miserable and dreadful one and she sustained it and her relationship with her son largely assisted by a passionate, successful, twenty-year relationship with another man.

PROOPS: Mm, mm.

CLARE: Even in these newsworthy days, that is still, it seems to me, the stuff of which tabloid journalism is made. I can see them fighting over it. If you were any other woman I'd say, 'Well, you're just naive,' but to hear you say that you were surprised by the reaction is very difficult to believe.

PROOPS: I was, you have to believe me.

CLARE: What does that say of you?

PROOPS: I'm not a liar.

CLARE: No, no. So what I'm interested in is not so much that you're a liar or you're not a liar, what I'm interested in is, what does that say of you because you've been in the heart of a tough street, Fleet Street, you know what they go for, you know what their eye for a story is and yet in this one your judgement about what is a good or a bad story seems to have let you down with a thump.

PROOPS: Yeah, it did indeed. Can I tell you perhaps what you may not be aware of and that is why this book was written in the first place. It was written because Maxwell wanted me to write an autobiography and I said I wouldn't and I asked him why he wanted me to and he said, 'You started from nothing, with nothing, knowing nothing and here you are, very successful and famous,' and all that nonsense and he related to people like that because that's how he was and he found that very exciting and very interesting and it fascinated him. I first met him when he was an MP and when I was very much involved in politics in the seventies and so on and he said to me, 'Write it,' and I wouldn't and he was very angry with me and he kept saying, 'Why won't you?' and I said, 'I can't because I can't bear the "I", the ego trip that it would be to do it.' I wouldn't do it. He was a very hard man to resist and I'm surprised that I actually resisted him. He then said, 'Would you agree to somebody else doing it, to being the subject of a biography?' and I said, 'Oh, all right, OK, I'll do it.' Now Maxwell knew nothing about my relationship with Philip, all Maxwell knew about was my career. He knew Proops slightly, he knew nothing about my marriage, nobody did and he wanted this book as a sort of testament to a successful journalist. And it was at that point that I then talked to Robert and said to Robert, 'Shall I do it?' I then told Robert the true story of my marriage, my relationship with Philip and so on, the whole thing.

CLARE: What age was Robert then when you did this?

PROOPS: Pardon?

CLARE: What age are we talking about?

PROOPS: Well, the book came out about six months, a year ago maybe.

CLARE: And Robert is?

PROOPS: Robert is now fifty.

CLARE: Right. So you told Robert about Philip?

PROOPS: Yeah, I told Robert.

CLARE: And what was his response?

PROOPS: He said, 'Well, I knew there was somebody else and I guessed it was him.' Now I don't know whether that's true or not.

CLARE: Some did suspect?

PROOPS: Oh, some knew, actually. I didn't know that they knew.

CLARE: So you're sure Robert Maxwell didn't know?

PROOPS: Oh, I'm sure Maxwell didn't. No, Maxwell, no, certainly not because Maxwell wasn't there then at that stage.

CLARE: No, but some journalists might have known.

PROOPS: Remember that Philip had died before Maxwell . . .

CLARE: Maxwell came along.

PROOPS: Came along.

CLARE: Yes. But you were saying the decision was made for a biographer to write this book and you told Robert.

PROOPS: Robert. I then decided that I had to make a decision then as to whether or not to tell the truth or whether to invent a blameless Marje Proops with a halo and not tell the truth.

CLARE: Or not have a biography at all.

PROOPS: Or not have a biography at all. And that was the point at which I discussed it with Robert and Robert said, 'Tell the truth and do it,' and he said, and still says, 'I think it would be good for you, it would get it all out of your system. It would be your confession and I think it would be therapeutic.'

CLARE: And what of that? Did you get it out of your system?

PROOPS: I think so.

CLARE: Did you feel a need to?

PROOPS: Yes, I do. I did.

CLARE: Because? Why?

PROOPS: Well, because by the time I did it, remember that both Philip and Proops were dead, I wouldn't have done it if either of them had been alive because I wouldn't have wanted to hurt either of them.

CLARE: No?

PROOPS: A few years before that happened, maybe three or four years before the book, I was having therapy, psychotherapy, twice a week. I started psychotherapy because I'd lost a lot of weight. I was very anxious and my doctor thought that I needed help and I got it. And I think that the result of that therapy for me was it developed in me, or encouraged in me, the need to tell, to reveal. Tom Kraft, who was the therapist who helped me, taught me in effect how to release the various feelings of terror, a terror of death that I had, a terror so intense that I couldn't bear to pass a funeral parlour. If I drove in the car behind a funeral I would come out in sweats and physical, awful physical fear, really horrible nightmares and the lot. But Tom taught me and helped me reveal these terrors and to cope with them, to face then and so on. And I think that it was partly, possibly mainly, due to that period of psychotherapy that I began to realise the value of therapy and of the need to tell, maybe even get rid of some of the guilt. I'll never, never ever lose it.

CLARE: Did the relationship with Philip come up in the pscyho-therapy?

PROOPS: Oh, yes. He knew everything, Tom.

CLARE: When you say the desire to tell, to tell whom?

PROOPS: Probably to tell myself, I don't know.

CLARE: You knew.

PROOPS: I think really that the desire to tell was perhaps based on the desire to cope with the guilt.

CLARE: You're a particularly interesting person in this respect because by virtue of your career you had relationships of a kind with a large number of people. Did you feel the need to tell them?

PROOPS: No.

CLARE: You know the people I mean, all out there writing the letters to you and so on?

PROOPS: Yeah, yeah.

CLARE: It wasn't there?

PROOPS: No, no, it wasn't there.

CLARE: And you'd told Robert as a result of this?

PROOPS: I told Robert only because of the book because I had to decide whether to do a truthful biography or not one at all.

CLARE: You say, 'I never imagined that other journalists would be interested in a twenty-year-old adulterous love affair during a sexless marriage.' Yet you know yourself the impact of it, and you knew from letters and things that there's nothing more traumatic than deceptions and so on. Now you realise that, was that a misjudgement of yours or that other people have been interested in the wrong things, or what?

PROOPS: Well, partly I think that other people are interested in the wrong things, yes. I think this sort of invasion, this need that people have to know about other people's sex lives is invasive. I'd never do it myself, never engage in that kind of journalism myself and never have.

CLARE: Though you've written speculative pieces about Princess Margaret or Charles and Diana in terms of their problems.

PROOPS: Well, yes but I wouldn't do any kind of invasive journalism to try to find out what they were doing.

CLARE: But I come back to this issue of privacy and so on. Your book is written and it's there but I suppose the thing I'm still intrigued by it is that the one area you are private about is linked with death. When you were talking earlier about age I was thinking of death actually, and now you've told me that one of the reasons you were seeing Dr Kraft was fears arising out of death. In that therapy, were you any clearer as to where that all originated from? Where does your fear of death come from?

PROOPS: I don't know. It may be because of a lot of illness that I've had. I've been at the point of death quite a few times. I've had a lot of serious operations. One many years ago when I had to have a thyroidectomy and they really thought that this was the end of Marje.

CLARE: And you've had a bypass operation?

PROOPS: I've had a bypass.

CLARE: Hips and so on.

PROOPS: Hips. The bypass thing was the most dangerous one because when it was diagnosed and I said to the doctor, 'What does that mean?' and he said, 'An operation tomorrow if I can fix it up.' And I said 'Is it dangerous?' and he said, 'Yes,' and I said, 'Is it life-threatening?' and he said, 'Yes.'

CLARE: Were you, as a child, fearful of death?

PROOPS: I think so.

CLARE: In your room?

PROOPS: Probably, I think so. I think probably my mother's timidity really was the start of it. If you have a mother who is so frightened for your life that she won't let you swim and you're a little tiny child, you are going to really believe that danger lurks on the seashore.

CLARE: Did your husband sense that in you, with that dispute over Robert and breaking his leg rather than his spirit? Did he see that you were very sensitive, perhaps, to the issue of risk?

PROOPS: He may have done, I don't know. I can't ever remember him talking about his feelings, ever.

CLARE: And now, what's the residual view of death that you have, how do you feel about death?

PROOPS: I can actually laugh about it now. In fact, the last page of that book, I think I'm right in saying, I think Angela who wrote the book, asked me if I think, thought about dying, how I would like it to be, happen. And I said, 'I'd just like to drop dead here in the office and have the cleaner sweep me up in the morning.' So I can laugh about it now.

CLARE: But I was struck by that image because that's the way I think I'd like to die too and a lot of other people I know, but what makes us rather frightened of death is not death, it's the slower death, or growing illnesses and incapacities. I'm struck that you're a very energetic, active, working woman still in full possession of her faculties. I wonder still about the fear of death, what kind of death did you think about?

PROOPS: I think the sort of death I was afraid of was a slow, painful one.

CLARE: That's still there, that's still a possibility isn't is?

PROOPS: Of course.

CLARE: And how do you cope with that fear now?

PROOPS: Well, I don't think it'll happen.

CLARE: Because you think you'll go the way you wish?

PROOPS: Yeah. I do.

CLARE: And afterwards, what's left?

PROOPS: Nothing.

CLARE: That's your belief?

PROOPS: Nothing.

CLARE: How Jewish are you?

PROOPS: If you mean, do I light candles on Friday night and have a ceremony at Passover and all that nonsense, the answer is not at all. I'm Jewish by race and birth. I identify with the Jewish minority as I identify with the black minority or any other minority group. I've got a ghetto instinct, definitely. But I never go into a synagogue unless I have to for somebody getting married or something and I don't pray to any particular God.

CLARE: Have you ever felt so despairing that you felt you couldn't go on?

PROOPS: Oh yes, I have. Because one of the reasons I started having therapy with Tom was this terrible depression, terrible depression. I was very lucky to fall into his hands.

CLARE: Had you ever had that before?

PROOPS: No, not even when I was unhappy, I didn't have. I learned then the differences between depression, clinical depression and the blues.

CLARE: And you'd sum up that difference how?

PROOPS: Well, I think that clinical depression in my own personal experience is despair and total hopelessness and, in fact, a desire almost mixed up with fear, but a desire not to wake up tomorrow and have to face it all again.

CLARE: Did you ever get to the stage of planning such a thing?

PROOPS: No.

CLARE: Looking back, what do you think saw you through?

PROOPS: Well, I think partly determination to get through. Partly Robert and my grandchildren. Partly the challenge of it because I'm the sort of woman who enjoys a challenge and in fact, seeks challenge and I actually seek confrontation, in my job, that is. And I think that there was some aspect of that in my determination to conquer this business. I was lucky to have help.

CLARE: Are you a risk-taker? When you look back was there something of that in the way you negotiated your relationships and your life, the very element that an outsider would see, the risk, the danger, that would be in a sense, meat and drink to you. You're a person who rides high on a challenge.

PROOPS: Yeah.

CLARE: On keeping the balls in the air?

PROOPS: Yes, I think so. In fact, I think that was an element in my relationship with Philip. Because Philip was a very secretive man and it was terribly important to him anyway that the relationship remained secret. It was more important to him than it was to me actually. In fact, there were times when I wanted people to know, I wanted people to know that this very special man loved me because it was something that I never thought I'd ever achieve in my life, so I did want it to be known. I knew it could never be because I knew it would be very difficult for him. But that whole relationship was a challenge which I went into knowing very well would really create all sorts of problems in my life.

CLARE: It is an interesting paradox isn't it, that our culture believes that it is better to let things out as part of, I suppose, curiosity to find out. Here I am interviewing you and there's the book. I think towards the end of this century more than ever, there's an assumption, a conventional wisdom, that it is better to have things out than in. Hence the search for counselling and the need to talk about post-traumatic stress, abuse, the horrors of life and so on. On the other hand, here I am talking to someone whose life survived by not letting something out, but by actually holding it in. In certain instances this passion for revelation itself may be a sickness?

PROOPS: Yeah, it's true, isn't it? And also I think that you can't generalise, can you, about people. There are fifty-six million people in this country, each one of them unique, with unique needs. And this is why I think my job particularly is so difficult, because I can only guess at what the people who write to me and seek help from me need and want. Reading between the lines, as Eustace Chesser used to say to me, is more important than reading the lines and I never have a chance to talk to the people who write to me. You, at least, have a chance to investigate your patients. Tom had a chance to investigate me.

CLARE: And if you had seen me all those years ago, would you have told me?

PROOPS: Yes, I'm sure I would, I'm sure I would because when I saw Tom it was such a tremendous relief to be able to tell him and also to know that he wasn't judging me and I think this is another very important aspect of counselling, people's fear of being judged and people's fear of moralising judgement. One of the things that I am very careful not to do when I write to people is moralise or be judgemental because I don't think it's my job to judge other people's morals any more than I think it's other people's job to judge mine. I think that what we do, all of us, we must take responsibility for and I take responsibility for everything that I've done. I'm not proud of it all and some of it I'm ashamed of, but I accept myself for what I am, which is human and fallible.

CLARE: Marjorie Proops, thank you very much indeed.

PROOPS: Thank you.

Esther Rantzen

Some people lead lives so public that they pose the question – what is left when the lights fade, the cameras are put away and the media caravans move off in search of the next coup and scoop? Esther Rantzen appears to be such a person. Not merely has her name become synonymous with consumer television and the public righting of wrongs but she has made public issues out of her own private experiences, family dramas and personal heartaches. She is one of the best-known women in Britain, instantly recognisable both in terms of her physical appearance and her voice.

During more than twenty years of her BBC television programme *That's Life*, she adopted with a passionate intensity such causes as dangerous playgrounds, tranquilliser abuse, laser surgery, flame-proof nightwear, sugar drinks and the plight of young children waiting for organ transplants. I personally can vouch for her fervour and determination, having worked with her on a programme exposing the deficiencies and weaknesses inherent in the policy of running down the large mental hospitals and developing community-based psychiatric facilities – the so-called community care programme. I witnessed the same utter determination, self-belief and single-mindedness as were brought to bear on her most famous campaign – the Childline Campaign on behalf of victims of child psychological, physical and sexual abuse.

Not surprisingly, given this degree of drive and determination, she has provoked intense critical responses. Her professionalism, that is to say the skill, expertise and energy she brings to her work, is rarely questioned. She has been described by admirers as the 'Lady Bountiful of the BBC', possessed of 'a heart of gold, a will of iron', a powerful campaigner for the underdog and ordinary, often forgotten punter, 'the people's friend'. Her admirers speak of her passionate commitment to her causes, her astonishing instinct for what will make a crusading campaign, her personal involvement with the administration and day-to-day concerns of Childline. But she has also been dubbed bossy, domineering and downright unpleasant. One detractor, the television critic Victor Lewis-Smith, went so far as to describe her in one memorable put-down phrase as 'a curious mixture of Mae West, Mother Teresa and Arkle!' – referring, I assume, to her particular blend of brassy sexuality, campaigning self-righteousness and public popularity.

But she has not been content with burrowing around amidst public failure, incompetence and waste, championing the needs of the ordinary and highlighting the oddities and eccentricities of men and women of all ages. She has quite deliberately exploited her own experiences – marrying a divorced man, delivering her first child, the problems of breast-feeding in public, suffering post-natal depression, the dilemma of career versus motherhood – these have all been described and analysed by her in the public arena. With her husband, Desmond Wilcox, she has talked in the tabloid press about their relationship, their mutual feelings, their lives together, right down to which of them does the flower arranging. Psychologically it is a performance not without its risks. One is that the very element that public life demands of you, namely the element of acting, of putting on a show, of adopting a public mask or persona oozes into your private, intimate, personal life. The dividing line melts away. Questions then arise including the thorny issue of authenticity. When I meet people like Esther Rantzen I, like others, have difficulty knowing when the performance ends and the real person begins. The difficulty is compounded if the individual concerned appears to draw no clear demarcation between what they actually do in public, for a living as it were, and what goes on in the privacy of their personal lives with their families, friends, their leisure, their own space, inside their heads. In the case of a Colin Blakemore or Bernard Knight or Lisa St Aubin de Teran, even in the case of a politician such as Bernie Grant, the differentiation between the public and the private can be made with varying degrees of success. Such individuals rarely accept the invitation or exploit the opportunity to turn the private into the public. When they do, it is usually within quite circum-scribed limits and occurs relatively infrequently. With someone of the make-up and status of Esther Rantzen it is extremely difficult because she immediately sees the private in terms of the public, and the opportunities afforded to her to make something publicly happen arising out of her own personal life are many, varied and tempting. With the eye of the seasoned veteran public broadcasting campaigner that she is, she quickly spots the media potential of her own everyday life. The public world of camera cables and arc lights, of microphones and clapper boards regularly invades the private world of hearth and home and holiday. In turn, the everyday, the minutiae as well as the dramatic moments of her life, become public property. Her husband, an accomplished media professional in his own right, is accustomed to it all and appears to flourish. Her children are as yet too young to be greatly inconvenienced. But the problem, of distinguishing what does not properly belong to the world and what does, remains.

She has the media, particularly broadcasting, in her genes and blood. Her father was head of engineering design at the BBC in the time of Lord Reith. All her professional life, following her period at university, has been in broadcasting. She is a doughty defender of public service broadcasting and the BBC. She is, too, a performer down to her fingertips. She did once have ambitions to be an actress. To a very obvious extent she is one. Her teeth, her hair, her smile that is flashed so blindingly on and off are public property. There is, not surprisingly, considerable curiosity as to what she is really like.

The commonest question raised about Esther Rantzen is whether she is as concerned about things as she looks? Is she sincere? It is a hellishly difficult question to answer about consummately professional performers. Was it not George Burns who quipped that the one thing a good actor needs is sincerity; once you can fake that you can fake anything. By definition, superbly faked sincerity cannot be detected save by comparing thoughts with actions and actions with thoughts. In the case of Esther Rantzen it is very much easier to assess the actions. Esther Rantzen is all action. She has helped raise millions for a plethora of good causes, has badgered and lectured and hectored the nation about its treatment of children, has made headlines over deficiencies in transplant surgery and the inadequacy of cancer screening. Her heart, judging by her actions, is in the right place.

And her thoughts? This is much more difficult. Right from the beginning of the interview we run into a problem. She insists she is not an introspective person. She is another of those many people who prefer to be constantly on the hop, moving from one issue to another, not pausing too long to think about motives or purposes or meaning. She instinctively identifies who she is with, what she is up to – there is a moment in the interview when she responds to a question as to what she is like by answering in terms of how she is doing. Her image of life is revealing too – a fast, dangerous and precarious car journey where she, the driver, is busy, preoccupied with focusing intently on the journey ahead and only has the occasional, snatched moment to 'look at the scenery as well'. It is an image of pressure, tension, concentration, movement. One slip could be fatal and everything would be over. But she is in the driving seat. It is all up to her. She does see herself in control – which indeed is as others see her. Esther Rantzen is often described as the boss, in charge, driving other people. Some of these other people quite like it. Others clearly do not. But, as she might say, that's life.

The problem is that within such a model of life everything, even a brief radio interview, becomes a potential hole in the road. And Esther Rantzen does come across as a very wary person. She does not relax. She concentrates hard on the task in hand. Words are chosen with care. There is a sense of someone who expects at every moment something to happen. There is much talk about looks, about being fat once upon a time, about vanity, clothes, attractiveness, appearances. But attractiveness, or how others see us, is as much a factor of what we let people see of what we are like inside as it is of how we appear on the surface. And if you are given to spending a considerable proportion of your life in the public eye you learn to keep your innermost thoughts to yourself. If the private shrinks and the public expands, it becomes difficult to reclaim the private. Psychiatrists and psychologists are sometimes accused of reducing everything to a relative handful of impulses, drives, desires, emotions. Perhaps that is why we are termed 'shrinks'. But it is not an entirely unreasonable thing to do. Ours is a narcissistic and voyeuristic world in which for some it can be difficult to be entirely sure one privately exists without some validation from the public world. Life can be lived in the full glare of the marketplace.

She does appear sensitive to the suggestion that she is controlling. She responds, like many career women, by defensively pointing out that men in equivalent positions are rarely taxed with such an issue. That may be so. Indeed it was often said of another powerful woman, Margaret Thatcher, that she was the focus of much bitchy comment about bossiness merely because she was a woman. There is some truth in the argument. But it is not the whole argument. There have been male figures – one thinks of Richard Crossman, Denis Healey, Robert Maxwell – whose bullying tendencies and arrogant manner have provoked public criticism. It seems reasonable to subject a tendency to bully and manipulate to analysis and criticism whether it be indulged in by women or by men, especially, if there is the view that for women to succeed in hitherto male preserves such as journalism, politics or medicine they have to behave like proxy machismo males.

But in the final analysis Esther Rantzen accepts the blurred divide between public and private. She relishes her fame and her fortune. The doubts are put away and it is back to Childline and the next campaign, perhaps about death! The ultimate programme one might say.

CLARE: Esther Louise Rantzen was born on the June 22nd, 1940 in Berkhampsted, Hertfordshire. She comes from a middle-class Jewish family. Her father, Harry, was a senior BBC engineer and her mother, Catherine, was a governor of a day nusery in the East End. She was educated at North London Collegiate School and Somerville College, Oxford, where she gained a Second Class Honours Degree in English. After university she joined the BBC and had a number of jobs in radio and television before she became a reporter/researcher on the then highly successful *Braden's Week*. The rest, as they say in Hollywood, is history. *That's Life* has made Esther Rantzen a household name.

In 1975 it transpired that, to quote the *Sunday Express*, Miss Ranzten was in love with Desmond Wilcox, then head of general features at BBC television, and, as such, her boss, who was living apart from his television director wife. After his divorce, they were married in 1977. They now have three children, two daughters, Emily and Rebecca and a son, Joshua. Love her or loathe her, and there are quite a few people who do both, Esther Rantzen is one of the most enduring top television performers and effective campaigners in Britain. After having been television personality of the year several times she was awarded an OBE in 1990 for her services to journalism.

Esther Rantzen, are you anxious about being interviewed about yourself?

RANTZEN: Yes. I think I am.

CLARE: Because?

RANTZEN: I'm not a very introspective person. I tend to think a lot about what I'm trying to do but not a great deal about my own responses to that and it worries me as a subject.

CLARE: Go on.

RANTZEN: I don't know what interests you about me. If you discover things which you will be able to take away and find useful, then that's a good thing.

CLARE: So why do you do it?

RANTZEN: Why am I doing this? Do you want the truth? Well the truth is that your producer Michael Ember is an old friend, that I worked with him in the wireless with great pleasure on a programme called *Start the Week* and that he told me that he thought I should do it and as I respect him a great deal as a producer I thought OK.

CLARE: The little I know of you does suggest to me that you don't do things unless you want to.

RANTZEN: I think that's probably right, it's true of most people, if you've got the choice you choose what you want to do but in this particular case, I also think that there's a bit of loyalty, a bit of friendship and curiosity.

CLARE: About yourself?'

RANTZEN: If I'm to be truthful, more about you. I want to see what you ask me. I'm very interested in why you're interested.

CLARE: Does that mean you're not interested in you? Or in what drives you, what keeps you going?

RANTZEN: Sometimes I do ask myself questions. I think anybody who has the kind of life I have, in which work takes up an enormous amount of time but there are other enormous emotional pulls in my life, has to say, 'Well, why am I doing this, have I got the balance right?' So to that extent, I do ask why I make the work choices I do and so on. But other questions I think about what my own motives are, I don't think I'm very good at analysing.

CLARE: Why are you such a worker, why do you work so hard?

RANTZEN: Because I find it very, very exciting. I find ideas and communication and discovering a story, in a journalistic sense, a tremendous challenge. I find the work very difficult, it never becomes easy so it never becomes boring and I think to be able to bring information and entertainment to a large number of people is such a challenge that if you get it right, and I don't believe I do get it right, but if I get it any where near right, then that's terribly exciting too. It's very rewarding.

CLARE: So what are you like when you're not working? Are you ever not working?

RANTZEN: Yes, absolutely. There are times when I take right off from work in the sense that I potter round a country cottage kitchen or I take the dogs for a walk, talk to my children, go to a school play whatever it is. But I would say that even those experiences sometimes get absorbed back into my work so that I'm very aware that I don't, if you like, put a damp proof course between my life and my work, it all seems to be melded into one.

CLARE: If we replaced work and non-work with private and public would that be true as well?

RANTZEN: I was actually just thinking, when I was thinking about this programme, because people said, 'Are you sure you want to answer questions about the private you,' and so on, and I was reflecting on how much of my life, my personal life, has been lived publicly. It's odd, it's an odd adult life I've had. But I don't really mind that. There have been some emotional upheavals in my life. I had post-natal depression after the birth of my first baby when I found the presence of journalists – I remember, I didn't know then, but I was just getting post-natal depression, and I'd just had my first baby and I remember looking at a phalanx of photographers who were all telling me how to hold the baby, 'Hold her up, hold her down, can you make her wink?' and I can remember the stress that was but that's quite unusual.

CLARE: You didn't have the privacy?

RANTZEN: You're right.

CLARE: Why?

RANTZEN: At that moment?

CLARE: Yes?

RANTZEN: Well, it didn't become public at the moment when the photographers were flashing light bulbs at me. That was just a picture of the baby. It was actually at the request of the BBC press office who were actually getting a lot of enquiries and once you've got that first photograph over then people get a bit bored with you so it was a good idea, I agreed with him. The fact that I had post-natal depression came out later and it came out actually because I was talking about it to a television producer friend of mine who decided to make a documentary about it. I think it was in the *Man Alive* series and she asked me if I would talk about it. I wasn't the only person who was, so to speak, comparatively well-known who had suffered from the illness but I was the only one who would agree to speak about it. I thought that was interesting. I hadn't realised up to that moment what a stigma mental illness is. And I therefore did think it was important to come out, so to speak. It was also a very educational experience for me because it taught me that there isn't a hard and fast line, as you know but I hadn't known, between so-called normality, and psychiatric illness. I realised that if you like, we're all somewhere on that scale and to be on the wrong side of that scale for a bit was actually a very salutary experience for me.

CLARE: Was that the first time that you'd been, if you like, the other side of the divide?

RANTZEN: Yes. It was the first time that my own responses and reactions surprised me and threw me. People would ring me up and say how are you and I wouldn't be able to speak because I'd find myself in tears, irrational tears. I should have been happy, lovely new baby and so on. My physical reactions were different. I remember putting a hand to my face, I remember this very clearly, and feeling my own fingernails and thinking, 'It feels like someone else's hand,' so I was thrown by all those natural responses that I wouldn't even think about.

CLARE: Were you thrown by having a baby? That was a decision you made quite late. You were in your late thirties and I wondered how difficult that was. You were, you are a very difficult, busy, competitive person. This is a disruptive event in the life of most people but particularly, I would have thought, somebody such as yourself who would have had to have a fair amount of control of your life prior to all of this just to keep you going.

RANTZEN: Well, in a funny way I haven't. I haven't ever planned my life. I never really thought that I would find someone who would love me enough to want to marry me. I never thought that I would have the enormous pleasure of a family of my own, although I always rated it an enormous pleasure.

CLARE: Why did you say that you'd never thought you would ever find someone who loved you?

RANTZEN: For a very conventional reason that when I was a teenager I was quite fat, quite plain – never have been beautiful – and even in those unpermissive times, when you know there wasn't tremendous freedom, nevertheless, there were parties, there was dating and I was aware that other girls my age were sophisticated and pretty and popular with boys. So although I had lots of friends, I never really thought of myself as the sort of girl that boys will fall in love with or a woman that men would fall in love with. I never saw myself like that.

CLARE: How do you think that self perception affected you? What would you see as the residue of that in your character? What did it mean? How did you cope in adolescence with that reality, with that fact, if that's the way it was?

RANTZEN: Well, one thing I did and maybe it's something that fat girls do, is I realised that I'd better be entertaining 'cos no one else would want my company otherwise. So I tried to be entertaining. We used to run clubs and enjoy jokes and enjoy drama and it threw me into having fun and being able to communicate fun and having friendships on another level.

CLARE: Did that mean that for example, at teenage parties in the fifties you would have been a bouncy sort of person, extrovert?

RANTZEN: I think I was.

CLARE: Energetic?

RANTZEN: Yes, Yes.

CLARE: You would perform?

RANTZEN: With my friends, yes, with my friends. But I was physically very unconfident and rather shy with the opposite sex, so at parties I would sometimes end up in the loo or on the stairs with my sister.

CLARE: What was she like? Would she have been dumpy and plain too or was she attractive?

RANTZEN: Very pretty young woman, very slender little girl. Very concerned about the fact she was so small, sometimes bullied for her size. Independent intellectually. She was a scientist where I was on the arts side. I valued then and value still her judgement enormously.

CLARE: Was she more confident than you?

RANTZEN: If you saw us together she's the introvert and I'm the extrovert.

CLARE: How conscious did people make you of this aspect of yourself that you refer to? Did people around you, family, friends, remark on your fatness. Did fatness become an issue?

RANTZEN: Not like it is today. In those days I don't think I knew anyone with anorexia, I'd never heard of bulimia, there wasn't that sort of dieting madness. This was pre-Twiggy. Even so, I hated it and it made me feel very unsexy, unattractive. People were nice to me about it. My family never referred to it but I think any fat adolescent is very aware of it.

CLARE: Which of your parents were you more like? Your father was in the BBC, your mother was a governor of a school.

RANTZEN: I suppose I'm a mixture. My father had a tremendous intellectual drive and he in many ways guided me when I was really very little. He told me that the object of life was to learn as much as you could as long as you could and he kept that going until he was ninety, when he died. My mum has a sense of fun, tremendous family loyalty, always put my sister and me first, as they both did. So I've got this feeling of a family where children were prized and both of them gave us both a strong emotional security I think.

CLARE: Was it very Jewish?

RANTZEN: Not very Jewish in the sense of orthodox Judaism because both my parents were rather unorthodox Jews. My father believed in God but didn't really believe in any kind of religious services much. I believe he probably prayed but prayed his own way in his own time. We're liberal Jews so that means that we didn't actually have a kosher home. I was brought up on an egg and bacon breakfast and I was brought up very, very English, British, English, to respect British institutions, democracy, parliament, the BBC, the royal family. My mum's a great royalist. So there was an absolute identification with Britain. But we felt very Jewish at the same time.

CLARE: And what Jewish memories do you have? What do you think of as the Jewish characteristics?

RANTZEN: Well, I suppose when I say I felt Jewish, I became aware of anti-semitism and racial prejudice quite early on in my life. I was born at the beginning of the Second World War. I was five when it ended and then the huge, hideous discoveries of the concentration camps and what really had been going on in Nazi Germany were proclaimed to the world. Of course, I didn't know that when I was five but I became aware of it as I grew up and I know that in my teens I read a lot of literature from survivors of the camps. I remember, we grew up in North West London, I remember seeing concentration camp survivors.

CLARE: Would your parents have talked about it?

RANTZEN: The first school I went to, before I went to North London Collegiate School, the headmistress was anti-semitic and I was moved from that school because of that anti-semitism and moved to North London Collegiate School where Jewish girls were treated as just ordinary pupils and there was quite a big community of them.

CLARE: What was Jewish about your home?

RANTZEN: Well, my mother was one of four daughters, all four daughters lived within five miles of their mother. My maternal grandmother was a dominant figure in the our whole family, not because she was a traditional, dominant matriarch. She was actually cuddly and gentle. She adored children. She was funny. She and I had a very close relationship. It was quite funny, really, looking back. By the time she'd had her first two daughters, she was trying for a boy. She loved her first two daughters, so she had a third daughter. She tried once more for a boy and she got a fourth daughter and the family story is that she called that daughter Jane because she was so furious and it was the plainest name she could think of and Jane was so lovely and such a beautiful little girl that Jane became my grandmother's favourite name. Similarly, I was her oldest granddaughter, and you would think of a lady that had had four daughters that she would have had enough of girls but absolutely not. She was delighted at long last to have a granddaughter and we had a very, very close friendship. I think, to answer your question, that it's quite Jewish for a family to be so cohesive and so close to each other physically, geographically, emotionally.

CLARE: It's very female?

RANTZEN: Very female. The daughters did actually get married and had sons as well but, yes, there was a very strong female influence.

CLARE: And how much did that affect you? You described yourself growing up in adolescence relatively shy, certainly of the opposite sex, there weren't too many boyfriends, or so I'm suspecting, but when you went to university, when you went up to Oxford, did you change or were you still the shy, reserved person that you describe?

RANTZEN: Well, I think, shy.

CLARE: Were you still fat?

RANTZEN: Yeah, I was. I wasn't actually shy and reserved – I joined theatre groups and wrote for reviews and performed in them and directed one and thoroughly enjoyed all the theatrical life at Oxford and I ran our college ball, things like that, but I always thought that was a very odd – I was voted to do that by my Somerville colleagues and I always thought that was very odd because, as I say, I was never a romantic figure and I was never invited to a great many balls myself. But I think it was because they thought that I could probably make it an entertaining evening because if you're not very pretty but you enjoy company then you do have to be entertaining. I did gain confidence as I got older and and when I was at Oxford I think that in some senses I was quite confident by then.

CLARE: The recurrent theme is an interesting one – that the exuberant, public, extrovert Esther Rantzen owes a great deal to a very deliberate attempt to cope with the social impact of being fat and shy and unattractive in adolescence. That it was almost a deliberate way of coping with that. Relatively non-sexual, a way of relating to lots of people, would that be so?

RANTZEN: I think that's right, yes.

CLARE: How much of that is tied up then with the sense that some people describe, namely that when they are engaged in the public activity that that's the only time they really feel alive, that, if you like, that when they stop, they don't quite feel comfortable. They don't necessarily go back to feeling shy and fat but there's a residue of that feeling of not being quite right?

RANTZEN: You mean only really functioning when there's an audience, is that what you mean?

CLARE: When there's an audience or when you're busy, when you're doing. What you said at the very beginning of this interview – 'I'm not a reflective person' – that that's not related to your intelligence or your genetic make-up or whatever; rather it's related to the fact that reflection, in a way, is the opposite of engaging. You're very wary of it. I sense that this is not really, to use that dreadful phrase, 'your bag', that you would much prefer to be writing a script before the camera than doing this. Looking at these kind of things is not something that makes you feel particularly comfortable?

RANTZEN: That's absolutely right. I would much rather you and I were engaged together in making a programme about an external subject that we both felt very strongly about. That I would much rather be doing. Yes, that's right. If I sit myself somewhere I need to be absorbed in a book or listening to a piece of music. My ideal is to sit with a child and my husband, quietly, but what I would not be doing then, I think, is reflecting. I would be reading or wrestling with some problem or both. I don't turn my attention inwards and I also hate being alone, I really hate being alone.

CLARE: Go on, because I sense you are not alone very often. I went to interview you once in your garden in Hampstead and the image I have is a table at which you'd been sitting and a television cable running across this grass and the sense that, attractive and all as this house was, it really was as public an arena as the BBC!

RANTZEN: Yes. My home has been compared with Piccadilly Circus, only slightly more traffic in my home, I think.

CLARE: And you like Piccadilly Circus?

RANTZEN: I rather do. My sister looked with some interest at my lifestyle and said it's really a commune and I like that, that is right.

CLARE: And being on your own, can you recall for me a time when you've been on your own for any length of time?

RANTZEN: Well, I went on holiday by myself once but then I immediately fell into company and so that doesn't count. I don't go for walks on my own. I need someone beside me, I need to share things. I find it very difficult to enjoy beautiful surroundings if there's nobody there to say, 'Gosh, look at that.' I find it very difficult on my own.

CLARE: You've never felt the need to be on your own?

RANTZEN: Very seldom. If Desmond and I have had a free and frank exchange of views between us I will sometimes try and stamp away somewhere else and sulk. He will not let me. I really think it's a marvellous trait in him because I think sulking is what destroys relationships. So he follows me and he says to me, 'Come on, what is this about?' and those are the only occasions in my life when I sometimes need a moment just to muster my own thoughts and I'm very grateful not to be allowed that moment 'cos I think it could turn into a sulk. But apart from that, I really don't want to be alone at all.

CLARE: Do you know what people think of you?

RANTZEN: Well, I read it occasionally when I can't avoid it.

CLARE: Do you try and avoid it?

RANTZEN: Yes, I try and avoid it. I do. I think people who say they can't be hurt by criticism are lying either to themselves or to other people. I've learnt that I can be hurt. I've also learnt that it's not necessarily constructive pain. Sometimes you learn things about yourself and you can put them right but only too often I find when people write about me, they are not things that I can do anything about. A gentleman columnist once started a column 'Hideous Esther Rantzen'.

CLARE: What about descriptions of your character? I've read a variety of things about you. It's not easy to get a hold of a consistent picture. I wondered how you would describe yourself? Some of the adjectives people use include energetic, driving, extrovert, demanding, perfectionist. Some would throw in the more critical ones – overbearing, very dominating. What would you pick out? I often ask this of people who come to me clinically – how would they describes themselves if they had to, if they had to write down a description. What kind of things would you say about yourself, now that you've got an opportunity? Because you, supposedly anyway, know yourself better than these people who write the public reviews?

RANTZEN: The problem is that I can't really describe myself. I can describe what I do and if you ask me how I rate what I do and what's the most important thing that I do.

CLARE: Yes, but I won't do that.

RANTZEN: All right, then.

CLARE: Because other people do it all the time.

RANTZEN: But it is very difficult.

CLARE: Don't they? People will talk to you that way. I've seen endless interviews with you. I've even done one myself about *Childline* and *That's Life* and your BBC career which is spectacular. I'm much more interested to know you, the person who is behind all of that and that's why I say to you, 'OK, well, how would you describe yourself?' and when you say you won't, is that because you can't, that you actually find it very difficult to back away from the image, because you're very good at describing what other people describe you as?' You used the word hideous. I would never, bad and all as this programme is, I wouldn't have done that, but you did it. I may have missed it, but I'm sure you're right, somebody probably did. They say awful things about people, but given that that's what they say and clearly it's untrue, what would you say about yourself?

RANTZEN: As a human being?

CLARE: Well, what else are you, Esther?

RANTZEN: Well, I'm a series of functions, aren't I? I'm a wife, I'm a mother, I'm a television producer, I'm a journalist, I'm a presenter, I'm chairman of *Childline*. You say I'm a campaigner. I'm a woman who is growing older. I've got to adjust my life and change. I've got to develop, if you like, into old age and all that. It's a bit like driving a car. Life is precarious and dangerous and goes very fast so you look at the road ahead and if you've got a moment you look at the scenery as well. You try and not crash into too many others. You try and get where you're going and suddenly the person, nice person who's sitting next to you looking with faint interest at your journey, says, 'Yes, but what kind of person are you, Esther? and I say to you, 'Ask me the end of this journey.' I don't know really. I can tell you that I'm trying to drive like this and I drive on the left. Do you see what I mean? It's very hard for me to say, I can tell you the things I would like to be. I can tell you that I would like to be a loyal friend. I would like to be the kind of mum that my children will remember with pleasure, maybe all their lives. I would love that. I would love to be a wife that lives up to my husband, who is a very extraordinary person. Those are my ambitions if you like. But don't ask me how well I'm doing because the answer is never well enough.

CLARE: But I didn't.

RANTZEN: You said what kind of human being am I.

CLARE: I didn't ask you how well you're doing, but taking that image, which is a very interesting one, of driving a car, I sensed that in a way you feel that to think about what we're doing is to risk messing up the doing of it. You said, 'Ask me it when we get to the end.'

RANTZEN: Yes. And the tougher it is and the more difficult it is, the less I want to know about my own difficulties.

CLARE: Was being fat very painful?

RANTZEN: Yes, but a lot of people go through it.

CLARE: True, and I interview some of them, but it's you who's here at the moment. How painful was it?

RANTZEN: Not painful enough to blight my life.

CLARE: No?

RANTZEN: I sometimes wonder if it wasn't the best thing that happened in the long run. Someone said to me, 'Why is it that beautiful women have tragic lives?' and I thought about that and maybe it's like being a beautiful flower that knows it's going to fade, knows that it can't be beautiful for ever, knows that the butterflies and the bees will go to the flower next door. Whereas, if you are a cabbage or a lettuce you're nutritional as well. I sometimes think that it's very useful for girls to go through an ugly duckling phase because then they discover who they really are, what their skills are, who they rate in terms of the people round them. I think to be fat from the age of fifteen to twenty-five is very tough because that's when you're most sensitive about what people think of you. Actually about the time I got a television job I really adored I suddenly looked in the mirror and I thought, 'Stop envying people, this is is what you're stuck with, this is who you are, live with it.'

CLARE: Was Desmond your first love?

RANTZEN: No.

CLARE: So when did you get a sense that you weren't fat and unattractive?

RANTZEN: Well, I've never felt attractive.

CLARE: Well, you said that you were surprised that you found a man who loved you.

RANTZEN: That's right.

CLARE: And that's why I assumed that Desmond was the first.

RANTZEN: Who loved me enough to marry me and commit like that. I stopped feeling fat when I lost weight and that was when I was twenty-five. I suppose up to then I had thought that that would solve all my problems. To my interest, I found it didn't. Presenting on television, in *Braden's Week*, meant that I had to look quite a lot at myself, more, I think than people in other jobs have to do. I changed my hair colour because it looked better on television to be blonde than brunette.

CLARE: You were a brunette?

RANTZEN: I am underneath. You're looking at a 10 stone brunette underneath this 8 1/2 stone blonde. That's who I really am.

CLARE: So in one sense, you have reconstructed yourself?

RANTZEN: I reconstructed my hair colour, that's right.

CLARE: What else did you change, if that's not too personal a question?

RANTZEN: No, it's not. I didn't think you minded about personal questions on this programme?

CLARE: Oh, there are boundaries to everything.

RANTZEN: Are there . . . another illusion shattered! Clothes. I changed my attitude to clothes. The real Esther Rantzen would live in a tracksuit. In fact for many years I did live in a tracksuit and my colleagues and friends used to get so bored because it was either the purple one or the pink one. But I got taken in hand by BBC designers who said, 'come on, you can do better than this,' and I was aware that people do judge you by the way you look. You know, they do for some unfair reason rate you more highly if you're neat and tidy and not in the same jumpsuit. When I first appeared on television on *Braden's Week*, I literally wore the same dress every week until a viewer rang in, a man, and said, 'Please can Esther wear something else?' So I had to do something about that. I still find it difficult to concentrate on looking good.

CLARE: Do you find it difficult to choose clothes?

RANTZEN: I find it difficult to choose clothes, yes.

CLARE: And so you'd prefer the casual?

RANTZEN: Yes.

CLARE: What was the difference in the way people reacted to you when you changed these various attributes?

RANTZEN: Oh, it was quite fun. Oh, it was really fun. Some of the people that I'd been at university with suddenly met me again and couldn't believe it. There was the dumpy, fat brunette and what had happened? I remember meeting a particular person in Television Centre and him stopping and staring at me and saying 'Esther, is that really you?'

CLARE: So they did behave differently?

RANTZEN: Absolutely.

CLARE: It has been remarked, apropos of *That's Life* in particular, that you control men and that those around you tend to be male. It's interesting the extent to which you have a certain style which exudes control, influence, dominance. Is that fair?

RANTZEN: No. But it's interesting. I've looked at that concept because journalists have sometimes accused me of being anti-women and never having women on the show which is factually not true. We have from Victoria Wood through to Molly Sugden. But it does interest me because as you've pointed out a little while ago, there was a quite strong female influence in my family – three generations of matriarchy and none the worse for that, but very nice men I did point out, married into it and enjoyed it and paid tribute to those women, my grandmother and my aunts.

CLARE: But would they have been powerful, Jewish matriarchs?

RANTZEN: Powerful people in the sense of intelligent and strongly holding their families together. Very committed to their families.

CLARE: As you are, as you would be?

RANTZEN: I hope I am, yes.

CLARE: So, continue, I interrupted you. So in relation to women and men now?

RANTZEN: Yes, well, the programme at the moment has a woman editor and a woman deputy editor and me so that is quite an interesting female triangle. The rest of the team – I haven't actually counted the number of people it's got, the men reporters working alongside me. Adrian and Gavin who are the main presenters with me are friends. I rely on their talent and skills. They are completely committed to the show and I don't care what gender they are and I don't think viewers do either. I think that what transmits from them is how good they are at their work. We audition men and women. We were consciously looking for women the last time, as it happened. The viewers voted for the presenter who is now with us, the newest presenter who is a Scot and a man. I'm aware that it's nice to have both genders on the show and I hope we will.

CLARE: So in fact, you are beginning to describe yourself and the characteristics, attributes you have. You bubble, you can be volcanic, you express your feelings, you like company, you're wary of isolation, being on your own. You've emphasised you're Jewish. Now, has that changed over the years? Have you, as we all do who come out of strong cultures, we go through phases and some go in one direction and some in others, but my understanding is that you still regard yourself not just as ethnically Jewish but as religiously Jewish. Is that right?

RANTZEN: Well, I'm an agnostic. I find it difficult to be definite about God and the afterlife and things but I will say that the only religion that makes sense to me spiritually is the rigidly monotheistic Judaism. Having been brought up in it and with that extraordinary, odd, painful, fascinating history behind it, I could never turn my back on it and my children are fascinated by it too.

CLARE: Have you brought them up as Jews?

RANTZEN: Yes, they're more orthodox than me now.

CLARE: But you married a gentile.

RANTZEN: He was. He's converted. He's now Jewish. I went to all that trouble to marry out and now look where it got me. That's a Jewish joke!

CLARE: I know. I'm stunned!

RANTZEN: You were surprised, yes. I was surprised.

CLARE: Were you?

RANTZEN: Yes, absolutely. Jews are not evangelical. We make it quite difficult for people to convert to Judaism.

CLARE: Perhaps you are evangelical?

RANTZEN: Do you think I am?

CLARE: I don't know. I'm asking.

RANTZEN: No, I'm not, excuse me saying so. No. But Desmond has actually married two Jewish women in his time. His partner was Jewish, created *Man Alive* with him. He has a tremendous feeling for Jews.

CLARE: Do you think people can become Jewish?

RANTZEN: Yes. It's difficult to become Irish, I admit, but you can become Jewish.

CLARE: How?

RANTZEN: Well, he learnt Hebrew. He studies all the Jewish festivals, Jewish observance. He had to do a little exam, had to write an essay. I went along. I had to keep my mouth firmly shut because I wasn't at all sure, being an agnostic about some of the things. He was much surer than me. But more than that, he has as much a feeling for family, for education, for the protectiveness, if you like, of children. He adores my family events and occasions. He even takes my mother on holiday. That's ever so Jewish. Would you take your mother-in-law on holiday? Do you do that?

CLARE: Well, she's eighty something or other now, but yes. I haven't taken her on holiday. She's come to stay with us on holiday.

RANTZEN: Not the same.

CLARE: No and if that's a criteria of being Jewish I think I've probably failed! But I'm asking you, a Jew, whether in your heart you believe it can be done?

RANTZEN: Someone become Jewish?

CLARE: Yes.

RANTZEN: I do, yes, I do believe that because I believe in the partnership of people. I don't believe that people are separate from each other. I don't believe there is something about black people, or Irish people which separates them and makes them fundamentally and in their heart and soul apart, divided for ever. I think we can cross those bridges.

CLARE: How important were you to Desmond becoming Jewish? You didn't become a gentile. He became a Jew.

RANTZEN: That is true but I did not want him to be Jewish. The last thing in the world I would want to do is convert my husband.

CLARE: Is that true?

RANTZEN: Yes.

CLARE: Why do you say that?

RANTZEN: Because religion is the most personal decision anyone can take. I wouldn't dream of trying to persuade him.

CLARE: But you see, interestingly enough, when you were describing him becoming a Jew, I wasn't struck by it as a religious decision. I was struck by what was almost a cultural, ethnic, historical tradition. They were the things you pointed to because you yourself are not particularly religious.

RANTZEN: No, but Desmond is. I've told you, he's more orthodox than me and he really loves Passover and Hanukah, the Jewish festivals. He loves the biblical stories. He loves the history of it. But he also is ferociously protective about the minority. He was terribly aware of anti-semitism. He's got into fights protecting Jews and I think he wanted, if you like, to stand up and be counted, not just on behalf of Jews but he wanted to be one too.

CLARE: Do you dream much?

RANTZEN: No, except when pregnant.

CLARE: And?

RANTZEN: Then I had completely wild dreams.

CLARE: Recurrent?

RANTZEN: Well, I'm not pregnant all that often! The pregnancy recurs and the dreams recur.

CLARE: No, I meant was it a similar dream or are they just all over the place?

RANTZEN: I can't remember.

CLARE: No?

RANTZEN: I can't really remember. They were pretty lurid I think.

CLARE: When you were depressed, were you more reflective?

RANTZEN: Yes, absolutely. I didn't know what was happening to me.

CLARE: Did you worry that you might lose absolute control?

RANTZEN: I worried that the depression would never lift.

CLARE: Did you worry that you might kill yourself?

RANTZEN: I worried that I would never be well again. I asked my health visitor, who is now a close friend, what was the difference between what I had, because she told me it was different, and the full psychosis and she told me how severe it could be and that sort of gave me some kind of comfort. But I never felt suicidal.

CLARE: You didn't?

RANTZEN: No, I was just completely miserable.

CLARE: Have you ever felt that you can't go on?

RANTZEN: Yes. Once at university I felt that.

CLARE: For long?

RANTZEN: It was during a period of a lot of exams and I just thought I couldn't cope with it.

CLARE: How do you cope? I'm told you work a ninety-hour week. How do you cope? What's driving you?

RANTZEN: Usually I'm responding to a set of deadlines, challenges, things I have to make or do. Maybe I create these but it's not a sort of internal clock, constantly ticking and pushing me forward. I feel as if I'm being challenged and pulled forward by the things that need to be done.

CLARE: Do you ever get the feeling that there is nothing you couldn't do?

RANTZEN: Sadly, no. I would very much like that feeling but I'm only too aware of what I can't do.

CLARE: Such as?

RANTZEN: I would love to be able to create a television programme so good that it would last in people's memories. *Childline* is the most important thing I've ever been associated with. I would love to have achieved a position where it was financially secure and answering all the children who need it. That would be wonderful. I would love to be in two places at once most of my life so that I can not only be here in the studio but I can be with my oldest daughter who's gone to a performance of a play tonight and that applies to most of my life.

CLARE: That last one, do you feel torn a lot?

RANTZEN: Yes, I really do. The more so since I've heard children on the *Childline* phoneline talking about their loneliness and a lot of them are children whose parents don't have time, either because it's a broken marriage and the new partner doesn't like the child, doesn't want the child, the child's in the way or because mum's at work a lot. I remember talking to a teenage boy who was telling me something very serious in his life and I said to him, 'Your mum would want to know, can't you find a moment to tell her?' and he said, 'Well when she gets home at nights she's so tired, she doesn't really want to listen.' So I said, 'What about the weekends?' and he said, 'She works weekends.' I have always wondered about Sunday opening hours since then. As a consumer journalist I ought to be campaigning for all the shops to open on Sunday but a bit of me wonders whether children suffer from the fact that mums more than dads are working on that Sunday in the shops.

CLARE: But when you heard that child, did it cause a pang in you?

RANTZEN: Absolutely.

CLARE: About the way you work?

RANTZEN: Yes, of course, and it worried me, and worries me very much. I am terribly concerned that all the pluses women have got now and, heaven knows, have fought for and heaven knows are deserved, the right to explore their own talent, their own potential to have equal terms in the workplace and so on. Who is putting the children first? Are the children falling between two stools now? Are men coming up alongside women to share parenting the way, actually, my husband does? And so while I'm thinking that about other children and other families, I'm very much worrying about it with my own family and my own children because, Dr Clare, there's no point being the most wonderful television presenter known to the British Isles if your children can't stand you and you've had no time to be with them. It's dust and ashes then.

CLARE: And does that worry you?

RANZTEN: Yes, of course, yes.

CLARE: But this is where our earlier discussion becomes crucial, the extent to which you drive in this car journey or are driven. You know, can you stop, get out, and look at the scenery or put the picnic out and talk to the children or do you have to keep going?

RANTZEN: I think I probably have to keep going a bit.

CLARE: Everyone says that.

RANTZEN: Mm.

CLARE: I hear myself say that.

RANTZEN: Yes.

CLARE: Everyone says, we have to keep going a bit.

RANTZEN: Well, let me give you a 'for instance'. There came a moment two years ago when I became aware that my children also had a five-day working week. Always, before, I was able to bring them into the office, I got knocked rotten for it and laughed at for it but they would come and have lunch with me in the canteen or whatever, but suddenly, they too were at school Monday to Friday and this meant weekends were terribly important and I was a person whose television programme on Sunday night had to be made on Sunday so I went to the BBC with some trepidation and I said, 'I'm sorry to ask you this but would it be possible for us to make *That's Life* on Fridays then I can have weekends with my children, that's actually something that we need as a family?' And they said yes. I think it was probably cheaper if the truth be known! I'm not denigrating their kindness. So that is what I have done. I have cut back, I will confess to you, though it means that I get less evenings with them than I did because the work that we used to do over the weekends has got to be squashed a bit into evenings.

CLARE: Taking your image, the car journey, do you think much about the destination, do you think much about death?

RANTZEN: I've had to recently a bit.

CLARE: Because?

RANTZEN: My father died in September. It was the first death I'd witnessed and been close to and I would love to die as he did. In fact, my father has in many ways been a role model, as has my mother but, bless his heart, he had his ninetieth birthday and the family was round him, the extended family, the cousins and aunts, and he sat there and I sat next to him and my sister had come back from Australia and he said to me,

'This is the happiest day of my life.' Imagine being able to say that at ninety and he was then quite ill and he spent the last two weeks of his life putting everything in order. There was some Mahler pieces of music that I didn't own that he cared about so he gave me CDs of them and we played them at his funeral. And he sorted out this and that and he wrote all his thank you letters and then he had a massive heart attack but he stayed alive long enough for me to get to him and we spent the last day. I wish doctors manage death better. I wish the doctor hadn't told me that I couldn't tell my father he was dying, that I had to keep the hope going, that I mustn't let him suspect because I wanted to say to him, really frankly, what he'd done for me all his life, what I felt for him and I had to sort of disguise it a bit. I had to say goodbye without saying goodbye. I said to him, 'You know you've created a wonderful family,' and he, who could barely speak, said, 'No, I didn't create it.' But he and my mother created it together. So I saw that death and I planned his funeral with the music, the Mahler, the *Songs of the Earth* and I put together some thoughts about him and I gave the eulogy for him because I knew I owed it to him, which was difficult to do. And then he was cremated, which is not very Jewish of us, we are not allowed to cremate really but we're liberal Jews, he was cremated and we miss him very much. But I look back at that death and I think that was a wonderful way to go, neatly and causing no pain to us. You know, it was what my father wanted, dignity and orderly death and if I could only achieve that, that would be wonderful.

CLARE: You don't fear death?

RANTZEN: I fear a long-drawn, bad death. I fear a death of the mind before the body dies. I fear senility. I fear all those things that distort your family's memories and your friends' memories, that's what I fear.

CLARE: When you were describing, just now, your father's dying and his death, there was a flash of public Esther as you suddenly emphasised the extent to which doctors kind of mess it up a bit. You talked earlier on about this porous boundary between private and public. I sometimes have this picture of you, Esther, that things that happen to you in your life, that you really have to resist the temptation to make a programme out of them, or a book or a public statement, that it could be said of you, something that I heard said of a rather public cleric back in Ireland, that he didn't have an unbroadcast thought in his head.

RANTZEN: Guilty. Guilty as charged. I haven't done a programme about the management of death. I've thought about it, because I think of it as something we have got to be looking at carefully, now that people in your trade can prolong life so long in a condition which really one wouldn't recognise as life. I think the moment of death is a very important subject and I have been alerted to it by my family experience. But fortunately, perhaps, for the British viewer and listener it is not my choice. You talk a lot about control and choice. I think it is because I'm female. If I were a man, you wouldn't think that I was dominating in quite this way. I'm actually an employee and that is all I am. If tomorrow the broadcasting authority, the BBC, ITV, decided I was box-office poison, then goodnight, dump her, hire a new one, they would do that without a backward glance. I understand that. That's the tightrope, the professional tightrope I choose to walk so I'm not in control. You use that word a lot.

CLARE: Esther Rantzen, thank you very much.

RANTZEN: Thank you.

Ruth Rendell

Ruth Rendell is one of the few people I interviewed whom I had met before. I first met her at a *Sunday Times* literary dinner and I was immediately impressed by her curiosity about people, her fascination for the unusual and seemingly irrational in human desire and behaviour, her ability to empathise and yet hold herself detached at once removed from the object of her interest. That is exactly how she seemed, at once enormously intellectually curious and alive while at the same time exuding a rather unsettling air of detachment and emotional control. I met her again when on the occasion of the publication of her then latest book, *The Crocodile Bird*, she accepted an invitation from me to talk about the mainsprings of her creativity in a programme in the *All in the Mind* series that I chair for BBC Radio 4. Her ability to slip effortlessly into the damaged mental states of her characters has long fascinated me. She does it well. Her maimed, disturbed, haunted characters are real. They do have their real-live counterparts in the people that I and some of my colleagues see.

Her theoretical framework interests me too. For Rendell, crime appears to start with the family. It starts with love or rather the lack of love. It starts with alienation. It is the family that is responsible for so much human misery and bitterness. Like so many who have had a somewhat loveless and fractured family life as a young child and adolescent she is pessimistic about the family as an institution capable of providing nurture and love. She herself is convinced that we need to find something better than the family although she is at a loss to know what that might be. She finds herself drawn to the dark side of human nature. All her own emotions, she insists, go straight into her fiction.

She is fond of quoting Arnold Bennett to the effect that humanity walks ever on a thin crust over terrifying abysses. The humanity that Ruth Rendell dissects in her novels certainly does. Her characters are the stuff of psychiatric clinics or, more accurately, forensic psychiatric clinics. In *A Demon in My View*, published in 1976, and *The Crocodile Bird*, which came out in 1993, the central characters are highly disturbed serial killers. In *Live Flesh* she explores the recesses of the mind of a sexual psychopath. In *Going Wrong* the central character is a murderous obsessive. Her world of crime is populated by rapists, child abusers, murderers but their seemingly bizarre, disconnected actions invariably have a coherence and a logic which only serve to make them more dangerous and frightening. She manages to make them comprehensible.

Where do all these dark, morbid fantasies come from? It is of course trite to assume that there is necessarily a strong psychological connection between the characters created by a writer and that writer's own personality, attitudes and beliefs. Nevertheless, given the intensity of Ruth Rendell's preoccupation with the obsessive, the psychotic, the psychopathic and her portrayal of the family as a place of secrets, untruths, distortions and defilements, it is irresistibly tempting to explore her own family experience and her own psychology for clues as to what it is that is going on when she starts to write. She herself is refreshingly open to such exploration. Indeed, she is disarmingly to the point when she declares that she feels that she has the ability to get under the skin of even the most repulsive of human beings. Making the irrational rational is what psychiatry is about. It is what Ruth Rendell is about in her own way too. It is not, she is at pains to make plain, the same as making excuses, even though, sadly, it is often mindlessly portrayed as such. Before the interview she told me that she does get letters from people who accuse her of being a monster because of her astonishing ability to get inside the head of a sexual abuser or a child murderer. It is the familiar confusion between the imagining and the act. Ironically, it is precisely this confusion which so tortures many an obsessional; he or she worries that the very thought of stabbing someone with a knife or shouting obscenities in a church or pushing a baby over a cliff *means* that this is what he or she wants to do and indeed will do. She says, 'To understand all is just to understand all.' She might as well have said to imagine all is just to imagine all. It does not mean to approve all or desire all or wish to commit all. Nor is it necessarily about forgiveness nor mitigation although neither is really possible without imagination and understanding.

At the present time, we are presented almost daily with some seemingly pointless act of violence – the Moors murders, Hungerford, the Gloucester serial killings, the James Bulger horror – and invariably, despite and after much public discussion and rumination, we are left as mystified and disconcerted as before. Rendell's novels serve to provide some kind of logical structure, some kind of philosphical framework within which such aberrations occur. It calls for a profound sympathy with the marginal, the outsider while at the same time it makes no attempt to reduce or simplify the horror and destructiveness of violence. She attributes this quality to her own outsider status, the only daughter of a Scandinavian mother and English father who did not make too happy a marriage and appeared to have left Ruth with her own personal array of fears and obsessions.

She is, for example, obsessed with time and agonises about being late. She is exceedingly obsessional too in terms of her writing, in the way she organises her writing, in the meticulousness with which she chooses the right word. She checks and rechecks. She worries about losing control. She is exceedingly sensitive. She finds it very difficult to make decisions. There is a compulsive aspect to her writing. She physically *has* to write. If she doesn't she feels unease, malaise, physically strange. She is in this respect like many a creative writer and like the obsessional who if he resists his particular compulsion, be it to wash his hands or count to a certain number, feels physcially unwell, anxious, threatened.

She feels she has inherited her pessimism, her expectation of the worst from her father, a man given to suspecting the motives of everyone around him. Her writing, she makes plain, is a process through which she can free herself, to an extent at least, of this paranoid tendency; it has also helped her realise the extent to which she is subject to it. And she makes an interesting distinction between the fairly orthodox detective fiction, the Inspector Wexford fiction, which she writes under her own name, and the 'psychological' fiction she writes under the pseudonym Barbara Vine. Whereas the classical detective story is about unravelling who has done what and in the process is about the restoration of stability and order to a disturbed world, the material she creates as Vine is concerned less with crime and detection and more with the mind, the motivation, the psychological profile of the perpetrator.

As with Colin Blakemore, Sir Colin Davis, Bernie Grant, Marjorie Proops and most of the other interviewees in this collection, I found myself touching on Ruth Rendell's religious beliefs. Her fiction conceives of a moral universe where virtue, whatever is being rewarded, is clearly preferred. Neither evil nor psychological instability is glamorised nor romanticised. We do not, it is true, discuss her particular beliefs. She is content to declare herself an Anglican and leave it at that. She is similarly fatalistic and matter-of-fact about death although this does not in any way prevent her from being anxious about dying.

There is, for me at any rate, a fascinating discussion of the extent to which writing for Ruth Rendell is essential for life, that she would in some sense die without it. It is clearly something of which she is aware. But what does it mean? Does she, for example, believe that the process of writing keeps an overwhelming fear at bay? She describes a recurrent dream whose content she cannot recall but from which she invariably wakes thinking that there is some medicine which is a matter of life and death and which she should have taken but hasn't. In the context of the rest of the interview it is hard to avoid the conclusion that it is writing that is the medicine that she cannot live without. In her conscious life she has never suffered from, let alone worried about, writer's block and indeed she is consistently productive. Perhaps it is only in her dreams that she can acknowledge the anxiety. But that particular speculative explanation only shifts the puzzle one station back down the line. What is it that she so powerfully fears as to make writing a compulsive therapeutic activity?

Ruth Rendell excavates her own past but she does it in the controlled and disciplined way of a creative artist. There are aspects of her past – the reason she left and returned and remarried her husband being one of the most important – which she prefers to leave covered up like some of the Victorian furniture she describes in one of her recurrent dreams. It will one day be uncovered, revealed, displayed, but not yet. Again and again there reverberates in the Rendell interview the motif of the past, of memories, of influences, which she is in the slow but seemingly remorseless process of analysing through her work. Her childhood sounds bleak and lonely. As a teenager she spent long periods of the day dreaming and splitting herself into the perpetrator of her actions and the simultaneous commentator on them. It can be a dangerous split but in her case it appears to have served her well, married as it has been to an exceptionally disciplined and creative imagination. She is one writer not at all reluctant to describe what she is about in her creative work as a form of personal therapy. In her dreams she does feel terrified by what she might discover, of what might lie under the sheets in the last room she enters. Her waking, conscious, creative fantasies do concern themselves with murderous impulses, with jealousy and deprivation, with lust, greed and pain. She worries about losing control but hardly ever does. She writes instead about ordinary people who for one reason or another are pushed over the edge. It could, she clearly indicates, happen to any of us. That is her terrifying fear about life. Given the right circumstances, the genes, the early childhood environment, the peculiar mix of neglect and abuse and deprivation and we could all do what her characters do. It is indeed a bleak vision. Who is to say it is not a true one?

CLARE: Much as she dislikes the journalistic soubriquet, Ruth Rendell is often referred to as the queen among the queens of crime. Whether she uses her real name or that of her alter ego, Barbara Vine, she is a highly prolific, imaginative writer who possesses a remarkable perception concerning the darker recesses of the human mind and the horrors of everyday life. She was born Ruth Grasemann on February 17th, 1930 in London, a Scandinavian mother, English father, both were teachers. She left school at eighteen and became a journalist on her local newspaper. At the age of twenty she married her husband, Don, a fellow journalist for the first time. In 1973 the marriage was dissolved but four years later she and Don remarried. At the age of twenty-three she gave birth to her only child, a boy and stopped working outside the home. For more than a decade she was a mother, housewife and unpublished writer. Her first book *From Doon with Death* was published when she was in her thirties and, since that time, she has written over forty books, most of them best-sellers, many translated into more than twenty languages and quite a few have been turned into films. She has an honoury doctorate from the University of Essex, is a fellow of the Royal Society of Literature. Among the many accolades she has received has been the Crime Writers' Association's Gold Dagger Award which she has been granted a record four times, the Cartier Diamond Dagger award and the *Sunday Times* Literary Award in 1990.

I admit I am one of her admirers. Indeed, I once wrote in a review that she has quite simply transformed the genre of crime writing. She deploys her peerless skills in blending the mundane, commonplace aspects of life with the potent, murky impulses of desire and greed, obsession and fear.

Ruth Rendell, you seem to me to be preoccupied with the sort of pulse beat of anxiety beneath the skin, the skeleton in the closet, the secret hidden within the smiling conspiracy of the so-called happy family, and so I wonder, are you a mystery to yourself?

RENDELL: No, I think, at the risk of sticking my neck out, I know myself rather well.

CLARE: Are you curious about what makes you do the things you do?

RENDELL: Yeah, I'm very curious. I have always been curious. I have a look and see what I'm doing when I do things, especially if I do something that I can stand aside and look at and think is strange and apparently inexplicable. I have a look and see why, or try to see why.

CLARE: That's been something that you've always done, as far back as you can remember?

RENDELL: No, that hasn't been something I've always done. That has been something I have done since I was an adult person. I certainly didn't do it as a child or a teenager or even as a very young woman. I did it later.

CLARE: There is an account I've seen somewhere that as a child you had a tendency to comment on your actions. Observing yourself doing things.

RENDELL: I believe that it's quite common among writers, because I read somewhere that Orwell did it and that he knew other people did it. When you are living your ordinary daily life you run in your head a monologue of description telling yourself, describing yourself in the third person as somebody else performing these acts and it seems to be the forerunner of writing, specifically writing fiction, with many people. And I did that. I did it a lot and I thought it was strange to do it but it didn't upset me. I wondered why I did it and it was a little bit of a relief when I read, not all that much later, that Orwell had done it and I thought, aha, I'm not alone.

CLARE: And how early do you remember doing that?

RENDELL: About seven, I think.

CLARE: And what kind of format would it take? What would you be saying or doing inside your head?

RENDELL: Oh, well, it would be, 'She got up from the table and went to the door and opened it and looked outside and saw that the sun was shining,' and, for example, if one is seven, 'That there was a rabbit on the lawn,' or something like that or that the cat had got up and walked across and so on, that stuff that is the stuff of fiction.

CLARE: And this would be as it was happening? This wouldn't be later on?

RENDELL: No, no, this would be while it was happening and then I would go on doing that until, of course, I would be interrupted by the intervention of somebody else coming to speak to me or something like that. But during my solitary time, a lot of my time would be spent doing that. I'm not saying all of it and it's very hard to calculate how much was spent, but quite a lot of it I think. I would say that it helped to make me happy.

CLARE: Helped to make you happy?

RENDELL: Yes, it made me satisfied. It made me feel that I was recording what I did without, then, a view to writing fiction, consciously, but it made me feel satisfied. It seemed to me to be the thing that one should be doing, telling oneself a story about oneself, or whatever one could, of course.

CLARE: You were an only child?

RENDELL: Yes.

CLARE: Did that mean you did spend large amounts of time on your own?

RENDELL: I think I must have done, yes, I think so. I seem to always have had a lot of friends, as I do today, and I think that is something to do with having been a solitary, an only child, seeking friends, but I must have spent a lot of time alone as any child does and much of that time I've filled with that kind of thing. Not only that kind of fiction, also, quite imaginary fiction telling myself stories about other things, of course, a long narrative voice would be there, proceeding in my mind for some time, half an hour, an hour perhaps.

CLARE: The account you give of recording your observation, should I say observing your behaviours, if somebody came into the room, would your narrative always be interrupted or would you then incorporate them? Would you ever describe in addition to what you yourself were doing, what other people were doing?

RENDELL: Oh, yes.

CLARE: How much did it become a kind of communal activity?

RENDELL: Oh, yes, anybody else would come in because they would simply be characters in the narrative. And so they would be described too and what they said, in fact, that would part of it. Expressing dialogue in some way with the intervention or interjection of 'he said' or 'she said' or whatever it might be or some exclamation and some change of expression or tone of voice.

CLARE: So from very early on you enjoyed observing people?

RENDELL: From very early on I enjoyed observing people. I think at that time especially adults, probably because I saw more adults then, at this early age, than I did children, although perhaps not, since I was certainly at school. I seem to have been, at that time, more interested in adults than in my contemporaries, though I'm sure that quickly changed.

CLARE: Did you tell anyone about that? You say you were reassured to read later that Orwell did it and other writers, but at the time, as a child growing up, did anybody know that going on in this little girl was this thought process, this commentary?

RENDELL: Oh, no, I wouldn't have told anybody.

CLARE: Because?

RENDELL: I would have felt that it was not a conventional thing to do and in many ways, I lived in a very conventional household and society. I felt, probably with justification, that what I was doing would be looked upon as unwise, perhaps even as unhealthy, so I wouldn't have talked about it.

CLARE: You say it was outwardly a conventional family, and inwardly, apart from this process that was going on in you, inwardly a conventional family or was it like some of the families in your works, not quite what it seemed?

RENDELL: I think it was not quite what it seemed. My mother, after all, was a Scandinavian, and we are speaking of something between fifty and sixty years ago. We're speaking of about fifty-five, fifty-six years ago and these things were looked on differently. Also my mother and her family, in spite of the fact that she taught in this country and she had gone to teachers' training college here, in spite of that I don't think she had become very English, whereas my father was very English. And this partly contributed to the great incompatibility between them. So, inside this apparently happy family, there was some dissension. This was not a happy marriage, though I was never short of love, there was plenty of that.

CLARE: For you?

RENDELL: For me.

CLARE: When you say your mother was very Scandinavian, what do you pick out as the characteristics that are Scandinavian, that were in your mother?

RENDELL: Well, she liked to speak her own language as much as she could, that is with her own family. She liked to read books in Danish because Danish was easier for her than Swedish though she was technically born a Swede. She liked to read Danish newspapers. She liked to eat Danish food and refer a great deal to the manners and habits of her family and her relations and this did not suit my father.

CLARE: It irritated him?

RENDELL: It irritated him. He, though a brilliantly clever, versatile man, and a most loving father, wanted everyone to be the same and of course he'd married a woman who was not the same.

CLARE: How had she come to be in England?

RENDELL: Her parents came here when she was fourteen and her oldest sister was sixteen and she had a younger brother and sister. My grandfather was always moving. I've written a book about this. In fact, he was always moving from country to country, trying to make some money.

CLARE: So, in fact, she was already an adolescent by the time she got here?

RENDELL: Yes, she was, yes. Speaking no English when she arrived and of course no great attention was paid to that as it is today. OK, you were plunged into a school where everybody spoke English and you did as best you could.

CLARE: You just got on with it. And what did she do when she left school, because she was presumably working when she met your father?

RENDELL: Yes, she was teaching. She was teaching and they taught in the same school.

CLARE: Oh, I see. And your father, you say, he liked everybody to be the same. In what way would that have affected you?

RENDELL: Well, I think that what I'm saying is that my father had very high standards. He wanted everybody to be very good at what they did. He wanted women to be specially good at those things which he would have thought of as a woman's province and men to be good, not only at their jobs but to be very good with their hands, such as he was himself. And he had wonderful manual skills. He used to say he would have liked to have built his own house. He never did but he could have, if he had the time. And my mother was totally undomesticated, so that was a hard thing for him. We had somebody, I had a nanny who also looked after us but my mother couldn't even boil an egg and he knew that when he married her, but yet, but yet. Whether they tried, I don't know but it made me a very insecure child because I loved all these three peple and I was afraid that one of them, or all of them would leave me. That is, I would be left with one. That I think was not an unrealistic fear.

CLARE: The three people, your mother, your father . . .

RENDELL: And my nanny.

CLARE: Yes.

RENDELL: Who was as much to me as my mother since she was with me from my babyhood and so I was afraid of losing one of them, I think as I say with justification. I didn't but I was always very, very frightened about this. So, I think that by telling myself these stories may have been a consolation.

CLARE: And when you say 'with justification', was that because occasionally threats were made by one or other to leave.

RENDELL: Oh, yes, of course, of course they always are in these circumstances, I think. Yes, they were always being made and you know, a child, of course, does not know how far to judge these threats, whether threats are real threats, whether they are idly uttered or, I think, they are mostly not idly uttered, I think that now and I thought so then, very much so.

CLARE: From which of them, if from either of them indeed, do you derive your imaginative talent?

RENDELL: Oh, from both my parents. My mother wrote poetry, she was a very good painter. She was very gifted. She had wonderfully good taste. My father wrote well and he was a great reader and he was a painter too, and very, very gifted in many ways. He was an extremely versatile man and, I think, he was the sort of person of whom is said, you know, anything they turn their hand to they would do well. So I think that if I have this I have it from them.

CLARE: Were they both very emotional people? Were the conflicts explosive and emotional or were they much more cerebral exchanges of disagreement. How was it verbalised?

RENDELL: Oh, it was emotional. You see, there again, it wouldn't appear to be so to anybody outside but inside, yes, and so I could never say that I was starved of emotion or that any of that was repressed. I saw plenty of that. There was always a great deal of arguing, quarrelling, shrieking, threatening and so on. Whether that is good I don't know but at any rate, there was no suppression of this kind thing.

CLARE: Has it made you a bit distasteful of that kind of emotional abreaction?

RENDELL: I don't think it has. Apart from saying that I don't think people ought to behave like that in front of children but that's a pretty usual reaction. I hope I didn't behave like that. I think they could have done better. Poor things, I think they had a hard time and I was extremely attached to them all but they had a hard time.

CLARE: What did they make of you, your parents? What did your father make of you? I wondered what kind of little girl you were. In the middle of all this, were you quite self-contained or did you give off the impression of weathering it all and taking it all?

RENDELL: I don't know, I don't know. I hated it, I think it may have been somewhat responsible for my living in the present now. I felt unable to look forward because I didn't know what would be in the future but . . .

CLARE: And looking back . . .

RENDELL: One thing I can say, when my father died, this is twenty years ago, after he died, he had, he had an extremely emotional deathbed, my father. A pretty good deathbed he had, I was very glad for him. After he died, a friend of his phoned and I said I hope you'll come to the funeral and I'd known him all my life and he said to me, 'Oh, yes, of course I'll come, you were a horrible little girl you know,' and I was flabbergasted by this and extremely distressed and angry, so there you are, perhaps I was a horrible little girl, that's what he thought I was.

CLARE: Did he say in what way it manifested itself?

RENDELL: I couldn't ask him, I was too upset. (Laughs.)

CLARE: And you were surprised?

RENDELL: I was astounded.

CLARE: Has that been a one off or has it stirred you to enquire in a surreptitious way as to what other people made of you when you were small?

RENDELL: I did tell my aunt, who was my mother's elder sister, who is still alive and who lived longer than anyone in the family, she'll be ninety-two. I did ask her and her response was, 'But you were a lovely little girl, darling.' So, what do we do about that one?

CLARE: When you say your father had a wonderful deathbed, how do you mean?

RENDELL: Oh, I mean that when he died (I would never have talked about this until my stepmother was dead, but she is dead now) he was fully conscious, I mean until he died and he died in my stepmother's arms and he actually said goodbye to us and he said, 'I'm a very long time dying, I'm sorry.' He was a dramatic man and he did it well, I mean it was great. I think he thought this is the way I'm going to die and then he just died and I thought that was wonderful.

CLARE: And your mother?

RENDELL: Oh, my mother had MS and she had it for years and she died, she had strokes and she was in a coma and she died.

CLARE: How disabling was it when you were younger?

RENDELL: Well, people didn't know what it was for a long time and so I was well grown-up before it was diagnosed. MS often just manifests itself as an unusual clumsiness and that's what that was.

CLARE: Yes, for years?

RENDELL: For a long time and various diagnoses were made and finally it was diagnosed as MS. It takes many forms and she was a slow MS patient. It was very, very slow and there were lots of remissions.

CLARE: And when she died, was that again, if you like, something that you felt had a natural aspect to it or was it very distressing for you?

RENDELL: It was very distressing for my father. I don't think it was all that distressing for me. I'd grown away from my mother, it was very hard to approach her in later years.

CLARE: She was difficult?

RENDELL: She was difficult and I hadn't been close to her for a long time. I was closer to my father and he was very remorseful when she died. He was very remorseful. He felt that he had not understood, as indeed he hadn't, and I think that my feeling about losing my mother was very much swallowed up in my feelings of pity for my father.

CLARE: He married again?

RENDELL: He married again about seven years later.

CLARE: And your stepmother died recently?

RENDELL: My stepmother died about six months ago.

CLARE: The central preoccupation I sometimes think of many of your books is really what's going on under the surface, what lies behind certain things. I'm rather intrigued that, presumably, the Rendell family looked from outside, pretty ordinary.

RENDELL: The Grasemann family of course.

CLARE: The Grasemanns.

RENDELL: Yes, in so far as it was possible when you consider that my mother was a foreigner, and we are speaking about the time of the Second World War, so there was always that. And, whereas now it would be very common to find a couple and a child and a nanny, it was not common then, not in that kind of middle-class suburban set up.

CLARE: Did it arouse suspicions? You would have been in your early teens as the war broke out. When you say 'foreigner', was there a sense that she was different or that you were all different.

RENDELL: One or two people, but literally one or two, suggested that my mother might have been German, but I don't think it was a very serious matter. I mean you would have had to have been extremely ignorant and very bigoted to suggest that. One of my uncles had a lot of that because he was a Dane but he had a very strong accent, also he spoke very good German, he was known to do this and he had never become a naturalised British subject. Whereas, of course my mother was naturalised before she met my father and it would have been automatic over there. There wasn't too much of that.

CLARE: Growing up for you as an only child, was your arrival in school, was school itself a particular challenge or did you find other children perfectly easy to get on with?

RENDELL: You know I think I did. As far as I know or remember, I didn't have those problems only children are said to have, such as difficulty with sharing and so on. I didn't have that and I always had a lot of friends. I still know, I still have friends that I was at school with. Friends are very important to me, I have a very strong, powerful attachment to my friends.

CLARE: And in your social life, does that process continue, of being observant whilst participating, of being a little outside while seemingly part and parcel of what's going on. Not quite necessarily going through the commentary but still observing?

RENDELL: I don't do the commentary any more and the commentary stopped not when I started writing fiction but when my fiction began to be published. I don't know quite why. I suppose it was something to do with saying to myself, now I am a real writer.

CLARE: Now that means it went on right into your thirties?

RENDELL: Oh, yes, but not so much, but it did go on, oh, yes, it went on quite a lot and I would think that in any writer who did that but never became a professional writer, never became a published writer, it probably would go on. It would be the substitute, the thing that you did instead of writing. When I began to be published, it stopped and it has never come again. The telling of stories of course is there because that is part of writing. The social commentary is only sporadic. For instance, if I were at a dinner party, say there were six people including myself, it switches off but if something happened that was of special interest, some remark were to be made, it would come, it would sort of swing in again and it would begin to work, would begin to roll, so to speak, and I would watch and wonder why and perhaps ask myself why afterwards and think about it.

CLARE: You said somewhere that the reason you left journalism, because when you left school you went into journalism, the reason you left was that it was irresistible to embellish facts. Fiction was what drew you. Fact was dull, boring. I wondered what that was about.

RENDELL: I think that I want to exaggerate the facts. I want to make them not necessarily better but more dramatically satisfying. And of course, I still find if I ever do any journalism, I still find this a nuisance though I am able to handle it, but I don't do much. It's mostly book reviewing, whereas in fiction I can do as I please.

CLARE: I'm interested in the fact that the people you write about, I accept that they're dramatic often because of the things that they have done or thought of doing or are thinking of doing, but I have to say, putting my cards on the table, that why I find what you write about so interesting is because you are one of the few people, it seems to me, who write about disturbed people in a way that matches my experience of them, as a clinician. I've talked to one or two of my colleagues about this and discovered that many of us are suspicious about the way in which psychological distress or strange, morbid fantasies and behaviours are portrayed in fiction. Somehow, it's always a tiny bit caricatured, stereotyped or exaggerated. Whereas, in fact, I often feel that just told as it is, it has a dramatic impact all of its own and that's what I often felt you did. So I was surprised to see that you felt that somehow you took something and elaborated it because it seemed to me that what you actually did was, you told it as it is and that's what gives it its power – not romantic, not caricatured, not exaggerated, which is the way in which a great deal of disturbed behaviour and thought and emotion is often presented on stage, screen or in fiction, but actually as it is, that you kind of creepily get into these people and just describe it as it is.

RENDELL: Ah, yes, but when I say exaggerate, I'm speaking really of action, not of people, not of characters, I think that when I was a journalist and I would be writing, I would be writing a description of something or some events that happened and it would seem to me the outcome was not perhaps as I would have it. Perhaps not so much exaggerated but I should have rearranged it. I would have arranged it better. But that's quite different with these people because with the people when I describe them I become them, that is, I get into them and I become them. I don't know exactly how this is done but I know that I do it. And I suspect a lot of writers do that.

CLARE: What attracts you about the people that you get into the skin of?

RENDELL: I think that it may be that I understand why they do these things. I'm not saying that I understand everything, there are a great many things that people do, of course, that I don't understand, probably never will but I also think that there are a lot of things that people say – 'Oh, you can't possibly understand how they did that' – I think I can and I try to and when I do, I can get under somebody's skin and I want to write about it. I want to try and work out why they did what they did and how they felt and then I have a feeling of rightness, 'Yes, it would be like this, this is how it must be.' This person who is for the time being me, would do that and, having done that, would do this.

CLARE: Now this isn't necessarily a justification for what they do, it's an explanation of what they do.

RENDELL: It's an explanation of what they do. I don't think that it's like saying to understand all is to forgive all. That isn't true. To understand all is just to understand all. I don't understand all but I think I understand some and I want to try to explain it on the page, if I can, and show how it is and if I do that, I think I can see when I have done it properly.

CLARE: When you see, then, contemporary real life morbidity, the Bulger case, serial killing, Brady, Manson, do you think that it probably is like that, that if you burrow around, that which seems completely abhorrent is less so, is just that little bit more understandable?

RENDELL: Some of it is, yes, I think some of it is but some of it is not. I said that I could understand a lot but not all. I don't think, and I really tried, I don't think I can understand the children who killed James Bulger. I cannot understand the Moors Murders either but I can come somewhere near to some of this. I can see how in stages of excitement and loss of will, certain things cease to be forbidden and they become possible and, having been done once, they become very much easier the next time and it's a cumulative effect. I can understand that.

CLARE: Does that mean you could imagine, in certain circumstances, you doing something morbid and violent?

RENDELL: I'm a very non-violent person. I can't imagine killing anybody myself but I can imagine getting under the skin of somebody else and doing it but for me because I never lose myself in these characters, I have a strong sense of identity, in spite of having two names, I don't lose that. Me, these hands, this person, this physical thing couldn't kill anybody but when my mind goes in this strange way it does, into somebody else, oh, yes.

CLARE: You see, supposing for a moment we elaborated a little on your own experience – only child, warring parents, a distressing sort of family situation which has made you very suspicious of families and family life, in different circumstances – that could be the genesis of one of your characters?

RENDELL: Probably will be one day. (Laughter.)

CLARE: How important, then, are the processes we've been describing? The process of observing, detaching, commenting and then transferring into writing. Do you think in terms of it turning you into somebody quite different?

RENDELL: Yes, it must be. It must be, but when I try to sort it out and split it up and find the stages, I don't find that very easy. But I seem to be able to do it without too much analysis.

CLARE: The comment of that friend at the time of your father's funeral is an interesting one because immediately it suggests, the possibility anyway, that Ruth Rendell as a small child, what was it again 'nasty and disagreeable'?

RENDELL: 'You were a horrible little girl.'

CLARE: So it's almost like the beginning of one of your novels.

RENDELL: Oh, yes, it is.

CLARE: Your own novels.

RENDELL: I don't know if it's relevant. I don't know if I was horrible. Remember my aunt – 'you were a lovely little girl,' so . . .

CLARE: That, too, is straight out of Rendell. Yes, or maybe Barbara Vine. How much have you put that behind you, your own personal experience of family life – because on the one hand you've been quoted many times as being dubious about happy families and the number of children and so on but on the other hand you did get married and you have a child of your own, now a grown man.

RENDELL: I have two grandsons.

CLARE: Two grandsons?

RENDELL: And I'm extremely fond of my family.

CLARE: So you are a family person in the end?

RENDELL: Oh, yes, yes I am. It's not that I'm not a family person. I am very, very fond of children. It's just that I become a little jaundiced perhaps with hearing about the ideal of a family because although I have known several very happy families, you note the word several, in my life, I have known very many more unhappy ones and I think that my experience, I couldn't say I had an unhappy childhood, I couldn't say it was an unhappy family altogether because, of course, they all loved me but it wouldn't seem to me to be an advertisement for marriage or the family at all.

CLARE: The fact that they all loved you, you've emphasised it a number of times, that it suggests, that whatever else about this experience, you grew up confident about yourself, that you were valued, that you weren't someone lacking in self esteem as the jargon would have it now.

RENDELL: No, I'm not a very confident person, though I am a shy person, although of course I've learnt to handle that but I have often thought that this may be due not to not being valued as a child, as I think I was very highly valued by a lot of people also in my extended family, but I think it was because we, that is my parents, knew so few other people so that I really grew up knowing my parents, my aunts and uncles and school friends and knew nobody else. I had no social life and so I think that that has made me shy. Whereas I can speak happily to an audience of 500 people without any problems, it is still highly unpleasant for me to walk into a party, a room full of people. And if it's unpleasant now after having been to hundreds and hundreds of parties, I don't see it getting much better and I have done my best to cure it.

CLARE: And what do you do to do it?

RENDELL: I just do it. I say, oh, you know, I don't think about it, be very calm and walk in there and you know very well that within five minutes all will be well. That's what I do and of course, all is well but I don't like it.

CLARE: Has it got worse as you developed a public persona?

RENDELL: No, it's got better. These things are said not to get better. They do get better because they simply get better when some of those people are going to be, or appear to be, very pleased to see you. Part of this is due to the fact that you're afraid that nobody will speak to you. Well, there are going to be some people to speak to me, so it's better.

CLARE: Yes. Because, the other interesting thing about what you've said about your family was that in those pieces you've written about families, there's always some kind of dark secret, something that's not as it would appear and I wondered whether the growing-up Ruth wondered whether there was a dark secret in her own family. How imaginative in terms of your own self were you?

RENDELL: Yes, there were dark secrets in my family, some of which I discovered the answer to. I think there are dark secrets in all families. I thought, of course, when I found the one or two in mine which were perhaps not so very dark that this was unique but of course, as I grew older, I found that most families have them.

CLARE: Did any of them concern you directly?

RENDELL: No, no they didn't.

CLARE: They concerned other members of the family?

RENDELL: They concerned other members of the family and not even immediate members.

CLARE: The other characteristic that you refer to, and it comes up in different kinds of ways, is obsessive. I don't know whether you mean that in terms of the way you write or in terms of the kinds of things you're interested in or your own internal life. Maybe it's imposed on you because I've learned to be suspicious of descriptions I read about other people, but anyway, that recurs and I just wondered, would you say, 'Yes, I have a somewhat obsessional personality.'

RENDELL: I would say I had, if obsessional is going to be the same as addictive or compulsive, is it? How different is it? I can get very easily addicted to things. I'm also a very determined person. I can bring these things under control but I do have them. I can get into compulsive ways. I can get obsessed with time.

CLARE: How do you mean?

RENDELL: With punctuality. In quite a serious way. I'm not a worrier, I don't worry about it and, of course, I'm living in the present but it causes me disproportionate distress to be late. I mean horrible. I've never missed a plane in my life. If I were to miss a train it's dreadful. It doesn't really matter what's at the other end. It's very bad.

CLARE: When you say it's dreadful, what's it like?

RENDELL: Oh, the panic is dreadful. It's out of all proportion. One shouldn't feel such a panic, distress and rage at such a thing as this that is basically, finally in the great scheme of things, unimportant.

CLARE: Would you take it out on yourself?

RENDELL: No, but let me say it's like this: I'm going in a taxi somewhere and I've got ten minutes to get there so the first five minutes is spent in an agony of, 'I'm ging to be late, I'm going to be late,' but when the taxi is making good speed, the second five minutes is spent in, 'I'm going to be early, what am I going to do.' Now this is true, and it sounds horrible and ridiculous, but it is true and it does this to me and it's very hard for me to handle it by trying to be deliberate, to take things later.

CLARE: How do you feel about being early?

RENDELL: Oh, well, you don't have to be early do you, you can walk round the block, you can, you can do all sorts of things. There's not much you can do about being late except be late.

CLARE: Was it ever so severe that rather like somebody I knew, lest he miss a plane, he almost invariably found himself in time for the one that went before.

RENDELL: Oh, yes, oh, yes, certainly. And certainly with trains. In fact I have caught many a train that was a train before the train I went to catch.

CLARE: Yes, and therefore arrived . . .

RENDELL: Oh, arrived ridiculously early but of course that doesn't always matter. I think it's an awful waste of time. Perhaps I shall be able to control it.

CLARE: Freud identified a number of characteristics, punctuality was one of them, of the obsessional personality, punctuality. I think a certain degree of pedantry, of care about words – now, one would expect that, I suppse, of a writer – are you very precise?

RENDELL: Oh, yes, if I do a review of a book it takes me a very long time because I write it and rewrite and rewrite it, and as for my books, I rewrite them over and over and over. I do spend a lot of time with a word, I always use a thesaurus and a dictionary and, yes, these things. I also do crossword puzzles.

CLARE: Are you a checker? In other words, do you check and recheck?

RENDELL: Oh, yes, yes, I do.

CLARE: What sort of things?

RENDELL: Oh, you mean, do I go back and see if I've left the gas on? I'm not very bad about that. I do a bit.

CLARE: When you say not very bad?

RENDELL: Some people are very, very bad about that. It's not unknown for me to go back once. I do it a bit. I don't do it every time I go out, I don't even do it once a week but I do it. I do search to make sure that I have a key, perhaps two or three times before I leave the house. I do check on other things quite a lot, yes, but I don't get up in the night to check on things but I might get up once before I went to sleep to check I'd turned off the computer, the iron, the video, or whatever it might be.

CLARE: Do you worry about things? Do you worry about disease?

RENDELL: No, I'm not a worrier. I'm a frightened person, I'm nervous but I'm not a worrier because I don't look to the future, you see.

CLARE: Frightened?

RENDELL: Oh, I'm frightened of things. I'm frightened of people.

CLARE: But your fear isn't of physical violence?

RENDELL: No, no, no, I'm not really frightened of physical things. I'm not frightened of disease.

CLARE: What is your fear of people?

RENDELL: I am afraid I need people's good opinion. This is something in myself I dislike because I even need the good opinion of people who I don't admire. I am afraid of them. I am afraid of what they will say to me. I am afraid of their tongues and their indifference.

CLARE: And does that mean that you would be very sensitive to what would be written about you?

RENDELL: Oh, yes, very, very. I am very sensitive. I find it's very hard for me to take a bad review or a bad article about myself. My behaviour, which will be happening to me this coming weekend of course since I have a new book, the *Sunday Times*, it will come and it will be lying on the kitchen table and I shall know which bit of it has this review in, probably, but I will have to think about whether I am going to open it now, later or never and probably what will happen is that having walked around it for a bit I will suddenly pounce on it, tear it open and read it.

CLARE: Quickly?

RENDELL: Yes, probably. If it's a good review I shall be immediately transported into ecstasy. If it's a bad review I shall be very unhappy.

CLARE: And this, I would remind listeners, is someone who's won four Golden Daggers, Cartier Dagger Award, *Sunday Times* Literary Award, books are selling in many languages.

RENDELL: Three Edgars and the Mystery Writer of America.

CLARE: Twenty languages.

RENDELL: A great many other awards all over the place, oh, yes.

CLARE: And yet, a single review! You will get reviewed in many newspapers. Would it be true that the single review that perhaps is lukewarm or even critical would dominate your thinking of the day if there were seven others, eight others who said this is a masterpiece?

RENDELL: No, I don't think it would be. And the next day, if I got a good one, the previous day's would be utterly invalidated, it would be annihilated pretty well. It might come back to me but it wouldn't much.

CLARE: In your personal life, does that desire to be liked or certainly sensitivity to being disliked, has that meant that you've been someone too easy to please, that you've said yes to things when you would have preferred to have said no?

RENDELL: Yes, I have, I have said yes to things. I am better at that, because of the kind of life I lead, I have to be. I am asked to do so many things that it wouldn't be humanly possible so I am learning, by talking myself into it and examining it, to say no.

CLARE: Can the people close to you, your husband, your son, can they reassure you in these moments of great doubt or panic?

RENDELL: I don't think they can. My son might be able to. My husband is very different from me. He has an equable, easy-going temperament. I wouldn't say he's insensitive, he's not at all and he's very sympathetic but it would simply be beyond his understanding. He simply says, 'Well, what does it matter to you?' and he will then list to me these things. 'Well, what does it matter to you, it doesn't matter, take no notice.' My son is very much like me and he would feel like that, yes, he would. But it would make him angry. Yes, it does make me angry, it would make him angry and so on.

CLARE: You've said the fear isn't a physical violence fear, it's a fear of people, in a sense, psychologically wounding you. You've also talked about a sort of spiritual fear.

RENDELL: What exactly do you mean by a spiritual fear?

CLARE: I don't know.

RENDELL: Have I talked about a spiritual fear?

CLARE: Well, it may not have been your words. Oh, in fact, I have the quote, yes.

RENDELL: You do?

CLARE: Yes, you said, 'I'm very interested in fear. I don't mean the kind of gothic fear of being alone in a churchyard, I mean a social fear,' and you've talked about that, a fear not of physical violence but of mental or spiritual violence, and I wondered quite what that meant.

RENDELL: Yes, I'm feeling like Robert Browning when I said that, only God and Ruth Rendell knew what I meant. Now only God knows. (Laughs.)

CLARE: I'm thinking back to you as a small child and I just wondered whether the kind of violence you mean is the violence, again psychological violence, that churns up your feelings, that means that you're not in control.

RENDELL: I suppose I might have meant the kind of thing that that man said to me when he said I was a horrible little girl. Yes, I think so. Probably something like that.

CLARE: Control is important?

RENDELL: You know, I don't think so. Control of me is important.

CLARE: That's what I mean.

RENDELL: Yes, but not control of those around me or my environment. There's no manipulation.

CLARE: No, I meant control of you.

RENDELL: Yes, control of me is important, yes. Control of me making me behave the way I think I should.

CLARE: I mean, being late for a train, that's what I meant.

RENDELL: Yes.

CLARE: That's a failure of your control. You're not blaming the railway station, or your friends, or the taxi driver, you're blaming you.

RENDELL: Yes. Oh, I do blame myself and I do want to be in control of myself and if I slip from this, I do castigate myself, I feel shame. If I slide away from quite rigid rules, yes, I do.

CLARE: And in terms of your writing, you're in absolute control. In the end you may take a great deal of time and change the words and so on, but in the end, you're running the show, that account, that description, what they say and what they feel and what they do, you're the master orchestrator.

RANTZEN: Yes, even though it may not always be as I would wish it to be, and often is not. I am. I can only say that with that I have done my best. If that is to be in control, yes, I am in control.

CLARE: And when it isn't quite what you want, how do you feel then?

RENDELL: I am able to accept that I have my limitations. After all, I know that there are things in writing that I can't do. I'm not a great writer. I'm an entertainer and I do some things well. I am not going to be able to write as the great writers have written so I accept that. I don't feel terrible frustration, I do the best I can and when I've done the best I can, I have to accept that.

CLARE: You say you have to, so it's a decision?

RENDELL: Yes, it is.

CLARE: It's difficult?

RENDELL: There's a lot of 'have to' and 'must' in my internal monologue.

CLARE: Is letting a manuscript go very difficult?

RENDELL: Fairly, fairly. Not very difficult because by that time I have handled it I'm sick of it by then. Yes, I'm sick of it. It must go and I've got used to letting it go. There have been a lot of manuscripts.

CLARE: Is it a physical thing, writing? I mean, do you have physical symptoms in the process of writing?

RENDELL: I'm a very physical person. That is, I'm very much in my body, I'm not somebody who can have a mind out there. So, yes, it is. I feel it in my hands, I feel it in my eyes, but pleasurably so. It's not a pain.

CLARE: It's not a feeling of malaise.

RENDELL: Never, never a feeling of malaise. It doesn't make me tired. Well, it might if I went on and on but I'm not that sort of writer. Again, the control comes in that I do write at pretty specific times

CLARE: Is there a feeling of malaise if you don't write?

RENDELL: There is a feeling of unease, yes, malaise, itchiness. It just depends on where I am. If I were at home and it were morning and I was not writing, I certainly shouldn't know what else to do and I should feel very strange. Not being a person who finds it easy to relax, so what on earth would I do?

CLARE: You never relax?

RENDELL: Well, I must do, I suppose, when I go to sleep.

CLARE: No, apart from that?

RENDELL: No, I read. I sit and read a lot but it's not relaxing. I'm very concentrated on it and I move all the time. People say to me, 'Oh, don't you long to have a holiday and relax?' No thank you, I don't. I don't like doing nothing and that to me is relaxing, doing nothing.

CLARE: And you don't like doing nothing?

RENDELL: No.

CLARE: And you finish a book, how long would it be before you'd start to write another book?

RENDELL: Well . . .

CLARE: Because you virtually have been writing . . .

RENDELL: Yeah, it might be a few weeks because I mean something else might intervene. I might go away. When you publish a book these days there's so much publicity to do and so many other things

CLARE: You've go to do the rounds and travel . . .

RENDELL: Yes, and also I do review books and I do write articles. There will be other things to do. There are all my letters to answer for one thing. And there will be things like proof reading and reading manuscripts and checking things and planning things, there will be that. I am in that state now because I don't intend to start another book until August. But that's all right because it's there in my head, you see. And although I'm not writing, telling myself the story is also a very pleasurable exercise.

CLARE: But it's underway already?

RENDELL: Oh, yes, of course.

CLARE: And how long has it been?

RENDELL: Since I stopped writing the other one, about three weeks. It's underway, yes, but it will be there, turning over in my mind for these weeks ahead I suppose. I say August, I don't know when it will be because I'm not really looking ahead.

CLARE: I'm wondering the extent to which there's an analogy here, not so much with obsession but with compulsion. The thing about a compulsion is that if you resist it, or if for some reason or other you're prevented from indulging in it, there is a tension, there is an anxiety, there is a feeling of not-rightness.

RENDELL: I think I would have that feeling if I were prevented, as you say, by something happening to me at the beginning of August to stop me. But I will be content, I think, until then with it in my head being mulled over, being thought of, being put into those first four or five chapters that I always think of before I begin to write anything down. I don't know how it would be for me if I were stopped, really stopped, by say, illness, then I don't know how it would be.

CLARE: It hasn't happened?

RENDELL: Never. But if I were to be really ill, so that I couldn't write, perhaps I wouldn't want to. But there again, this is a hypothetical looking ahead stuff that I don't really go in for.

CLARE: So why do you want to?

RENDELL: Why do I want to? It's what I like doing better than anything else.

CLARE: The actual process of writing.

RENDELL: Yes, I like to write, I like to write a sentence and hear it in my head and think, that sounds right. It conveys exactly what I want to say. It also gives a good strong suggestion of the place. It's good English prose, it sounds well. Right, we'll go on to the next sentence. That is very satisfying to me, to do that. And then to have a page, and then to read it, and then to think, is it doing what it should be doing, is it presenting this character in this setting, thinking in this way, doing in this way, behaving as it should be and yet, in good English prose without superfluous words, without a lot of adjectives, unnecessary stuff. Is that, is that as it should be? Good, we can then go on to the next page. Why that should be to my personal taste, I don't know, except that it is.

CLARE: And the dark side draws you.

RENDELL: Yes, the new book is about the hidden and the secret and it is about the unravelling, or it will be, about the unravelling and the unfolding of a totally unsuspected secret thing. But I wouldn't say that it was particularly dark, not yet. I think that the secret is, just at the moment, totally unlooked for, unexpected.

CLARE: Does that mean that at the centre you're a wary, a suspicious person? That you suspect motive. That things, things are not what they seem, people are not what they seem.

RENDELL: I'm afraid it does. Yes, I do think it does mean that and I think that I owe this directly to my father who though a very witty, amusing and clever man, and I think popular with people, suspected people very much, suspected their motives. I think that I have that from my father so that I have had to resist it in my social life for years, of not expecting the worst from people. That is I suspect that people will not be pleasant, that they will not like me, that they will not be congenial, that they have in fact bad motives. And of course, I now tell myself,

'No, it very likely is not so, remember last time when it was not so and these people were charming and pleasant and pleased to see you and it was all good and from this came these friends.' And this helps me but I'm still very aware of it and I think I put it into my fiction because that is what we do, we put it into the fiction and a great blessing it is and this may be something to do with why it is so nice to do, because, no fantasy life for the fiction writer, it all goes into the fiction. None of this stuff, it can all go into the fiction. It comes back, but it goes into the fiction.

CLARE: But it's the real-world experiences that you tend to latch on to, to correct yourself. The fiction doesn't do it, the writing isn't therapeutic, it's the living in the real world that's therapeutic.

RENDELL: Writing is therapeutic, partly.

CLARE: How?

RENDELL: Yes.

CLARE: In this instance, for example, how would the writing make you any less suspicious?

RENDELL: I think the writing showed me that I was suspicious. You see, it's part of not having a mystery in you but knowing yourself. And when you start writing a lot of things about suspicious people you say, 'What is this stuff about being so suspicious?' and then you begin to think – this has happened to me quite a long time ago – and I realised, yes, I did suspect people, so then comes back the fiction into the real world. The real world went into the fiction and out of the fiction it comes back into the real world and is, so to speak, tested and looked at and used, I hope for benefit.

CLARE: A colleague once observed it to me, that to be any way a good psychiatrist, you have to be a touch paranoid, a touch suspicious, always on the lookout for that which is not so. Are you curious about people? I know you've described a process of observing, of watching, of noting, and I suspect like the best writers of fiction, you've a good ear, you can recall things. Are you inquisitive?

RENDELL: Yes, I'm inquisitive, I am curious about people. I want to know, I want to know their secrets. But, of course, strangely enough, because I am the last person to whom I would tell a secret, people tell me their secrets and they confide in me. Perhaps they know that I will not tell them, they will find their way into my fiction but in so disguised a form that they won't be recognised. But yes, I want to know what they're doing, I want to know what they're thinking, I want to know about them, lots of things about them, of course.

CLARE: Do you hoard in your head, or do you actually have all sorts of places that you put things that you'll come back to?

RENDELL: No notes, no notes, no plans, no hoarding, all in my head, in a kind of great pool to fish it out of. Not deliberately, not consciously, but of course, by association, something happens and out it comes.

CLARE: And is that why the actual process of writing itself may not go the way you think, because something comes into your mind unexpected while you're writing?

RENDELL: Oh, yes, all the time that happens, that's why I do my first four chapters in my head, four or five, I can have an idea of the end but all the rest has to come as I go along. It unfolds out of the characters, out of association, out of the place, out of dialogue, out of things I see. I don't know what it will be but it will happen like that.

CLARE: Why did you choose to write under your own name and as Barbara Vine?

RENDELL: With Wexford it's a detective story. With the Ruth Rendell psychological, so called, mostly it is a perpetrator, it is some serial killer or, somebody who is seriously disturbed. With the Barbara Vine books it's everybody. You do have a murder, but it's either in the past or it's peripheral or it's an accident or it's somewhere but it's all the other people and their secrets and their thoughts and how they interact that I wanted to do.

CLARE: And you chose Barbara Vine because if you'd continued to write as Ruth Rendell it would be judged that way, whereas under a different name you would start afresh in a sense. Was it to do with the reception or was it to do with the creation?

RENDELL: It was to do with the reception because I had an idea that was so different and I wanted my readers to know it was me. It was never concealed, my identity was never concealed, but under a different name I thought they would understand then that they should expect something different and apparently they did and it worked and I liked it and went on with it.

CLARE: It's important to say that it was the same you! You actually chose names that are part of you. Vine is your great grandmother's name and Barbara is your second name so you weren't necessarily making a statement of splitting yourself but merely indicating that this was a different aspect of yourself.

RENDELL: Different aspect of myself. Also so many people in my family and among my friends call me Barbara so if either of those names is called in the street I'd look round to both of them, you see. I do like the idea of being split.

CLARE: Are they slightly different manifestations of you? Your great grandmother was it on your father's side, was it the English side?

RENDELL: Yes, yes, it was. Well, you know I've thought about this a lot and I don't think of myself under names. Do we think of ourselves by a name? I don't think so. In my internal monologue, I am 'you'. I don't know if this is true with other people but I am, now. I wasn't always as a child, of course I wasn't, I was that third person. But now I am 'you'. I don't think I am Ruth or Barbara, that is what other people call me. So I don't sit down at that machine and write and think, 'Now I am Barbara, oh, now I am Ruth.' I am writing one or the other books and I write.

CLARE: Would you always know which it was going to be?

RENDELL: Oh, yes, yes. When the idea comes then the decision is made, that's it.

CLARE: You would regard the way in which you treat morbidity as a moral way. Usually, I think it's true to say, in your books, I won't say badness gets punished, that's wrong, but sickness rarely leads to health, let's put it that way. It has an inexorable often awesome finish, completion or understanding but no one could ever see it as immoral in the sense that something pathological becomes reinforced, rewarded or encouraged. And because you identify with certain things, your desire to understand pathology seems rooted in a feeling that that's what it is, it's not romanticised. It is pathology and our need to understand it is in some way to make ourselves more whole. Would you say you are in that sense a religious person, that your morality stems from some kind of religious belief?

RENDELL: Oh, yes, yes I am a religious person. Not some kind of religious person – I am a religious person and my morality stems from that and that's all it is.

CLARE: Would it have a name? Are you Anglican or Lutheran or what?

RENDELL: I'm an Anglican, yes.

CLARE: How important is that to you? For example, does it affect your perceptions of the future in terms of the next life or death or what all that means?

RENDELL: Well, yes, it does. Sometimes it does and sometimes it doesn't. I think that in this respect I am like most people who aren't seeing a lot of pie in the sky. I would like to think there was an afterlife, sometimes I think there is and sometimes I don't and really I vacillate between these views. I would hope to be enlightened, but I don't know.

CLARE: Again, you take it as it comes, in a sense. You're in the present. You don't think too much about the future.

RENDELL: Well, I do think about death. I just think about it because I think it's a good thing to think about it and I wouldn't hide away from it.

CLARE: Why is it a good thing to think about?

RENDELL: Because I must die and I don't want to come to death quite unprepared. Not even unprepared at all. On the other hand, it is quite hard for me because I don't think much about the future but I know I must die so I think of it and it's not particularly unpleasant or unwelcome to me to think of it. I'm not a shier away from it.

CLARE: When you think of it, is it the process itself or the things that surround it? Is it the physical dying?

RENDELL: It's the immediate annihilation and whether there is anything after it I think about. What that is like? What it is like simply to cease to be alive. Whether it is just a cessation of consciousness like sleep or whether, as some people say, it is not, that it is going on to something else, to a next stage. And I hope that I may know. Of course, I shall know one day.

CLARE: Do you enjoy being alive?

RENDELL: Do I enjoy being alive? I don't want to die, at least, I don't want to die now or for a while. I enjoy it sometimes and sometimes I don't. I'm very healthy. I think that's a wonderful thing and something we don't appreciate until perhaps we lose it so I physically enjoy being alive very much. I very much enjoy looking at things, not just at things, cities, countryside, specially cities, just walking and looking. I like the things that I am accustomed to in London, for instance. When I'm here, the things that I've always known. I wouldn't like not to have them and yet I like change, I enjoy it.

CLARE: Have you ever felt on the edge?

RENDELL: Yes, but I shall not talk about it any more, but I have, a long time ago.

CLARE: But not recently?

RENDELL: No.

CLARE: Do you get morose, gloomy?

RENDELL: No, not particularly. I might be a little depressed for a while but there's not much of that. On the whole I am, I think, a person of enthusiasms and a lot of vitality and energy and go. I'm not inclined even to low spirits very much. I always think that if I feel like that I can always get out of it by losing myself in reading, or in writing, of course.

CLARE: And you must spend a considerable proportion of your waking life writing.

RENDELL: Well, I spend about five hours, perhaps six, and only four of those are creative writing. The rest is all the other things, the peripheral things that go with being a writer. And then I spend a lot of time reading and thinking about it.

CLARE: What would be the peripheral things that go with being a writer?

RENDELL: Ah, well, they would be reading proofs, reading manuscripts, doing corrections, writing letters, that stuff. I don't have a secretary.

CLARE: But the actual writing would be four hours a day?

RENDELL: Yes.

CLARE: Is that very organised again?

RENDELL: It's very organised. It's possible to do some more in the evening, a couple of hours perhaps, it sometimes happens.

CLARE: I was struck, watching you when you were imagining what goes on when an idea's germinating and you kind of looked up and I sensed that somewhere, I don't know, the back of your brain, that's where the ideas were floating around. Do people, let's take your husband or your son, do they know that something is happening to you when you're particularly preoccupied? Do you become remote?

RENDELL: My husband says yes. I don't know that my son, he probably doesn't see me doing that, or hasn't done for years anyway. But my husband says he does. He knows it, he knows that I'm doing it and that's all right.

CLARE: Has that ever been a problem?

RENDELL: No.

CLARE: No?

RENDELL: No, it's never been a problem. I think that that is because he not only accepts what I do but actively likes it and I think I could say admires it. And since he is in any case rather inclined to be silent man, I don't think it bothers him.

CLARE: You married him twice?

RENDELL: Yes.

CLARE: You've been interviewed many times but I've never seen a satisfactory explanation for that very interesting fact.

RENDELL: Well, I don't think I can give you one. That is not to say that I don't know it but I do know it but I cannot give it. I don't think that to give it would be a very good idea, particularly for my husband. Some day I suppose I shall have to write my autobiography to stop people writing a biography and then I will be inclined to talk more about it.

CLARE: That's perfectly reasonable. What has it been like, therefore, for the name Ruth Rendell to become a sort of public name, to have a public projection of your private person?

RENDELL: Well, of course, a lot of this social fear is fear of humiliation, is fear of ridicule, is fear of being ignored, is fear of indifference. So you might say that becoming famous does away with a great deal of that. You are no longer going to be ignored, people are not going to be indifferent to you so in a way it helps. Up to a point it does, and with celebrity it's something that you may say that you find annoying but then of course, I don't think you'd like it if it wasn't there. I mean I wouldn't like it if it weren't there. Some of it is very nice.

CLARE: What do you make of the current preoccupation, political preoccupation, with the issue of the impact of disturbing material on people's behaviour, on the people who read it? That to read about graphically described, disturbed thoughts, behaviour, impulses, affects the people who read it?

RENDELL: I think it does, I think it affects. People who say that books, literature, whatever, have no effect should only look at the Bible I think and ask whether it has, has any effect. I'm sure it does. That is why I am careful that these people I create should not be the kind of people others wish to model themselves on. So that I do not have macho, Rambo-like characters, very strong and handsome and so on, charging through the streets of Los Angeles firing off Kalashnikov guns and so on. But, as you said earlier, these people are not happy, their morbidity does not lead to success and happiness. So I think and hope that my readers don't want to be like my characters and the feedback I get from letters shows me that this is so, that people are not being, so to speak, led astray by what they read in my books.

CLARE: Can you shock yourself?

RENDELL: No, but I can be shocked, of course. I can't shock myself and I cannot frighten myself. Although there again I can be very frightened by what I read. Strangely enough, although I do not believe in ghosts at all, I've been very frightened by ghost stories, and they frighten me terribly. I couldn't read them if I were alone in the house at night, and yet I don't believe in ghosts. I find this very odd. But that's by the by. I do not frighten myself.

CLARE: Are you frightened, disturbed, distressed by, say, accounts of violence on the news?

RENDELL: I am not disturbed by accounts of violence. I am disturbed by sights of violence. I am very disturbed by accounts of the killing of children, for instance and helpless people and indeed, that I can't watch or look. But the sight of the sort of violence that you get when you see two men knocking each other across a room or shooting, that doesn't bother me.

CLARE: Do you dream?

RENDELL: Yes, I do dream, I have very interesting dreams. I have a recurring dream. I am in a very old, old house, I am very keen on houses you know, I've had a lot. I'm moving through this room and it's full of furniture and it's Victorian furniture and all, all very old and it's all covered up. It's a huge jumble and it's all covered up in sheets. I pass through it and I look at it and it's a huge mêlée and I pass on into another room and there's even more and as I pass on I become more and more and more frightened of just this inanimate stuff. And at last, the last room I make myself wake up because I don't know I'm dreaming but at some point I realise I am. Then I have another dream where I'm not aware of dreaming but I wake up convinced that there is some kind of medicine I should have taken and have failed to take and it's a matter of life and death and I haven't taken it. Indeed, I haven't taken it for weeks and what will happen to me? Well, I don't take any medicine. I never worry about these things as far as I know and this is dreadful because I wake up shouting or sweating or in a horrible state over this wretched pill, or spoonful of something I haven't taken. That I've had a lot of lately, I don't know why. That's only just two of my crazy dreams.

CLARE: And they'd be recurrent? You would dream them several times?

RENDELL: Oh, yes, both those are recurrent dreams. I haven't had the furniture one much lately although I did in fact go into an Elizabethan house near me which had an attic just like that, and that was a strange experience.

CLARE: I wondered, in the house, did you move from basement to attic?

RENDELL: No, I just moved through a series of rooms up on the top floor somewhere. As for the medicine, I've had that a lot lately.

CLARE: And can I ask you, is your dreaming related to your

writing? Would you dream more when you're not writing, would you dream less when you are?

RENDELL: It seems to make no difference and I don't dream about what I'm writing. In fact, I have never been a writer in any dream. I've never written a line in a dream and I've never used my dreams in my writing.

CLARE: As we talk, your past, it's not as if it's a closed book, yet it hasn't been fully excavated. I mean, there's furniture there but it's covered up and I am struck by the fact that at some stage you expect you will take a closer look at it.

RENDELL: Yes, I think so, because of course, nobody can live entirely in the present. Unless, I suppose, you can if you've got some sort of abnormal brain function. I live in the present to a large extent, but of course, this is in the past, of course there is all this old furniture stuff and whatever it may mean.

CLARE: Would you be somewhat wary of it? When I met you the first time some years ago and I said to you I'd be interested in interviewing you at some stage, I was surprised when you said yes. The reason I'm surprised was I sensed that you were a person who in a way was a bit wary of all of that, of looking too much at the past, that there wasn't much point, so I was surprised when you said yes.

RENDELL: No, I don't really think that that is so. I've no objection to looking at the past. I get tired of being interviewed in some ways when I'm always asked the same questions, but that is not at all this kind of thing that this is, which is why of course I said yes, because I knew it wouldn't be.

CLARE: But the actual elements in your past, I sense there are moments, bits, that you could go back to and uncover quite a lot, that you know they're there.

RENDELL: Oh, yes, lots of things, yes, that's right.

CLARE: So, like the dream?

RENDELL: Yes, yes, all that furniture is there and it's covered up with dust sheets and some of it isn't.

CLARE: So then the question is, why might it frighten you?

RENDELL: I don't know, if I knew that I might not have it any more. It's a very nasty dream. It's very, very frightening. Much worse than the medicine really.

CLARE: But they're related to each other, those two dreams, are they?

RENDELL: No, I don't think so. I've only been having this thing where I've forgotten to take this tablet or pill thing for about six months.

CLARE: Well, again, I don't know why it suddenly comes into my mind, but the notion of writing, I wasn't thinking of it quite as a medicine. Do you remember when we talked about whether there was a certain sense of unrightness or illness, we didn't use the word. I used the word 'malaise' because it's a better word. That's what I suppose I was getting at. I wondered the extent to which, and that's why you interest me, the extent to which writing keeps you alive?

RENDELL: Well, I think writing does keep me alive. I think I write to stay alive in a way. It's a great motive for writing but I haven't stopped writing. The dream doesn't come when I'm not writing, the dream comes any old time.

CLARE: But, some people, some writers, they write and then there's a long gap and they go away and it doesn't quite sound like the nutrient of life for them.

RENDELL: That's right.

CLARE: They do it because they have a talent and they do it because they're good at it and they do it because they like it and they may do it because they don't like it, but they do it because they need it. Some of them would say to me, 'I just have to, doctor, I just have to. I'd rather I didn't sometimes but I just have to.' But you've described it almost like breathing, really.

RENDELL: Yeah, breathing or food or something like that. I need it. I love it. I enjoy it. It is everything to me. It is what I do.

CLARE: But it's essential?

RENDELL: I think so.

CLARE: That's the point.

RENDELL: Yes, it's essential.

CLARE: You wouldn't live without doing it?

RENDELL: So is this pill thing that I haven't taken for a brief instant in my dreams, it's essential?

CLARE: Yes, it's essential. Have you ever worried that you couldn't do it? That nothing would come?

RENDELL: No, never. And this has been a great blessing to me because I've never been short of ideas, I've never been. And since I know what I'm going to write down before I go to it, I don't have this writers' block, blank page stuff. Never.

CLARE: And it happens all the time, it cycles, it's like the heart beating or the lungs inflating, the ideas are there, they come and then at a moment when it's appropriate, you start to transfer them into writing and then that process, it's completed, and so the cycle is completed.

RENDELL: Yes.

CLARE: Is there some kind of goal you want to achieve? That's the kind of question I'd ask of somebody for whom writing is not life itself. The writing is rather like a career, a vocation, or something that has goals and achievements. Whereas for you I feel that you're going to tell me that no, you just write, that there isn't something you want necessarily to do, some great opus you want to complete. Am I completely wrong?

RENDELL: No, I'd like to write a very, very good book that I thought was very good, a sort of crowning thing, but no, I write because I like writing, I love writing. It is what I do and I just go on. There is no special goal

CLARE: Would the crowning book be something completely different from what you're doing or would it be the kind of distillation of all that is the very best?

RENDELL: I think so, that's what it would be, yes.

CLARE: So it would be perfecting what you're doing.

RENDELL: It would be, if I could do that. Yes, that would be it. I would like to do that. I would like to write this book that satisfied me and I felt this is it. I can't say that I think that I would then stop, I'm sure I wouldn't, but it would be nice. But if I have a goal, that is the goal I have, but I don't really think in terms of goals. I just go on doing it.

CLARE: And when you say you go on doing it, am I to understand that, illness apart which might affect the very wish to do it, which I concede . . .

RENDELL: Mm, it's true.

CLARE: That apart, you would anticipate that you would go on doing this till either an illness developed that would take away the wish or that you died.

RENDELL: Yes, yes I think so. Of course, if I become very, very old, there does come a point with most writers where they simply can't. They lose their grasp on contemporary life. But you can usually manage to write something though, even in those circumstances. Or they become very weak and feeble or, goodness, their mind goes or something, but those things apart, if they don't happen, I will write until I die. I'd like to write until I die. I would ideally like to die while I'm writing. I have never thought of that before but I think that would be very good

CLARE: Ruth Rendell, thank you very much indeed.

Lisa St Aubin de Teran

It is often said that writing, and other forms of human creativity, can exercise therapeutic effects. Writing, for Lisa St Aubin de Teran, as for Ruth Rendell, would appear to have acted, at least in her early years as a novelist, as a form of therapy. In the course of this interview, Lisa suggests that she turned to writing because of an inability to communicate verbally. She unquestionably forces her characters to cope with their fears as she coped so extraordinarily with her own as a newly-married young woman on an Andes plantation in a violent, male-dominated society with not an English-speaking soul in sight. Indeed, most of her novels are concerned with matters that constitute the raw material of her own fears. In this interview, she talks about how *The Bay of Silence*, a novel concerned with child abuse, schizophrenia and grief, and regarded by some critics as her least autobiographical work, is based at least in part on her own experiences of teetering on a nervous breakdown during one of her three pregnancies. Writing it she found 'extremely therapeutic'. Here art, the process of writing, helped her come to terms with her own mother's illness and her own personal, suicidal fears and in writing the book she conquered the terror and the nightmares which threatened to engulf her.

There is nonetheless a degree of danger in taking Lisa St Aubin de Teran's work and life experiences and reading this or that 'explanation' of who and what she is from them. It can of course be provocative and stimulating but it may also accentuate any tendency to self-doubt on her part, as she herself is at pains to point out. The media attention and comments which Lisa attracted with the publication of her first few novels tended to see her in a light in which she did not see herself. 'I felt', she said to me, 'I don't exist because everybody sees something, they see my past, they don't see me as I am'. Yet she herself is aware of the extent to which she has used writing as a *means* of discovering herself, that as she has moved from relationship to relationship, from house to house, place to place, escaping from herself, and experiencing degrees of contentment and unhappiness in the process, she has slowly been pulling together and integrating the various strands within herself. She has analysed in her writings, with a detachment and a thoroughness which would have graced a series of psychotherapeutic sessions, her mother's remarkable mixture of strength, affection, ambition and despondency, her father's flamboyance, romanticism, creativity and detachment, her childhood of separation from the one and intense identification with the other, and her own persistent idealisation of personal relationships.

The story of Lisa St Aubin de Teran's life is itself like one of her novels. On her mother's side, the St Aubin of her name, she comes from a once-wealthy Jersey family who fell on bad times. While her great-grandmother and grandmother lived in reduced yet still relatively comfortable circumstances, Lisa's mother gradually came down in the world and regarded her impoverished state as something to be ashamed of. She married four times, bore four daughters and suffered from recurring depression. She ended her working life as the headmistress of an approved school for girls. Lisa's father, who left her mother one month after Lisa was born, is a rich South American academic, novelist, diplomat and playboy. She admits to wishing that she had inherited everything from her mother because she was much closer to her mother throughout her childhood and her adolescence. But genes will not be denied. It is her father who is the hugely romantic figure in her past, from whom she appears to have inherited her skill as a writer and her passion for travelling. Given such parentage, it is perhaps not surprising that Lisa believes she came from a family that lived on its illusions so that to fantasise is a part of everyday life.

The causes of mental instability are these days attributed to genes, environment or a mixture of both. By such reckoning, Lisa St Aubin de Teran is a candidate for serious psychiatric difficulties and she has in fact experienced them. Her family history for psychiatric disorder is rich. Not merely did both her parents suffer psychiatric ill-health but her maternal grandmother died in an asylum, certified insane. Her own mother was seriously and suicidally depressed when pregnant with Lisa and spent much of the pregnancy in a psychiatric hospital. Lisa's childhood was a disjointed and fragmented affair, so that when Jaime de Teran, a young Venezuelan exile, picked her up in a London street, pursued her relentlessly, frantically bombarded her with declarations of love in fractured English, married her (she was only sixteen) and swept her off to South America, the whole bizarre experience seemed only a fraction more eccentric than living a semi-Bohemian existence with her depressed mother in a flat in Clapham.

To suggest that the themes in her novels owe much of their inspiration to the key figures and events in Lisa's own life is to understate. Fact and fiction are inextricably interwoven. A character in her novel *Nocturne* remarks that memories 'drain through me as though I were a pasta sieve'. It could have been said of Lisa herself. Her first novel, *Keepers of the House*, published when she was twenty-nine, is an account of former splendour and inexorable decline and draws on her own personal experience as a child in England and as an adolescent bride in Venezuela. *The Slow Train to Milan*, which she has admitted to be autobiographical, tells of a teenager on the run and involves murder, theft, terrorism and exile. But it is the novel *Joanna*, published in 1990, which is arguably the most revealingly autobiographical of all the fiction she has written. Joanna is the daughter of a disturbed Jersey woman who spent most of her life locked up in a psychiatric institution but not before she had inflicted on Joanna a catalogue of horrendous physical and psychological abuse. The book, written in tribute to Lisa's mother, sticks closely to her own personal family experience. In an interview given at the time of publication, Lisa was quoted as saying 'mental illness is taboo and much misunderstood. I wanted to show the lines that exist between insanity and strangeness and to ask, if our circumstances were different, would we, too, be insane?'

She is not only fascinated by mental illness but also by travel, moving on, journeys, particularly railway journeys, which is hardly surprising given that for much of her life that is precisely what she has been doing – physically, maritally, psychologically.

Of her passion for trains, she once observed, 'Sometimes I stand in wonder at the lengths to which I will go for fostering my dreams about them'. She does not appear to have felt any pressure to put down her roots nor to have found any place where she wanted to stay, at least not until Italy. She lived with Jaime de Teran for seven years on a South American sugar plantation, running the family estate as her husband deteriorated psychologically and ended up in a state of chronic depression. She was surrounded by feudalism, poverty and disease, found herself acting as unofficial doctor, nurse and social worker to the estate workers' families and immersed in the lives of the larger-than-life characters that made up the inhabitants of the plantation. For reasons she discusses in this interview, she eventually left her husband, 'escaping' with her daughter Iseult back to Europe. Once more in England, she met and married the poet George MacBeth, bore him a son, Alexander, and together they lived in a partly fifteenth-century, crumbling gothic mansion which they lovingly restored.

This marriage too disintegrated and after six years ended in bitter recrimination. Neither of her first two marriages are described with much passion but both appear to have appealed to her exceedingly romantic view of people and of places, a personal tendency she attributes to the effects of her early childhood reading! Not alone did she as a young, impressionable girl, read and admire figures like Byron, Stendhal and Shelley, she positively identified with them and the dramatic and colourful lives they led. She aspired to living just such a life, of making a great, definitive, passionate personal commitment of her own.

After the break with George MacBeth she again moved, this time to Italy. When I interviewed her she was living in Umbria with her third husband, Robbie Duff-Scott. He too is a colourful and romantic figure, a painter who shares Lisa's passion for extravagant clothes. There are suggestions that with the death of her mother she has been released from a sort of emotional bondage and is now able to engage in deeper and more sustainable relationships.

Lisa St Aubin de Teran's life and her writing both raise and illuminate questions concerning the relationship between fact and fiction, life and art, identity and show. Elsewhere she has remarked that it is easier for anyone born of two or more nationalities or even classes to belong abroad, away from home. 'There is', she has been quoted as saying, 'no guilt attached to feeling different when one is a tourist'. There is in this interview a consideration of what it is like to be the foreigner in the family, 'the one with the dark skin who doesn't look English'. Given her background, one might be forgiven for assuming that she might yearn after stability, roots, predictability but the truth would appear to be that she has been infected with her own brand of restlessness and an acute fear of boredom. There are constant references in her writing to an anxiety about boredom and dullness, to boredom as a disease and to the scary prospect of leading a dull and safe life. She confesses to feeling intensely shy, 'a fairly quiet person', and in the interview with me spoke with a soft, whispered reserve and care which only served to highlight the dramatic content of her personal story.

If much of Lisa St Aubin de Teran's creativity is fuelled by the psychological turmoil and conflicts of her childhood, will her writing dry up as she resolves her own problems of identity and value? One reason why many artists are wary of therapy, be it lithium or psychoanalysis, anti-depressants or behaviour therapy, is the belief that, as Kay Redfield Jamison in her enthralling book *Touched with Fire* has noted, 'turmoil, suffering and extremes in emotional experience are integral not only to the human condition but to their abilities as artists'. A typical exponent of this belief was the manic-depressive artist, Edvard Munch, responsible for the great painting 'The Scream', who once replied to someone who had suggested that he could rid himself of his troubles, 'They are part of me and my art. They are indistinguishable from me and it would destroy my art. I want to keep those sufferings.' Lisa St Aubin de Teran does not want to keep her sufferings but she does want to consolidate her work as a writer of fiction and a teller of tales. She insists that all her work is not autobiographical and certainly her travel writings stand separate from her psychological excavations. Not every artist needs to suffer like Munch, and who is to say in any individual case that suffering and art are indivisible? For Lisa St Aubin de Teran, however, the question is not an academic one and the answer will be provided in its own time. I personally will follow her writing career and indeed her own life with particular interest having met her and participated in an interview which even now, many months later, I recall with much appreciation and gratitude.

Lisa St Aubin de Teran is an award-winning novelist whose life story appears to be as strange as her fiction. She was born in London in 1953. Her parents met in a psychiatric clinic while both were recovering from nervous breakdowns. Her mother was an impoverished English woman from a well-to-do Jersey family with three failed marriages already behind her and he a novelist and professor of Afro-Caribbean studies, from what was British Guyana. That marriage broke up when Lisa was one year old. Lisa herself has three children from three different marriages and is now a grandmother at the age of thirty-nine.

Her first husband, whom she married at the age of sixteen, was Jaime Teran, a thirty-four-year-old Venezuelan political exile. They spent two years on the run from Interpol all over Europe, but mainly in Italy, before moving to his isolated sugar plantation in the Andes. For seven years she was kept a virtual prisoner until she managed to escape with her daughter Iseult. She came back to England and wrote her first autobiographical novel, *Keepers of the House*, which won the Somerset Maugham Award in 1983. In 1982 she married the poet, George MacBeth, twenty years her senior. They lived in a Norfolk castle and had a son, Alexander. The marriage collapsed two years later and Lisa herself had a nervous breakdown. She moved to Italy where she now lives with her third husband, Robbie Duff-Scott, five years her junior and her two-year-old-daughter, Florence.

Lisa has published seven novels, a number of short stories, a book of poetry and her memoirs *Off The Rails* which is a kind of monument to her obsession with trains and train journeys which in her own words is 'bordering on the insane'. Indeed, mental illness seems to be very much in Lisa's family. *Joanna*, another of her autobiographical novels, is devoted to the psychological impact of her maternal grandmother's insanity on her own mother.

CLARE: Lisa St Aubin de Teran, judging by your novels, you clearly like writing about aspects of your own life. How do you feel about talking about yourself?

ST AUBIN DE TERAN: I suppose I find it quite easy to talk about myself. If I had to say what I really like writing about, I like writing about aspects of lives of people who are close to me so a novel like *Joanna* isn't really autobiographical – it's biographical. It's about people I knew or knew about but not about myself.

CLARE: The reason I'm interested in you is because you're whole essence, background experience, raises a variety of questions which to someone interested in psychiatry, psychology are very central. For example, the whole question of identity, of who a person is. In your description for example of your father, you describe him as such a mixture of things – poet, painter, actor, diplomat, playboy, a colourful man with a variety of traditions, of bloods in him. And then there's your mother, likewise an extremely interesting and complex figure. The question arises, how do you see yourself? How do you decide what you are in terms of your ethnic background? What are you? Who are you?

ST AUBIN DE TERAN: I think I could say who I was. As a person I feel who I am, but what I am in ethnic background is almost impossible for me to feel because it's so mixed. I come from a really, truly mixed ethnic background and I've never consequently probably felt quite at home in any of the places that I've lived unless I live in a so-called foreign country. I'm not at all Italian. I feel at home living in Italy because I know I'm a foreigner and it suits me to feel at home somewhere where I don't have this ambiguity of not quite belonging. I feel I do belong because I am a foreigner. That's how people see me and so I don't have that odd sense of being out of place.

CLARE: How do they see you? You live in an Italian village?

ST AUBIN DE TERAN: I live just outside of a very small Italian village, yes.

CLARE: And do you know how they categorise you, other than the foreigner?

ST AUBIN DE TERAN: Well, we've been very lucky, living where we do, for two reasons. One, I've got an Italian passport, which with three children is a great help and secondly, we've bought a house that had been derelict for 100 years and which used to be the centre of all kind of village festivities and after we'd bought this house, there was nowhere big enough for the scattered population of 400 of the village to dance in winter and so they use our house still for all their winter festivals so we've been very lucky making friends on a good basis with virtually everybody in the village and I'm sure that that's helped us to feel as much at home as we do where we are.

CLARE: Do you know what they make of you?

ST AUBIN DE TERAN: I think it's one of the really nice things about Italians is that they don't necessarily make anything. They just let people be eccentric or different. I think you have to be really horrible to fall out of that sort of net of hospitality and kindness which is there as a part of a kind of community spirit, so I don't know what they make of me. I think there must be some quite bizarre aspects to the way that we live and the way that we're perceived but I don't feel it interferes.

CLARE: Did this feeling of not quite belonging – does it or did it extend right back? Is it something that you've, in a sense, as far as you can remember, always been conscious of?

ST AUBIN DE TERAN: Yes, I think I've always been conscious of it. Not least because I come from a family of three sisters but they're all actually half sisters, although I feel very close to them I know that they're my half sisters. I know that I'm the foreigner, as it were, in the family. I'm the one with the dark skin who doesn't look English, who would arouse comments when we went anywhere. So from a very early age I was aware of being different, of not quite fitting in.

CLARE: And does that mean that you yourself were curious about what made you the person you were? I suppose your father being the figure that was different – he was there and then he was gone – but he must have left, to judge by what I hear, from what you said elsewhere, what I read – a trail of experience, an aura about him and he came back from time to time.

ST AUBIN DE TERAN: Yes, I was always curious, more curious to see my father than to know him, really, because he made very rare appearances.

CLARE: What did he actually look like?

ST AUBIN DE TERAN: Well, he's sixty-seven and very big, you know, he's not just tall he's actually big and he's got a very, a very sweet face. He's got a very charming smile which has actually been the downfall of many a young lady but he has a very charming smile and he looks, I suppose when you say what does somebody look like it's more like who do they look like. I don't know really how to describe him. He's dark in the way that I am. We're actually the same colour. That's the one thing that I've inherited, his colour and his hands.

CLARE: What else?

ST AUBIN DE TERAN: What else? I don't know, I suppose because I've been so much closer to my mother all my life, I've always wanted to think that I inherit everything else from my mother but I don't really know. My father was a writer and I'm a writer so I grudgingly say I inherited that as well.

CLARE: He was also something of a mover, he moved, he travelled. He didn't seem to stay long anywhere.

ST AUBIN DE TERAN: No. Yes, he kept himself a moving target, I think.

CLARE: I wondered about that in the sense that you yourself have a fascination for moving, for going from place to place.

ST AUBIN DE TERAN: Yes, I think probably to a certain degree that that is something that I inherited from him. Both sides of the family, my mother was a mover, she could never stay in the same place for more than a few months without wanting to pack everything up and move on to somewhere else.

CLARE: Really? It often goes hand in hand with a pretty low threshold for boredom.

ST AUBIN DE TERAN: I don't know, I think really I've got a pretty high threshold for boredom. I don't know, I'm one of those people who at a party, I will stand for hours and hours cornered. I'm quite shy and I find it impossible . . .

CLARE: But you wouldn't enjoy that.

ST AUBIN DE TERAN: No, I wouldn't enjoy it but I would be able to tolerate it whereas a lot of people I know just could not tolerate it, they'd be gone, they'd get out of the situation whereas I can't seem to do that.

CLARE: You're shy?

ST AUBIN DE TERAN: I've always been so.

CLARE: Not a characteristic I associate with your father. He was a man socially quite skilful.

ST AUBIN DE TERAN: Socially very much at his ease, yes, yes.

CLARE: The shyness, what do you attribute that to?

ST AUBIN DE TERAN: I don't know. I feel quite lucky because I'm not nearly as shy as I used to be. I used to be so shy it was sort of ridiculous. Until I was about twenty I virtually didn't speak at all and in fact my first husband's friends that I was living with, used to endlessly play jokes on people, if we were staying with them, saying I was deaf and dumb because three or four days would go by and I wouldn't utter a word and then there'd be this great surprise at the end because I'd say something. I just was terribly shy and I don't really know why.

CLARE: Was it linked with the sense of not being quite at ease, not quite belonging and also of course being different, visually, visibly different, physically different. Did people actually pick on you because of difference?

ST AUBIN DE TERAN: I grew up at a time when there was a lot less racial integration in Britain than there is today and so I was not aware of being picked on. I was aware of people finding me quite a sort of exotic person. It wasn't until I think I was about eight or nine that it dawned on me that this could be looked at as something that was, you know, a social disadvantage. I was in a playground at school and having an argument with a girl and she said, 'What are you doing, chocolate face?' and I just fell off this climbing frame! I thought, 'Oh, what has she said? Why is she saying that to me?' and then I thought about it and I thought, 'Oh, I see, it's all about being dark' but that's actually the only time either before or afterwards in England that I've ever been aware of any colour prejudice, so I don't think it would have been in any way to do with that. I think I'm just naturally a shy person. I have two very, very gregarious, extrovert daughters and a rather shy son.

CLARE: Your mother, what is her temperament?

ST AUBIN DE TERAN: My mother was one of those people who is shy and masks it up by being very extrovert but she was actually, I think, really quite a shy person underneath, afraid of meeting new people, not really much confidence but exuding a sort of false confidence, if you like.

CLARE: When I read about you, I wasn't sure whether I would meet somebody deep down very shy or who would be fairly exuberant, because sometimes you've said things like you see yourself as the heroine of a great opera or best of a bad play. There is the sense of you really cutting a dramatic figure and dash. There is your interest in Edwardian clothes and style. So I had thought that perhaps I'll meet a great dramatic persona. And then at that same time, cut against this, were descriptions of you as you've just said – shy, quietly spoken, socially careful. Are there those two aspects to your character or did I just pick it up wrong from what I'd read?

ST AUBIN DE TERAN: I think circumstances of my life have rather cut the dash rather than me personally. I'm a fairly quiet person really unless you know, a certain very sudden swing in the mood will make me be sort of extrovert but it happens so rarely I guess I'm quite a quiet, shy person.

CLARE: So how do you explain this extraordinary series of events? If I just take your very first marriage. You were at school at south London up to mid teens. How did you come to meet a Venezuelan political exile who was going to have you on the run through Europe for two years? How did that happen?

ST AUBIN DE TERAN: I went out to do a spot of shopping in the local high street and he just followed me home and followed me upstairs and put his foot in the door and, and that was really how I met him. He didn't speak to me or offer any violence but he did force his way into the flat where I happened to be on my own and he just sat there for a couple of hours and then he got up and left, but he knew where I lived and he began to follow me quite, sort of, regularly and systematically, proposing and saying how desperately in love he was with his little dictionary, because he couldn't speak any English. And after about eight months he wore me down. He kept saying he'd die if I didn't marry him and I thought I'd never been to a Latin country, so I didn't know everybody says that to you, so I thought, well, I better marry him, so I did.

CLARE: At that time, you were living on your own?

ST AUBIN DE TERAN: I was living with my mother.

CLARE: You were living with your mother. What did she think of him?

ST AUBIN DE TERAN: Well, she was out at the time that he first came round and she got back. I sort of called her up and told her what had happened, and that there was this chap who'd forced his way into the flat and she was absolutely horrified and came rushing back. He had a very kind of charismatic effect on people and she thought he was rather wonderful. In fact most people who met him seemed to think that, probably far more than I did and I was very influenced by everybody thinking what a wonderful person he was.

CLARE: And what was he doing at the time, over here in London?

ST AUBIN DE TERAN: Absolutely nothing! He was sort of in exile. He'd just been a political prisoner for two years in Venezuela and he was in exile and he was doing absolutely nothing, sleeping eighteen hours a day.

CLARE: Living on what?

ST AUBIN DE TERAN: He had a private income. He was very wealthy.

CLARE: But his English was poor.

ST AUBIN DE TERAN: His English was non-existent.

CLARE: Non-existent?

ST AUBIN DE TERAN: Yes.

CLARE: So was it a grand passion?

ST AUBIN DE TERAN: I didn't feel a grand passion at all. I felt literally this man's going to die if I don't marry him, how awful.

CLARE: But your mother – just tell me a little bit about her? The relationship between you and your mother – how close was it?

ST AUBIN DE TERAN: Very close, looking back, because my mother died twelve years ago, I think I had an almost unnaturally close relationship to my mother and maybe this was due partly to the fact that she'd had a very difficult life up until the time I was born. And just when she was a few months pregnant she'd tried to commit suicide and spent almost her whole time that she was pregnant with me in a mental hospital and came out to have me, and she sort of seemed to need me more than a mother often would need a child and she was very, very close. It wasn't a closeness that was in any way oppressive, as a child I was very happy to be that close to her but I was aware from I think the time I was maybe three or four that she really needed me, I had to prop her up.

CLARE: What had led to that breakdown? Had there been personal disasters for her?

ST AUBIN DE TERAN: Well, I think it had quite a lot to do with my father. Living with him had been too traumatic for her and then she had suffered from depression for most of her life and it linked back to when she was a child herself. She was a battered child but had never really been able to come to terms with the cruelty that she'd suffered as a child and the rejection. Gradually she got into a situation of quite serious poverty, not severe poverty in the sense of third-world poverty but never having enough money not to worry continually about how to pay the rent or how to buy the shopping or things like that. So life was quite hard for her and she was unable to cope.

CLARE: Would she talk to you about these things?

ST AUBIN DE TERAN: A lot, yes, yes she used to.

CLARE: When you were quite small?

ST AUBIN DE TERAN: Yes; because she had these terrible depressions. I used to share a bedroom with her and often she couldn't sleep and so she would talk all through the night about the way she was feeling and how, you know, she would be trying to cope.

CLARE: How did you cope?

ST AUBIN DE TERAN: Well, when I look back I remember those nights like that and I always felt they were preferable. When she didn't talk to me she used to sort of just pace around. She would walk around and make herself very, very tired and I hated it when she did that. I preferred her to sort of stay and talk than to completely wear herself out, not least because she used to work very hard and would always have to go to work the next day even if she hadn't got any rest.

CLARE: What did she do?

ST AUBIN DE TERAN: By the time I was about five, she'd gone into teaching maladjusted children.

CLARE: When she'd be talking, would there be a central core preoccupation? Did it revolve around one or a number of things or would it range far and wide about life in general?

ST AUBIN DE TERAN: It would range far and wide about life in general and actually a lot of the time, although she would start being very sort of depressed and tearful and distraught about things, she would intersperse these monologues with anecdotes and sort of bits of biography and so it wasn't a kind of totally gruelling process. It was mixed. It was like watching a good film where you got a sort of emotional shock but it would be sweetened by other things.

CLARE: Did you ever worry that she would ever harm herself, that it would all overwhelm her? Did she ever harm herself while you were growing up?

ST AUBIN DE TERAN: No, she never did. I knew because she'd told me that she'd tried to kill herself when she was pregnant with me and I felt that she wouldn't try to do that again. She always used to say that she wouldn't try and do that again and that she felt she had a reason for living because she had her children. She'd sort of given up men and turned to kids really.

CLARE: Perhaps you didn't realise it at the time but you did actually carry a heavy responsibility. You were her reason for living.

ST AUBIN DE TERAN: It was a heavy responsibility, but I also felt that I had a privilege, if you like, in that I did get very much the bulk of her affection and time and her love. I had an unfair share within the family of that.

CLARE: You felt special.

ST AUBIN DE TERAN: I felt special, yes.

CLARE: Did she have, as parents sometimes do, an ambition for you?

ST AUBIN DE TERAN: She was very ambitious for me. Her first

ambition was just that I would get out and not have the kind of life that she'd had, that was ambition number one. I think that was why when she saw what she thought, mistakenly, was this very nice Venezuelan chap, that this would be OK because I would get out. I would not have to live in sort of penury. But she had great ambitions for me, literary ambitions. I think she would have liked to have been a writer herself and she'd hoped that I would be a writer. She wanted me to be very famous and very successful and she always convinced me that I would be.

CLARE: Why writing? Why did she pick on that?

ST AUBIN DE TERAN: I think it was what she admired most.

CLARE: Really?

ST AUBIN DE TERAN: Yes.

CLARE: And so very early on you picked that up from her.

ST AUBIN DE TERAN: Yes.

CLARE: Would she encourage you to write?

ST AUBIN DE TERAN: She didn't actually, funnily enough. She didn't encourage me to write, she encouraged me to read and I used to read an enormous amount from a very early age. When I started writing I realised that I'd done the thing that sort of absolutely would please her most because she was very, very thrilled about that and for me it was great because until I was twenty-nine she was my audience of one.

CLARE: Did she live long enough to see your success?

ST AUBIN DE TERAN: She never saw anything of mine published. No.

CLARE: She died shortly before your Somerset Maugham Award for example.

ST AUBIN DE TERAN: She died before my first novel was even accepted by the publishers so I'd never even published a short story or anything. I'd written several novels by then and she was convinced that I would break through, but she never actually saw my success.

CLARE: How much do you think it was a conscious factor in you being a writer, that she wanted you to be?

ST AUBIN DE TERAN: I don't know really, because with my father being a writer and so many family friends being writers, I feel I grew up in a sort of reasonably literary, artistic household.

CLARE: What did he write?

ST AUBIN DE TERAN: He wrote novels and plays and poetry.

CLARE: So, when Jaime followed you, wooed you, pursued you, she saw him as someone who represented a cosmopolitan world, talented, financially secure. Where did the financial security come from, what did he own?

ST AUBIN DE TERAN: Actually at the time that I married him, I was unaware of the fact that he was an immensely wealthy person. He merely seemed to have a supply of money and I didn't know where it came from. It didn't seem a particularly lavish life. He was living in Clapham after all, in a rented house, so I didn't think, you know, this is a Saudi prince. I thought this is someone who has come to London and is living in Clapham, which in those days was a pretty odd choice of place, but his family had owned sugar and coffee plantations in the Venezuelan Andes for getting on for 400 years and that was his background. It was old family money.

CLARE: It still is extraordinary. You were sixteen when you married this man. Was he your first boyfriend of any real note?

ST AUBIN DE TERAN: Well, I was very shy, absolutely.

CLARE: Then he was?

ST AUBIN DE TERAN: Yes, I just used to read books.

CLARE: The big question mark concerns your mother. Clearly she was very close to you, you were very important to her and you described it. The bond was a very intriguing and rich one. I can see that one of her motivations would be that at least this would in some way see you into a life that she would have wished to have had herself but it had eluded her. However, on the other hand, you would be very precious to her. Wasn't there are a great risk? What did you know about this man, really?

ST AUBIN DE TERAN: Absolutely nothing, that was the big mistake. But from the point of view of her and her losing me, we'd always had a sort of pact that at a certain point when I settled in any way, got my career sorted out as a writer, we would live together, so whoever I was living with, there would be a mother-in-law living there too. So she didn't feel when I left that Lisa's leaving. She felt that this was a step on the path of our going and living somewhere very nice, always abroad because she didn't like living in England.

CLARE: Well, what about more bourgeois preoccupations like A-levels? You went to James Allen Girls School in Beckenham.

ST AUBIN DE TERAN: Yes.

CLARE: A school with an academic emphasis, a fine record and so on. You would have been a bright student I would have thought and so they would have had ambitions for you, there would have been teachers who would have liked to have seen Lisa really become a star.

ST AUBIN DE TERAN: Well, from a very early age at school I was a sort of compulsive truanter and so I didn't spend a great deal of time at school, but I did spend a lot of time in the public library and so I got ahead with my school work. I left James Allens by the time I was fifteen but I'd already got my ten O-levels and was well on to getting my A-levels then; and then I went to a crammer because they wouldn't let me take my A-levels so quickly and I was in a great rush to have everything behind me. So I went to a crammer so that I could get my Cambridge entrance at sixteen but I married Jaime and left for Italy instead.

CLARE: Do you think back and about how it might have been different. That was an extraordinary turning point, as it turns out.

ST AUBIN DE TERAN: It was. One of the reasons I wanted to go to university was because I wanted to study archaeology and I wanted to study archaeology so that I could go and live in South America and earn my living. This was my rather immature plan. I don't know how many archaeologists manage to do this but that was my aim and since through meeting up with these Latin Americans I was getting an offer to go to live in Latin America anyway, in the long run I felt that it wasn't too much of a hardship to miss the intermittent stage of the university.

CLARE: The Latin America link would again be an echo of your father's background?

ST AUBIN DE TERAN: Yes.

CLARE: Were you intrigued by that background?

ST AUBIN DE TERAN: Very much, yes.

CLARE: What was it that appealed to you about it?

ST AUBIN DE TERAN: It just seemed to be completely exotic. There was the allure of the unknown because I saw my father maybe once every three years for a couple of days or a couple of hours. I didn't really know him very well but he seemed to me a very exotic person and I liked the idea of this hot country. I've always suffered from the cold and I just loved the idea of this hot country where people would be sort of very open and friendly and there'd be palm trees. I didn't think much beyond that at the time. When I wanted to study archaeology I wanted to go to the Andes. I loved the idea of going to the Andes or going to Patagonia and I'd read a lot of books about Patagonia and I didn't have a very clear picture of what it would be like.

CLARE: Why was Jaime a political exile, what had he done?

ST AUBIN DE TERAN: Well, he'd been involved in the guerilla uprising of the late sixties in Venezuela and he was exiled but because he came from such a grand family he wasn't actually on the run from anybody. He just couldn't return to Venezuela or they would have killed him. His two friends he lived with were actually actively wanted by Interpol and so there was a kind of solidarity with him. He was on the run and since I was with him I was on the run, but we weren't wanted for anything. It was his friends who were at risk.

CLARE: You would have been about eighteen when you went to South America with him.

ST AUBIN DE TERAN: I was eighteen, yes.

CLARE: Where did you go?

ST AUBIN DE TERAN: We went to a place in the Venezuelan Andes and that's actually the only place we went to.

CLARE: And there you were.

ST AUBIN DE TERAN: And there I was.

CLARE: With him. And what was that like?

ST AUBIN DE TERAN: Well, the first six months were just an horrific bout of culture shock, it wasn't at all what I thought, if I thought at all where I was going. It just was a complete sort of shattering of all my dreams and expectations.

CLARE: What was it like?

ST AUBIN DE TERAN: I arrived on this very isolated sugar plantation and it was in some ways quite primitive. It was run in a sort of semi-feudal way. All the workers and all their families, fifty-two families of workers, lived in extreme poverty. Upon arrival, literally as the ship was pulling in to the port of La Guida, Jaime suffered what turned out to be his first sort of schizophrenic episode and didn't realise who I was which was pretty serious for me. I wasn't a member of his family, I wasn't accepted by any of the people who lived and worked on the plantation because the family had intermarried for 400 years. Nobody would speak to me at all. He wouldn't speak to me, he didn't know who I was! Just occasionally he used to say, you know, was I still there and had we met and things like that and apart from that, nobody spoke and, and it was too isolated to leave. There was no public transport. There seemed to be no way out. I just had my passport and sort of a few belongings in a bundle and I thought the first car that comes through here I am getting out, but no car came through and so I stayed there because I began to grow very attached to the place. I've often grown attached to places, perhaps because I feel rootless. I have a facility of dropping roots rather quickly but I began to feel attached to the place and within a year of being there I was pregnant. I mean, we were sort of reconciled at a certain point for a couple of months and I became pregnant and once I became pregnant I then became an honorary Teran because I had a blood link to this family; so the minute the pregnancy began to show that I, too, had Teran blood in me, everyone came down terribly friendly and nice and I became very close to the peasant workers on the estate. In fact, the next sort of six years my whole life was really taken up with their lives and running the estate and far more than a marriage. I didn't really have a marriage after that.

CLARE: During this time did you stay in contact with your mother?

ST AUBIN DE TERAN: Yes, she used to write to me about four times a week. I used to write to her about three or four times a week too.

CLARE: But during the first six months there was never any attempt to get you out or send somebody for you?

ST AUBIN DE TERAN: Well, I didn't feel I could tell my mother what was happening because I'd never told her the difficulties that I'd have because I always felt she was quite frail and, sort of, her stability was quite frail and it would have just broken her heart to have found out that this apparently lovely person wasn't that lovely and that I was not living in wonderful style on this great plantation that she'd heard about and so I didn't tell her that I had any difficulties.

CLARE: Is that very much a characteristic of you, that you keep your problems to yourself, that you sort them out yourself?

ST AUBIN DE TERAN: A bit, yes, that has been a bit the way things have gone. I always felt as a child that I couldn't burden her with my problems.

CLARE: What did you do with them?

ST AUBIN DE TERAN: I hated school, I actually really hated it but I didn't feel I could say to her, 'I hate school,' because it would have just distressed her and upset her and she had her own problems. So I used to play truant but I used to play truant very skilfully and I didn't actually, for a long time, get caught.

CLARE: How did she take it when she found out that you weren't exactly a diligent attender at James Allen?

ST AUBIN DE TERAN: She was terribly upset but it was a sort of mixture of the shame and the thought of my wrecking my chances of going to Cambridge and having this brilliant career.

CLARE: But she didn't react by feeling betrayed?

ST AUBIN DE TERAN: Maybe she did but she never said she did. I think as a mother part of what she wanted for all of us girls was for us to be happy. Also she was working with a lot of sort of disturbed adolescents in her work and so she had quite an understanding of people's problems, maybe more than any other normal middle-class parent. She knew the problems that would arise with people who feel alienated in school.

CLARE: But it meant that when you were in the Andes you contained this disaster inside. You just lived with it and, with the pregnancy, things eased a little bit. But it must have been a miserable time.

ST AUBIN DE TERAN: It was a miserable time but there were certain other factors. There were no telephones in that area so I had no chance of speaking to her directly, and letters, my letters, always arrived opened from the post office and I knew if I wrote letters that there was a possibility that these letters were being opened on their way out and being read. I was living in a neighbourhood that was entirely dominated by the family I'd married into. Only two people, two wives, had ever made the decision to leave their marriages and both of them had been killed as a result of it. They'd been shot and I'd been warned that I would be unable to get out of the marriage. So I felt, you know, it would be very unwise to write in a letter that he's an absolute beast and this and that because I could have got caught out and I felt a certain sense of danger there. But the main thing was I wanted her to think I was blissfully happy. Like when I went to live in Italy she thought I was having a two year honeymoon and having a wonderful time and everything was fine and I wanted her to think that because it was what she'd never been able to have. I wanted her to think that I was, so I used to send her photos, I used to go and stand in front of people's villas and have photographs taken of me whenever friends were around with a camera and we used to say, you know, I'm staying here and I'm staying there and she loved that myth. She wasn't having a wonderful time but she thought, well, you know, Lisa is, that's great, that was important.

CLARE: I've got this picture of you off there in the Andes feeling very much an island, surrounded by this sea of foreign difference, slowly coming to terms with it because of the pregnancy. Yet, as you talk about it you're very matter-of-fact, I don't know whether you realise just what an extraordinary story it is.

ST AUBIN DE TERAN: It was probably twenty-one years ago that I went there and that's for me a long time, so when I left Venezuela I was sort of feeling very bitter and twisted and upset.

CLARE: Angry?

ST AUBIN DE TERAN: Angry, yes. But I've lived a lot of life since then and I don't feel that way about it at all, so I see as though I'd sort of taken a sieve and sifted things out. I've sifted out the things mostly that I want to remember and want to take out from that experience.

CLARE: Do you feel you did learn something about yourself in that experience?

ST AUBIN DE TERAN: Oh, absolutely, yes.

CLARE: What?

ST AUBIN DE TERAN: I did.

CLARE: What would you point to?

ST AUBIN DE TERAN: Well for me one very noticeable thing was I turned from being somebody who was so shy that I sort of literally couldn't speak to people, I could hardly communicate verbally with people at all.

CLARE: Verbally?

ST AUBIN DE TERAN: Verbally with people, I could only write things down but I got so lonely living on the estate that I reached a point when I just wanted to talk to anybody about anything at any time and so when I left the estate I discovered a part of me that I just didn't know before. This very communicative side to myself became quite strong and I became tough. I'd always been a bit of a wimp really and, you know, living in a completely male-dominated society, it was violent – I mean, you know, you went into a bar and somebody said something and someone didn't like it and they'd stand up and just shoot them dead and everybody just stepped over the body and the barman would drag him out into the sawdust and just go on having a drink. I saw that three times when I was there. People would be just sort of shot in bars where I happened to be having a drink.

CLARE: Did you ever feel in imminent danger of your life?

ST AUBIN DE TERAN: Yes, on several occasions. Whenever I went off the estate I was armed but everybody was armed and you know, not to be was actually foolish. If your car broke down, you know, you're virtually dead unless you know how to fix a car and you've got a gun to protect yourself on a country road. It was rough in a way that I just had no preparation for and I coped with it and that gave me a lot of confidence for other things in my life. I felt I had actually dealt with this. I was running this estate. When I first went out there I'd never even seen a stick of sugar cane. I didn't know which way it went in the ground or what to do with it and the estate was just crumbling away really. Because from the time that we went back the foreman who'd been running it felt unable to make any decisions because *el padrone* had come home, but *el padrone* was having a nervous breakdown of some major description and would not make any decisions at all, wouldn't even be there. For the first few months, there was virtually nothing to eat. In the first two or three months when I lived there I was the hungriest I've been, hungrier than when we were in Italy and I thought we were starving because there was just nothing to eat. In fact, one of the real friends that I made out there was a lady, much older than myself, whose family had a sort argument with Jaime at some point and she was trying to woo him back to visiting their family again and she used to send her chauffeur to the estate every other day with a little plate of some delicacy. Venezuelan delicacies are quite heavy but you know, they were very, very nice and this was actually the only food that I had for sometimes weeks on end. There would be this tiny little sort of crème caramel or something. I'd sort of try not to pounce on it as the chauffeur delivered it on a tray and then wait until he'd gone.

CLARE: How did you come to leave?

ST AUBIN DE TERAN: I realised I was going to have to leave about three years before I did because by that time my relationship with Jaime had broken down. Really from the time that Iseult was a tiny baby, just a few months old, our relationship was deteriorating and he was becoming increasingly more unpredictable, more violent and there were a lot of very unpleasant incidents on the estate in which he was involved and I felt, I've got to leave while I still can. Because I think sometimes when you live with somebody who is very mentally unstable you can wind up becoming quite mentally unstable yourself. I felt this was a danger for me. I was living with somebody who was round the bend and I worried that I was going to end up like this myself. I also felt in physical danger from him. He'd two or three times caused me quite serious injuries and he never had any recollection of anything he did, but I began to be quite frightened, physically frightened of him and that made me much less able to cope with him being around, because he could sense that I was frightened, so I was becoming a sort of victim which is not a good position to be in. I was frightened for my daughter and I realised it was going to be very difficult, physically, to get away. I had to make a journey through almost the whole of the place to get out and his family was a very dominant family there, you know. There were road blocks, there were all sorts of things and he was known, his name was known enough to make it very difficult to leave. I was just incredibly attached to a number of the families and people who were living on the estate and I realised that if I left I would be leaving them in the lurch so I wanted to make some kind of arrangement so that they wouldn't be turned off the estate or lose their couple of acres of land. I wanted them legally to be able to keep that because I knew I wouldn't be able to go back and look after them if I made a run for it. I'd had a lot of health problems, I had a very serious kidney problem when I was there and they were getting worse and I gambled really. I thought if I let them get so bad that they become untreatable here, I'll be sent abroad for treatment and so I waited until I was very ill and then I was recommended to go abroad for treatment. So I had all my papers signed for me to be able to legally take my daughter out of the country because she's Venezuelan and I have no legal rights over her, or hadn't at the time, and I went on an aeroplane that went via Berlin and at Berlin we sort of jumped the plane and went on the run.

CLARE: How long did that last?

ST AUBIN DE TERAN: It lasted for about two years, until I felt that I wasn't being pursued in any way, that there wasn't the imminent risk of Iseult being kidnapped and taken back.

CLARE: You said you felt bitter?

ST AUBIN DE TERAN: I did for years after I left Venezuela. I did feel very bitter.

CLARE: What did you direct the bitterness towards?

ST AUBIN DE TERAN: Well, I felt mostly bitter about Jaime himself, about the system that had reared somebody and allowed him to live and behave in a way that was completely lawless, to have the power of life or death over other people with no kind of moral or social intervention.

CLARE: Did you ever feel bitter or angry that you'd either let yourself or had been let get into that situation?

ST AUBIN DE TERAN: I used to feel, I've been such a fool, I've wasted so many years of my life, I've allowed myself to be worn down by this and I felt that it was through my own stupidity.

CLARE: You blamed yourself?

ST AUBIN DE TERAN: I blame myself for marrying a complete stranger, you know, with an interpreter at the wedding for goodness' sake. I thought why did I do that, I had to be crazy.

CLARE: But you'd no one to advise you?

ST AUBIN DE TERAN: Well, I was meant to be the adviser. Ever since I was sort of four years old I'd been advising my mother, you know. I used to advise her about what jobs she should take and what she should do and I used to do the accounting and run the housekeeping and sort her out at the bank and all these things. I was the adviser and so I felt, I had been able to advise all these other people about their lives, I'd been a complete idiot about my own.

CLARE: You describe it without too much ill-will but it was a lot of your mother to ask of you.

ST AUBIN DE TERAN: I think in some ways it was a lot of my mother to ask of me, but she gave me a lot and I think that to have survived the kind of traumas that she survived in her life I think it was a lot for anybody to have asked of her to have been even half as good and as giving as she was.

CLARE: Are you very maternal? As you speak about your mother you sound positively maternal towards her. From very early on you were looking after her. The arrival of Iseult in the Andes, did that make an enormous difference? You now had someone else who depended on you. Did that give you a way of surviving out there?

ST AUBIN DE TERAN: Yes, I think perhaps that's true. I never thought I'd have children. I'd had glandular TB in my own childhood and that tends to leave one sterile. I'd been told I'd never have children and so it was a complete surprise to find myself pregnant.

CLARE: How did you feel about it?

ST AUBIN DE TERAN: Well, I didn't believe it. I was five and a half months pregnant before I knew it. I thought I had worms which was quite common out there. I didn't think this was possible.

CLARE: And when you discovered it was?

ST AUBIN DE TERAN: I was very happy. That's what I wanted. I had wanted for a long time but I just didn't think I could. Iseult was very ill from the time she was born until she was five years old so she didn't have a sort of normal babyhood or childhood and perhaps the very protective way I feel about her is because she had such a difficult beginning. I felt I was always struggling to keep her alive, rather than sort of keep her happy or occupied. She had a series of tropical diseases which she just seemed unable to shake off.

CLARE: How much do you think you define love in those terms?

ST AUBIN DE TERAN: In the terms of looking after?

CLARE: Yes.

ST AUBIN DE TERAN: Probably quite a bit. I think probably quite a lot.

CLARE: So, you would be very experienced in looking after. How are you in terms of being looked after?

ST AUBIN DE TERAN: I like being looked after.

CLARE: You do.

ST AUBIN DE TERAN: I do. I like a lot of attention. I think if I'm greedy for anything in my life I'm greedy for attention. I like actual being looked after and attention.

CLARE: In what way do you do it? In one sense you're quite independent. You move. You survive break-up. You often describe yourself as rootless.

ST AUBIN DE TERAN: Perhaps it's more an emotional being looked after than a sort of actual, you know, having things done for me. I think of myself as somebody who emotionally is quite insecure at heart. I think I'm quite insecure.

CLARE: Your mother didn't emotionally look after you in that sense.

ST AUBIN DE TERAN: I don't know. You see, in some ways I think that she did and that I always felt that she completely loved me and that provided an emotional security more than any other. OK, if I had a nasty accident I wouldn't tell her but I knew, I actually knew, I could have told her. I just didn't want to cause her that pain but I seem to need a sort of total love from people, for people to feel completely dedicated emotionally to me, which is, when I think about it, a kind of greedy way of feeling but I'm aware of feeling that, of needing this kind of high level of passion and involvement in my relationships.

CLARE: Did you seek that in your second marriage?

ST AUBIN DE TERAN: No, I didn't, no. I was just aware of needing that and wanting that.

CLARE: It didn't affect your marriages, certainly not the first two. When you married George MacBeth it did not seem to be the act of somebody looking for a profound, rich, committed, supportive, loving relationship.

ST AUBIN DE TERAN: I think I was just always looking for this immensely romantic, passionate, almost purely motivated Byronic love affair. I was always looking for that. I was always looking for it – I didn't used to find it but I was always looking for it. Often I could talk myself into being almost half-way there on the very flimsiest of pretexts, because I so much wanted it that I would will myself into believing that this was what I'd found.

CLARE: And was that so of that second marriage? Did you, for a brief period, believe that this was what you'd found?

ST AUBIN DE TERAN: No, not really, but I found something else, if you like. I came to know George and to be close to him through his writing and because writing has always had a huge importance to me, and I feel very passionate about it, we had a kind of, a communion at that level. In fact, it was one way at the beginning because when I first knew George he didn't like the way I wrote at all and was very critical of it, which, you know, made me feel, 'This is not my perfect partner because he doesn't like what I write and I would die for what I write.'

CLARE: It wasn't a marriage that lasted long?

ST AUBIN DE TERAN: No.

CLARE: Because?

ST AUBIN DE TERAN: I think for a number of reasons. In some ways George was tremendously supportive to me, he was very supportive. But he was, I would say, very supportive to the idea of me rather than me as a person so that when my nervous breakdown began, for instance, he was quite unable to accept anything at all was happening. So, although I would say, 'I'm quite desperate by now and I think I might kill myself and I don't want to go on living,' he would say, 'You must be very tired, have an early night,' because his idea of me was of a sort of almost perfect person who couldn't possibly be feeling like that. So there was a failure to communicate which gradually came to disturb me. It coincided with my having published my first books and getting a great deal of media attention, getting a great deal of magazine interviews and profiles and things, all seeing me in a light in which I did not see myself, leaving me feeling very disturbed that actually I didn't exist. I felt, I don't exist because everybody sees something, they see my past, they don't see me as I am, and I was feeling very desperate and in need of a centre.

CLARE: What particularly had brought that on, because you'd been through a lot?

ST AUBIN DE TERAN: Well, my mother died. I think it was really that as much as anything. She had a very gruelling death by cancer and then she died and after she died I felt my reason for living in England had gone and my reason for staying strong had gone and well, my best friend really, the closest person in my life had gone and I just added that to not being happy at all in my marriage, not being happy by then at all in my work. I was unable to work any more. I felt very out of place, living as I was this very artificial, superficial life in this castle in Norfolk, all laid out for, sort of, magazines to photograph but with no real life in it.

CLARE: What happened?

ST AUBIN DE TERAN: I left. I left and I went to Italy.

CLARE: You call it a nervous breakdown. Did you have to see someone?

ST AUBIN DE TERAN: No. The nervous breakdown came really after

I'd got to Italy. I thought, if I leave, I'll be all right, I'll go somewhere else. But of course, it was me who was going and it was me who was having the head fits so by the time I got to Italy and had been there for a couple of months I felt aware of having a real nervous breakdown.

CLARE: How would you describe it to someone, what was happening to you?

ST AUBIN DE TERAN: I felt completely out of control of myself. I felt unable to live with my thoughts and feelings.

CLARE: Would you have been out of control with your emotions? Would you have been weeping?

ST AUBIN DE TERAN: Oh, yes.

CLARE: Great surges of emotions?

ST AUBIN DE TERAN: Great surges of weeping and sobbing and collapsing in the street and shaking and, you know, the works, really.

CLARE: Panic?

ST AUBIN DE TERAN: Panic, feeling the buildings were all falling on top of me and anxiety attacks, terrible anxiety attacks about my children, feeling that something terrible was going to happen to my children.

CLARE: And they were what age, at this stage?

ST AUBIN DE TERAN: They were two and twelve.

CLARE: You'd had a second child.

ST AUBIN DE TERAN: Yes.

CLARE: Were they with you?

ST AUBIN DE TERAN: My daughter was at boarding school at the time so she was with me for holidays and Alexander was with me all the time.

CLARE: When you say you went to Italy in this turbulent state, did you go to somebody or to somewhere?

ST AUBIN DE TERAN: I went to somewhere but it was somewhere I didn't know, I'd never been to. I was just trying to rent a place to go and live and Sestri Levante came, pulled out of the hat and so I went to this place called Sestri Levante.

CLARE: Was there anybody there that you knew?

ST AUBIN DE TERAN: No, and that was, I think, a big mistake. It was a big mistake. Probably, one of the biggest reasons for the breakdown was the birth of Alexander. Something happened when Alexander was being born and I actually became aware of something that was unhinging in my brain.

CLARE: What, snapping?

ST AUBIN DE TERAN: Yeah, I just felt something sort of almost like a sort of chemical change. I was being given enormous quantities of drugs to force me to have him by natural birth and I was actually incapable of doing that for some physical reason that I don't know, but all my children have had to be born by caesarean. But with this second one, my doctor was off sick or skiing or something and another doctor came in and he tried to force me for the best part of a day to have the baby normally, so I was in a sort of very, very severe pain but also being filled up with a drug. And after about eight hours I felt something going in my head and I didn't feel it come back until probably about two and a half years later.

CLARE: But in Italy, when you got there, you still felt dreadful really?

ST AUBIN DE TERAN: Yeah, I felt very lonely, terribly lonely. And I made friends on about day one with a chap who worked in the ticket office at the station and that was really where a lot of the sort of resurgence of my train travelling came up because under any pretext I would just turn up at the station and the best pretext was to make a short train journey and then a longer one and a longer one so the first person I kind of latched on to was the ticket man. But it was a very difficult, that was the most difficult time that I've ever known. I hadn't told any of my family that I was having a breakdown.

CLARE: You never tell anyone really when you're in bad straits?

ST AUBIN DE TERAN: No. I've regretted that subsequently. I think I should have told, I should have told.

CLARE: Did you seek help from anyone? Did you seek any psychological help or medicine?

ST AUBIN DE TERAN: No, I wrote a novel. I wrote *The Bay of Silence* when I was living in Italy and in it, created a woman who was going mad.

CLARE: Breaking up . . .

ST AUBIN DE TERAN: . . . and breaking up and who had a terrible fear that something would happen to her child and I actually exorcized my own fears through sitting down and working, you know, sort of six, eight hours a day, day after day after day, writing that book. I found that extremely therapeutic.

CLARE: But when you were writing it, you were . . .

ST AUBIN DE TERAN: I was gibbering, I was barking!

CLARE: There would have been times when you would be fearful of going out, for example?

ST AUBIN DE TERAN: Yes.

CLARE: Or thinking that something terrible might happen to you?

ST AUBIN DE TERAN: Yes. I'd got the door barricaded up with furniture sort of every other night and I was really in a very strange state, but by making something happen to the child in my book I lifted the fear that something would happen to my own.

CLARE: Did you at any stage during that time think that you couldn't go on?

ST AUBIN DE TERAN: I was very frightened of committing suicide during the whole time. I just cut off and closed down. In fact, subsequently friends and family said, 'You know, you were very strange, you just didn't seem as if you were there at all.' But from the time I went to Italy and things got out of control, I was frightened of committing suicide. I actually left Norfolk because I felt convinced that I would commit suicide if I didn't, because I felt I'd reached the point when I just could not go on any more the way I was. I didn't want to commit suicide and I was frightened of doing it. I felt, you know, I really don't want to commit suicide but I'm feeling so desperate I wonder if that's the sort of state you get into when it happens but I didn't actually . . .

CLARE: Do anything . . .

ST AUBIN DE TERAN: . . . . Do anything.

CLARE: No. The state you experienced, would you describe it as pain?

ST AUBIN DE TERAN: A sort of torment, really. It was more like a torment; not, I think, a pain because I think of physical pain as something else.

CLARE: What did keep you going, apart from the writing?

ST AUBIN DE TERAN: Children, and this sort of inane optimism which I somehow always had a sort of streak of, even then. Even then I felt, I've got to get over this time and it will be all right. I'd seen my mother have several nervous breakdowns as a child and I realised that you could get out of them and life could go on.

CLARE: Did you worry about that, that you had, in a sense inherited something?

ST AUBIN DE TERAN: When I was a child, I, and I think all my sisters, used to worry ourselves silly thinking, you know, we come from a family of lunatics and it's all going to be hereditary and that's terrible. But by the time I got to about fourteen I felt, maybe wrongly, I don't know, but I felt this isn't a worry. I thought, I worry about it so much I must be completely sane because I'm sure people who are absolutely crackers don't worry it about it at all, so I must be OK.

CLARE: And then in Italy, in the middle of barricading the doors, not being able to go out, worrying that you might harm yourself, recalling your mother's states, did you at any stage think this is a family curse as some people sometimes call it?

ST AUBIN DE TERAN: No, not really. No, I didn't think that. I was very aware of my mother all the time that I had the breakdown, I was very aware of my mother. I felt she was displeased with me. I felt that although she'd died, she was actually very displeased with me and she'd never been displeased with me in all my life. I felt she was. I used to have terrible nightmares in which she'd sort of come back and talk to me and shout at me and say horrible things and that I sort of let her down and betrayed her. And that I had to make something of my life and I had to do something and that I had to be honest with my emotions and I had to look after the children and give them a better life and not be this kind of depressed zombie. I felt as if I'd really let her down terribly badly by pretending to be something I wasn't. So living in Italy was, I think, when I managed to get my centre back. It was very important for me because I felt she would have really approved of my living in Italy. She would have loved the thought that I was living in Italy and that the children were being brought up there.

CLARE: What was the something that in your dream she felt you were pretending to be that you weren't? It's quite interesting to hear what you feel you are not, because, of course, that immediately, that does tell you a lot about what you feel you are. What was this person that was beginning to emerge in Norfolk and clearly was so disturbing that it led you to flee in a sense. What sort of person would I have found if I'd gone to Norfolk?

ST AUBIN DE TERAN: I think I lived a life that was very locked away from any kind of contact with other people, other than a very small group of people who were working in the house and there was no kind of social mixing. There was no giving out to other people, there was a lack of generosity, if you like. I mean I would throw great big parties but they were all very orchestrated, there was a lack of contact, a lack of real generosity of spirit rather than of tables groaning with food and I felt she would have disapproved of me, that she would have disapproved of the artificiality, of the lack of any real feeling, this sense of order rather than of emotion.

CLARE: When you were writing the book, did the nightmares ease, did she still stay around but change? What happened to all of that?

ST AUBIN DE TERAN: I wrote that book, *The Bay of Silence*, and I began to find myself again, I began to feel in touch with myself again and the nightmares eased and just disappeared.

CLARE: Did she disappear too?

ST AUBIN DE TERAN: No, she's . . .

CLARE: No? Do you dream much about her?

ST AUBIN DE TERAN: I do, I still dream now, I have conversations with her in dreams. From the time that she died and all during her life and ever since that one bad period, I've always felt very close to her, very close, as though we had an enormous amount in common; so it was, I think for me, the most disturbing thing, this sense of her anger.

CLARE: You've spoken about the sense of her in your dreams. Do you have a sense, or did you then, have a sense of her in waking hours?

ST AUBIN DE TERAN: Mm, yes.

CLARE: Would you have ever felt she was speaking to you, heard her speaking to you?

ST AUBIN DE TERAN: I sort of sensed her speaking really, yes.

CLARE: Or would you find yourself speaking out loud to her?

ST AUBIN DE TERAN: I managed to avoid that one.

CLARE: But she's the most powerful person in what's made you what you are. Would that be true?

ST AUBIN DE TERAN: Yes, I think that's true.

CLARE: You know really what she would like you to be. Is it what you are now, living in Italy, writing and about to commence on a rail journey in South America for television. What would she make of it? What do you think she's saying?

ST AUBIN DE TERAN: I think that what she always really, genuinely wanted was for me to be happy, not sort of happy all the time, but just to be able to be happy and to be completely honest with myself and I felt that when she was angry with me it was because I was neither of those things. I'd been pretending, I'd been living in a way that was a pretence, a sort of sham. I feel that now she would see that I've managed to get in touch with my emotions in a way that I don't think I was able to do for a very long time. I always wanted to fall in love with someone, I always wanted to have this grand passion. I never was able to because I think I was just completely sort of locked in emotionally in myself. It's only in the last seven years that I actually feel fulfilled as a woman, as a person. I didn't before. I knew I owed it to her but I couldn't somehow do it before and now, I think that I can.

Robert Winston

In Britain at the present time, it is estimated that around one in every ten couples is childless. What is not known is what proportion of these childless couples are so by choice and how many are infertile. One of the most dramatic and impressive developments in so-called high-tech medicine has been the growth of the speciality of reproductive medicine. It has developed with such startling rapidity that today much more can be done for infertile couples than at any previous stage in human history. The technique of artificial insemination with either the husband's semen (AIH) or that of a donor (AID) has been used with success for over two decades. Artificial insemination involves obtaining semen by masturbation and injecting it into the neck of the women's womb. It is a relatively straightforward procedure. Artificial insemination involving the husband's semen is essentially a matter of building up the semen and helping it on its way. It is also used if semen is preserved by freezing for use after a vasectomy or indeed after the husband's death. Artificial insemination involving a donor is usually only employed when a husband's semen is seriously deficient either in terms of fertility or genetically.

More recently, the complicated, time-consuming and expensive technique of *in vitro* fertilisation (IVF) has been developed. It is concerned in the main with female infertility. In IVF, an egg is removed by a minor surgical procedure from the woman's body and then fertilised with semen in the laboratory – *in vitro* means 'in glass', that is to say, in the laboratory dish. For this reason, babies conceived through such a process are often referred to as 'test-tube babies'. The fertilised egg, termed an embryo, is then implanted in the womb of the woman from whom the egg was taken in the first place (so-called embryo replacement) or on another woman (embryo transfer). The semen used, as in artificial insemination, may be that of the woman's husband or of another male donor.

The development and use of these techniques have been accompanied by intense professional and public debate concerning the moral acceptability, the ethics of what is involved, and there have been a number of public statements made by such bodies as the British Medical Association, the Medical Research Council, the Council for Science and Society and, most notably, by the Warnock Committee chaired by Dame Mary Warnock. The Warnock Committee first reported in 1984, by which time the number of babies born in Britain as a result of IVF was over 200. It rejected the argument that such treatment was either unnatural or inappropriate in an over-populated world and argued that infertility came within modern medicine's proper concern with 'remedying the malfunctions of the human body' and hence was 'a condition meriting treatment' for which provision should be made within NHS priorities. This was a particularly robust response to those who, perhaps not unreasonably, doubted whether not being able to have a baby could be legitmately termed an illness and questioned the assumption that the health to which every citizen increasingly believed he or she was entitled included the ability to produce as many children as they would wish to have.

The development of reproductive medicine has been one of the great boons of the scientific revolution in modern medicine but, like so many of these, it has not been without its problems too. Professor Winston in the course of this interview refers to a Greek patient whose fallopian tubes had been blocked and were unblocked by a new surgical technique. She observed what a mixed blessing this was; before the treatment, when the tubes were blocked, she *knew* she was not fertile; with the tubes unblocked, she no longer knew whether she was infertile or not. IVF can also cause enormous heartache for couples both in terms of the demands it places on them as they wait for ovulation, the surgical removal of the egg, and implantation, and during the couple of months before successful implantation can be definitively confirmed. And then there are the failures. Unless one has known a couple who have progressed through all the stages of IVF only to lose the implanted embryo after a few weeks or for whom implantation just will not occur, one cannot imagine the loss, the grieving, the lamentation that ensue.

But the very existence of a potentially effective treatment of IVF has also served to intensify the issue of infertility so that often it comes to dominate the couple's relationship in such a way that without a successful outcome to treatment the relationship stands a very good change of being permanently jeopardised. Many people attach such importance to producing a child that in every marital or equivalent relationship in which they find themselves it assumes the highest priority. This brings with it the worry that couples who become obsessed with the idea of producing a child as the goal of their lives may end up investing and surrounding any offspring of the procedure with intense and unrealistic hopes and fears such that its subsequent healthy development may be put at particular risk.

Virtually every doctor working in clinical practice has witnessed the anguish of couples who for one reason or another find that they are infertile. Listening to a couple who have fastened with desperation on to the possibilities inherent in IVF, I invariably find my mind turning to the issue of what it is that makes having children such an important, sometimes the most important, desire that people, men and women, can have. It is only in this century that human beings have gained a reasonable degree of control over procreation. In turn, this has presented new problems, not least the fact that infertility is less and less seen as an unfortunate deficiency of nature and more as a defect to be remedied by medical science. But, as Professor Winston reminds me in this interview, there has always been a stigma attached to barrenness. To be declared sterile brings with it connotations of shame, inadequacy and failure.

Professor Robert Winston is one of the leading figures in reproductive medicine. I invited him to be interviewed not merely to discuss his own path through a Jewish family to medicine by way of the London Hospital School, but also to discuss some of the key issues provoked by the nature of the research work that he and his colleagues pursue. The obvious question to put to him is just why it is that being unable to have children causes such desperation, such pain, in infertile couples.

As one of the most vociferous, visible and pugnacious champions of the infertile in the country, he is particularly well-placed to answer. But my main reason for asking Professor Winston to sit in the psychiatrist's chair is that he is a man in a field of medicine concerned with women's health, he has made his lifetime's work the study and treatment of infertility and he is himself a family man who places a particular value on the importance and the impact of family relationships in the formation of an individual's temperament and personality.

Implicit in so much of the work that I and others do in the fields of psychology and psychiatry is the belief that our genes interacting with our environment shape the way we develop and mould who we are. Not surprisingly, most of the dozens of interviews in this interview series over the years have involved individuals from a variety of walks of life, exploring, amongst other things, the influence of their parents, for good or ill, on their own characters and lives. In the case of babies conceived through *in vitro* fertilisation where the egg or the semen comes not from the father or mother who rears them but from anonymous donors, what is the impact on their self-understanding of the realisation, later on in life, that their biological and their actual parents are not the same? It might be said that the issues raised are no different from those occurring in adoption and that indeed is a persuasive argument, but the fact remains that in cases of IVF where the egg comes from an anonymous donor the confusion between the genetic mother and the mother bearing the new infant is of a different order from that involved in normal adoption. The fact also remains that whatever the emphasis on anonymity of donors in the field of IVF, the offspring manifest the same intense desire to know about those who have genetically contributed to their make-up as people who have been conceived in 'natural' ways.

I am not at all sure that the ethical discussion concerning IVF and anonymous donors has kept pace with the scientific, the technological developments, and this interview with Professor Winston does not particularly reassure me. But what is impressive is Robert Winston's willingness to share his uncertainties and doubts and to admit that he does not have all the answers.

He is honest too about what it is like to be a senior scientist in a respected research institute who believes that he has a responsibility to involve himself in the wider public debate concerning aspects of medical research. Involvement with the media has still the connotations the great Sir William Osler conjured up when he warned doctors about the hazards of consorting with the harlots of publicity and the press!

It is ironic that so much of the interview with the man who more than most is responsible for *in vitro* fertilisation in Britain should concern itself with his reflections on the influence of his own father and mother on the way he developed his personal beliefs and attributes and his Jewishness. Professor Winston comes from an extended Jewish family with an orthodox Rabbi as a grandfather on his mother's side and a proud, supportive Jewish mother. He is one of many doctors in British medicine who has had more than a passing interest in the theatre (even if there is only one Jonathan Miller). His award-winning production of Pirandello's play *Each In His Own Way* at the 1969 Edinburgh Festival serves to remind us, if we need reminding, of the extent to which the clinical practice of medicine even in these scientific, rational days of audit and accountability involves some of the skills of a theatrical producer, including the ability to organise and motivate a disparate group of individuals, to inspire them by flair, leadership and example, to fight on their behalf for their work and their professional integrity and to sell the value and worth of what is being undertaken to those who have money and influence. What he did all those years ago for Pirandello and his theatre group he now does for infertile couples up and down the land.

CLARE: Professor Robert Winston is a pioneer of international renown in the treatment of infertility. He specialises in the controversial area of *in vitro* fertilisation, indeed is often referred to by the tabloids as Britain's number one test tube baby boffin. The oldest of three children, he was born on July 15th, 1940, into an orthodox Jewish family in North London. His father died when he was nine and he was brought up by his mother, Ruth, a prominent figure in the Jewish community with a distinguished record in social and welfare work.

Robert Morris Winston went to St Paul's School and was educated at London Hospital Medical College. He is now Professor of Fertility Studies at London University's Institute of Obstetrics and Gynaecology and Consultant Obstetrician and Gynaecologist at the Hammersmith Hospital. He has been married to Lira, a history scholar and school governor for more than twenty years. They have three children, two sons and one daughter. They maintain an Orthodox Jewish way of life.

Professor Winston, you said somewhere, 'Although I'm perceived as very clever, I don't think I am. I'm a fluent talker, which means people often don't see through me.' Does this mean that you feel there's quite a gap between how you're seen and the way you think of yourself?

WINSTON: I must have been particularly perceptive on that day. I don't remember saying that but it's very much how I do see myself, really. I think I am quite fluent. I don't really think of myself as being clever in any sense. It's very difficult to quantify what is meant by intelligence anyway, really.

CLARE: Well, for example, have you been seen by others as clever?

WINSTON: Well, I think the only time I experienced genuine unpopularity at school I think was when I was top of the form. I remember coming home from school when I first started at prep school seeing '1' against my name in the four subjects we were taking and I wasn't clever enough to realise that that meant that I was first, I thought that that was the marks I'd got and I used to tell my mother that I'd not done very well and then one fortnight I got a 1, 1, 2, 1, and I said to her that I'd done slightly better, which I don't think really denotes much intelligence, simply that I was working.

CLARE: Does that mean that you might have been one of those medical students, for example, that I recall who tended to underestimate just how good they were and often plagued the rest of us as a result by worrying about how they would do when the rest of us knew they would do very well indeed?

WINSTON: I didn't do well as a student. I don't think anybody would have thought that I would have become, for example, an academic, let alone a professor. My track record was one of doing a lot of outside activities. That's why I think I'm fluent. I'm a bit of a butterfly and that has always been, I think, one of the things that somewhat directed the kind of professional areas that I've been interested in. I was quite taken with the idea, possibly, of doing psychiatry. I think partly because psychiatry, it seems to me, and this may sound presumptuous, but as a psychiatrist really nothing human is alien to one because anything of the human experience can be used and is of importance. I think of course there's an element of that in all medicine. I think that was perhaps why I did medicine, because originally I wasn't going to. Originally I was going to read natural sciences and the idea of doing medicine was quite a late decision.

CLARE: Just sticking with the issue of fluency. Sometimes fluency in medicine is slightly suspect. Sometimes I feel that people are a little suspicious of a doctor who speaks too fluently. They say of them, really, what you were really saying about yourself, they're nothing like as clever as they seem. I wondered have you sensed that it's your fluency that makes people wonder about just how good you are?

WINSTON: Yes, I'm sure that's true. I'm conscious rightly or wrongly that certainly I've created a lot of jealousy for myself I think in the profession.

CLARE: Why have you done that?

WINSTON: Well, I think it's partly being on the media a lot and partly being rather fluent in what I'm expressing and I think many colleagues, I may be wrong, but I suspect many colleagues are quite jealous of that and feel almost threatened because I'm presenting a case which I feel, often, quite passionately about. You don't have to be intelligent to feel passionately about things and certainly I've tended to be led, I think sometimes, by my heart rather than my brain over issues which I've felt worth campaigning for. I don't think many professions tolerate people that have a high profile that well, and I sometimes think that that may actually still affect my relationship with people. When I've published some research which I think is quite worthwhile, I sometimes feel that perhaps it's not appreciated in the way that it perhaps might be.

CLARE: Does this mean that you, too, have therefore, reservations about being so public?

WINSTON: Yes, I do have reservations about it and I've always had those reservations. But I think it's been tremendously useful to be public. For example, there have been occasions when I think it's really been positively helpful when parliament was debating the human embryology issue. I think being public and being fluent probably was quite helpful because it did enable one to get to the people who were going to legislate and impress them that this wasn't something which they should look at in quite the way it was being presented.

CLARE: Where does this fluency come from? What's the background to it?

WINSTON: My mother was a brilliant public speaker. My grandfather was a fine public speaker with a very good command of English.

CLARE: What did he do?

WINSTON: He was a rabbi. He could give a sermon in the most elegant language – rather unusual for rabbis who are usually very intelligent people but don't always use the English language particularly well. He did, and he was very widely read and I certainly came from a home that was full of books. I think my father was probably quite fluent actually, too.

CLARE: What did he do?

WINSTON: Well, he was actually a diamond craftsman. He ran, by modern standards, a rather small firm. But he was almost a renaissance sort of person. He played the violin particularly well. He was a fine competition standard chess player. He acted, I remember him playing in *Hamlet*, for example, when I was a kid, watching him on stage. He used to flit rather like I do from thing to thing, not always doing it terribly well but enjoying it.

CLARE: He died when you were quite young.

WINSTON: He died aged forty-two. Yes, he was very young but

people said of him that he lived life remarkably fully for his age.

CLARE: What did he die of?

WINSTON: Oh, well, I think rather typically he neglected his health. He got a cold and then he got an abcess on the lung and then he got a brain abscess and in the days when antibiotics perhaps were not given quite as readily as they would be now he suffered in consequence.

CLARE: What sort of man was he?

WINSTON: He was a vibrant personality. I remember the most flaming arguments at home with my mother but they were, I think, a deeply loving couple. It was a very stable relationship but I remember he once threw a cup of coffee at my mother in the dining room which left a huge stain on the wall and then at breakfast some weeks later he said, 'You know, I've been thinking, it's about time we had this room redecorated.' And I remember one of his passions was archery and he used to practise archery in the dining room, so he'd put the target up on the wall, you know, when the weather wasn't good enough and fire arrows off. He was rather unusual. He was an interesting man.

CLARE: Do you remember his death?

WINSTON: I remember my reaction to it. When he wasn't well I was in my grandfather's house and my grandfather was very formative in my upbringing. He certainly taught me my religious education and I think, to some extent, some of my, sort of, non-religious, literary education came from that household. I was actually staying with them when my uncle came through to tell me that my father had just died and I remember crying a bit, but not crying over much about it because really it wasn't something I could really entirely grasp at the age of nine.

CLARE: Since then?

WINSTON: Oh, I have to say I've deeply regretted not knowing him better and I think I've always rather missed having him around. I think I wouldn't have liked him enormously, because he was profligate, he was wasteful. He used to buy things on impulse and do things which probably weren't terribly sensible.

CLARE: Do you sometimes identify bits of yourself and think, 'This is him?'

WINSTON: I don't know. I find myself to be quite good at the same sorts of things sometimes. I've played competition chess myself a bit, and bridge too which he also did rather well. I'm a fairly musical individual but I don't play an instrument as well as he did.

CLARE: But you talked about him being profligate?

WINSTON: Oh, I spend, I spend money, yes. I'm wasteful. I'm actually even wasteful at work. I'm wasteful I think even in the way that I probably run the unit. I don't expect people, for example, to be defined with their research role. I would prefer to have a unit where ideas are bounced around and people perhaps waste six months and if they don't publish, they don't publish, but we've done something interesting. That is very much something which I think is perhaps a characteristic which, well, it's not genetic but it's a characteristic perhaps I share.

CLARE: I'm interested in speaking to someone who in a sense lost a father just before a father would start to really make a certain kind of impact and so I'm intrigued to know what you feel you missed and what it did to you. How different would you be, do you think, had he lived? What did it do, losing a father at nine?

WINSTON: I think it's very difficult to know, isn't it? When you haven't had something it's difficult to say, but I think probably relationships with women were much more repressed as a teenager. Probably if I'd had a father they wouldn't have been, I suspect. Because I didn't have any kind of role model, there wasn't anybody else to talk to apart from my mother who was left not quite destitute but certainly impoverished by his sudden death. He didn't plan financially so she had to suddenly work. She had been doing local politics but she hadn't worked. She was quite capable of working and she turned out to be highly successful at the job she did.

CLARE: What did she do?

WINSTON: Well, she worked as an adoptions officer. That's an odd,

odd thing, I don't think my interest in infertility in any way relates to her work. But certainly she became, at one stage, the person who'd placed more children for adoption than anybody else in the United Kingdom.

CLARE: Did she talk much about it? Were you conscious of what it was all about?

WINSTON: Well, I mean she used to do quite a lot of visits at weekends, so on Sunday we would get into the car and she would go off to families and I would sort of trot around and stay in the car quite often with her. I did sort of see her indirectly at work and met some of her colleagues. But I really don't think that her work in any way influenced my career. I think that was quite different, quite different.

CLARE: And the dynamic with your mother, you were the eldest of three, so in a sense you were the eldest in that family when your father died.

WINSTON: Difficult position to be in I think, in some ways. A feeling of responsibility perhaps.

CLARE: Have you got that?

WINSTON: Yes, I think I have. I think I probably do have a sense of responsibility, perhaps a sense of social responsibility. I hope that doesn't sound arrogant. One of the things that pleases me most about my own children is that I look at them and I think that they're very responsible individuals, even at the young age that they are. They're very caring and perhaps if one leaves that behind one that's really probably worth doing.

CLARE: What was your relationship with your two younger sibs? You had a younger brother and a young sister.

WINSTON: Yes, my sister has always been a fairly fiery character. She's an artist and very passionate. Highly intelligent.

CLARE: Do you clash?

WINSTON: Yes, and we used to play cricket together and she'd walk off, you know, if I bowled a ball that she didn't like and would stump around and generally make an appalling show. My brother's a much softer individual, I think, than she. He's a scientist. He works in the States.

CLARE: Was it an extended Jewish family, the sort that non-Jewish people often rather envy or are intrigued about? Warm and emotional and passionate and full-blooded and committed.

WINSTON: I don't know that it's particularly passionate. Indeed, I think in some ways it's quite Anglo Saxon in its relationships. My father was much more Anglo Saxon, much less religious in his background than my mother.

CLARE: The rabbi grandfather was your mother's father?

WINSTON: Yes.

CLARE: Right.

WINSTON: And an orthodox rabbi, but extraordinarily openminded actually. That was quite interesting in the way that I think most orthodox rabbis now probably have difficulty with. For example, you know, he would read Dante in the original, he would read Balzac in the original, and, you know, I guess they're both writers that perhaps you wouldn't think of a Jewish rabbi as reading first hand but he was equally fluent in Talmud. Clearly he would have to be.

CLARE: And your father's relationship with him?

WINSTON: Was very good. They obviously respected each other.

CLARE: How important was your family life to your subsequent development? Would you see that as a time of stability, despite the loss of your father, or were you an anxious person?

WINSTON: No, I think it's been a very stable background to come from. I think its stability is evinced by the fact that for many years after my father's death my mother, who had a very close friend, didn't actually remarry. She finally remarried when I was a late teenager, about eighteen or nineteen when she felt that it really didn't much matter what we felt any more. But actually, he was a very nice man and I think a great sadness, really, is that she then lost him subsequently. He died relatively young, in his sixties, which I think was a pity for my mother.

CLARE: Is your mother still alive?

WINSTON: Yes, she is. She's in her eighties. She's a bit frail.

CLARE: What does she think of you?

WINSTON: I think she's proud of all her children. I mean Jewish mothers are, aren't they, really? I suppose all mothers are. I think she exaggerates what we've done, rather.

CLARE: Had she ambitions for you?

WINSTON: I suspect she probably did have, yes, I think she did. I think she saw me as being somebody who should be aligned in the Jewish community. I think she was very happy when I went into academic medicine. I must say neither of those choices, either being an orthodox Jew myself or actually being an academic were automatic for me. In fact there was a period of my life when I was totaly unorthodox.

CLARE: Tell me about that.

WINSTON: Well, once I suppose half-way through medical school I had serious doubts about faith. I still do have, actually. I suppose I spent a number of years not conforming in any kind of religious way and mixing almost entirely in non-Jewish company. I suppose really I came back largely because it was a philosophy that I understood. It was an anchor. There wasn't a great sense of faith about my return, more a sense of commitment and a sense of belonging to a long cultural tradition. Being able to speak, well, not speak but read, classical Hebrew and Aramaic was important, understanding a bit of Talmud and so on. I think my mother was pretty relieved actually but it was by no means certain that I would necessarily even marry somebody Jewish, I think.

CLARE: But she would have been anxious about that?

WINSTON: Terribly, I mean she would have been mortified had I not. As it turned out I married my wife who came from a deeply religious family but by that time I was already committed I think to really maintaining my Jewish origins.

CLARE: The equivalent in my culture, when people in the middle of medical school throw off Roman Catholicism is that in a sense they may also for a period of time move away from its moral position. It's a time when people become sometimes sexually quite liberated or excessive or they even mix in a quite different cultural milieu. Did it take that shape with you?

WINSTON: Well, I think all medical students are a bit sexually liberated anyway. An awful lot of them are, aren't they? It was almost the norm in the sixties, well, late fifties and sixties. I don't suppose I was much different from most of my colleagues. But I don't really think I lost what are the real moral values. I mean, the importance of relationships and the importance of dealing honestly with people. I don't think I lost those things in any way and I would rate those as being, I think, quite important to me all the time really, and still are of course.

CLARE: What, what did take you into medicine? You've several times already referred to it as if it was something that really might easily not have happened.

WINSTON: Well, I was all set to read natural sciences at Cambridge and it was suddenly the thought that I was going to be staring down a microscope and looking at fungi and probably not doing anything which was terribly interesting and realising that actually what I liked most probably was people, though now I sometimes wonder! This is a terrible admission for a clinician to make – I think it's partly because clinics in reproductive medicine are incredibly stressful – but there are times when one really wonders if one's always made the right decision. It's quite difficult to deflect anger, both one's own anger and one's patient's anger sometimes. And there's a lot of anger in people who are unable to reproduce. But none the less, I think I've chosen an area which really does depend on human relationships and that's what I think really finally fascinates me.

CLARE: So you said, 'I'll do medicine?'

WINSTON: Yes.

CLARE: And you went in to the London Hospital Medical School?

WINSTON: I went into medicine without thinking very clearly what I was going to be doing.

CLARE: Had you had any experience of illness?

WINSTON: No, no.

CLARE: Hospitals?

WINSTON: No, I'd not met any doctors either.

CLARE: No family commitment to medicine?

WINSTON: No, no. Nearly all my family were academic. There were a few academics, people like historians and so on, quite a few of those, or rabbis.

CLARE: These days on your UCCA form you have to indicate your involvement with a mental disability unit, or geriatric nursing home. Had you done anything?

WINSTON: No, no work experience. I think it was easier in our day. First of all you didn't have to get particularly brilliant grades. It seems to me now that people taking A-level really have to get straight As and everything. I think there was a bit more flexibility. But you know, I didn't like the bit much before clinical medicine. I loved the three years of clinical medicine and hated being a doctor. I found it totally frustrating being a doctor for the first four or five years. I wanted to get out and, indeed, I did actually give up medicine at one point and did my other sort of love, which was theatre.

CLARE: You hated it because?

WINSTON: I found it very, very confining. I think it was the fact that it stultified any kind of originality. I used to direct plays quite a bit and act a bit and I decided that I wanted to do that. I decided I wasn't good enough at writing so I couldn't write poetry. I wasn't a good enough musician. I could act a bit. You could put all those together as a director and you could be imperfect in all providing you understood them and that really seemed to me to be very creative and, and for a while, I really thought about doing that seriously, professionally.

CLARE: Now, you say you enjoyed the three clinical years. Medical education splits into the pre-clinical years, which is largely, or was then anyway, basic sciences and biology and you didn't get too much patient contact. It's changed a bit now, but that's the way it was. Then there were these three clinical years when you rotated right through clinical medical school and saw all sorts of patients in all sorts of settings and then you qualified. Now, when you say it was stultifying, let me press you about that. Was it the people you worked with, the hierarchy of medicine that was stultifying? Was it the patients that were stultifying?

WINSTON: Yes, certainly one's chiefs changed completely from being fascinating individuals who were extraordinary characters and brilliant teachers and often most amusingly egocentric into being people who were self-centred and authoritarian. My first six months on the house at the London I think I got one weekend off. The second job pretty well killed quite a precious relationship because I couldn't get away from the job, and the hierarchy, registrar, senior registrar hierarchy I found very difficult to take. It doesn't matter which boss it was now but I remember one boss who used to do a particular operation which would leave patients without a particular hormone. He would remove the adrenals and he was convinced that you didn't need to supplement hormonally, the hydrocortisone, the cortisone and I used to give patients injections of that hormone after the operation for days, knowing that if I didn't they would collapse and he used to say, 'See, patient's perfectly well, we've done an adrenalectomy, she never needed cortisone, you're quite wrong.' And I found that very difficult to accept. And there was an element of slave-driving. One didn't have time to really talk to one's patients. I think there was that and, also, the stresses of being a house surgeon. I nearly killed a patient on my first day. I gave an overdose of insulin because I didn't know to check the bottle. I left it to the nurse to check. I didn't realise that you had to check the bottle so I gave a quadruple strength of insulin intravenously and as it happened, the patient was so sick it saved her life. But I felt very emotional about that and I wasn't well treated by my seniors either as a result of that. They thought I'd been very careless. But the truth was that nobody had actually taught one the practicalities of practising medicine at all. One was completely unprepared. Things are a bit better now.

CLARE: Do you think it is?

WINSTON: Well, I hope it is. I don't work in an undergraduate teaching hospital so I don't perhaps see. All my house surgeons have done at least one or two or three jobs beforehand and we don't work in an authoritarian atmosphere. I expect staff to call me by my first name. I don't want to be called Sir! So there is that change.

CLARE: But it was so intimidating or circumscribing that you actually got out, you left for a while?

WINSTON: Well, I did a path job which is the best thing to do because you're not on call and you can leave at four o'clock when you've looked at the slides.

CLARE: Yes, and there are no people, interestingly enough.

WINSTON: And there are no people except there was the most engaging consultant pathologist who I worked with who was one of the most real people I'd actually met as a chief and who was absolutely forgiving over the fact that I was not primarily interested in path. It was a very useful thing for me to do because, of course, I subsequently ended up in research and of course, being able to do histology, that's looking down a microscope at things, turned out to be a most useful skill and it's one I still use. But it gave me a lot of time off to do theatre.

CLARE: They're interesting people, pathologists.

WINSTON: Yes, they are. They are very interesting people. They have a different view of life and they are actually closer in some ways to the science of medicine as well. And surprisingly, they're not cynical. I mean, to watch a good pathologist, it sounds a bit curious, doing a post-mortem is very revealing. They actually care. That's extraordinary but most of the pathologists I've watched doing post-mortems, actually care about what they're doing and they're not at all uncouth.

CLARE: Did he understand your difficulties that you were having with medicine?

WINSTON: He encouraged me.

CLARE: In what way?

WINSTON: We used to sit at the bench looking at slides, and he would say, 'Well, you know, it's about time you went off and went to this rehearsal,' and he would talk about the play that I was interested in or the one that I was reading.

CLARE: That is pretty unusual.

WINSTON: Yes, he was a good chap, actually.

CLARE: And you had always had an interest in drama. That was so through school, was it?

WINSTON: Yes, I never really got much change at school.

CLARE: You were at St Paul's.

WINSTON: Yes, that certainly runs in the family. Both my father and mother used to act a bit. I did act a bit at school. I played in operations at school. I really came into my own when I went to university and then I acted quite regularly and picked up big parts and got a chance to direct, wrote scripts for reviews and so on and that seemed to go well.

CLARE: And you did these reviews where?

WINSTON: Well, we went all over. Mostly of course they were local but occasionally we got to the Edinburgh Festival.

CLARE: You did?

WINSTON: With the odd review, yeah.

CLARE: And was there ever a moment when Robert Winston might have become a fully-fledged actor?

WINSTON: I don't know about an actor but a director possibly. I actually won a director's award at the Edinburgh Festival and did think about it quite seriously.

CLARE: Now were you still in pathology at this time?

WINSTON: No, I'd actually by that time ceased all paid work.

CLARE: So there was a period when you were not a doctor.

WINSTON: I was living on the proceeds of what we were earning at the box office at that stage.

CLARE: How long would that have lasted?

WINSTON: About five or six months out of medical work. I was doing a play by Pirandello which was actually at the Edinburgh Festival and that was a great success. It played to packed houses. What Pirandello is interested in is in relationships, the relationship between reality and illusion but also in the relationships between people, and the leading actress has to play the part of a leading actress being deluded into believing that she's real when she's not. And she has to play this for real and of course, I had a professional actress and in the green room afterwards, at one point, I said, 'Well, that was a brilliant performance but of course, totally superficial, as it has to be.' And she said that I was a real Svengali! It was only after the end of the production that I realised that my difficulty would be that I would be living with people who didn't actually have, necessarily, an understanding of real life. That's how it seemed to be at the time. I think that's not true of good actors actually but certainly in the circles I was moving. And that really put me off. I felt, well, really, looking at people who might be ill is probably much more important than looking at people who are pretending to be ill. And, do you know, I still have that problem, even when I go to the theatre now. I passionately love Shakespeare but I still have some difficulty watching people playing Shakespeare because I think of them playing the emotions. The player-king in *Hamlet* sums it up rather well.

CLARE: Whereas the real life drama of the medical theatre, that's authentic.

WINSTON: It's absolutely authentic.

CLARE: And you missed that?

WINSTON: I missed it and I think I rather deprecated the fact that people were copying it and doing so imperfectly because we do those things imperfectly, and that I was in some way involved with it. I still have that problem in my relationship with the media actually. For example, going in to the coffee room, waiting for a breakfast time television and listening to the media people around one, I actually find quite off-putting because it's so superficial. Not always, of course it isn't, it would be disgraceful to suggest that people in the media are superficial because that's wrong but there's an element certainly, which I find rather sad.

CLARE: Do you find yourself sometimes wishing that you could take them into your own arena of life?

WINSTON: And show them?

CLARE: And show them.

WINSTON: Yes. I have taken them to clinics sometimes. They found it quite difficult to take, too.

CLARE: How much then of you, the director, is in your medical life?

WINSTON: If I'm really honest and I think one has to try to be, if one's going to play this game, I think inevitably you know. It's politically very incorrect to suggest that you manipulate or that you are authoritarian, but actually doctors do manipulate patients, and I think I do too. If I'm really honest I'm sure I do. I hope the manipulation is honest. It certainly tries to be.

CLARE: How can manipulation be honest?

WINSTON: Well, that's a very interesting question, isn't it? I think you can be honest and manipulate. Indeed I think doctors inevitably manipulate by the very nature of the job. For example, if I see a desperate couple in front of me who want to do *in vitro* fertilisation, and I really feel that they've got a one or two per cent chance of success, and I'm also concerned that they're being totally unrealistic about the chances of success, and I also feel there's a real chance of emotional damage because they're going through a bereavement process and that probably the best thing is that they come to terms with the infertility by a period of mourning and then actually being happy again, i.e. not going through further treatment, I think it's almost impossible not to manipulate that situation. I can't believe that one can avoid taking a stance, even though one tries not to.

CLARE: So in that situation you would play it such that a period of time would elapse?

WINSTON: Yes.

CLARE: No decision would be made. You'd let them mourn?

WINSTON: Well, absolutely. I try not to take decisions for patients. Many patients, particularly who are well, want their doctor to take the decision for them, and one tries not to do that because that actually is very manipulative. But, nonetheless, you do by body language, by signs, I think, manipulate patients. I think it's very difficult not to and I think I don't have a particularly good track record in that respect. I suspect that I do that, like most of my colleagues do. It's quite a dreadful admission, really.

CLARE: You work in a team. I know myself because so do I, it's the feedback you get from members of the team that often tells you how you appear and it can be sometimes a bit of a surprise.

WINSTON: Oh, yes.

CLARE: Is that what you pick up from that? That they see you as someone who actually is quite a skilful manipulator?

WINSTON: Well, I don't know. I know this from patients, too. I remember once, there was one patient who I'm dearly fond of who I've treated for years, fortunately successfully, who I met for the first time many years ago and refused to treat her, I thought on really good grounds.

CLARE: This was for infertility?

WINSTON: Yes, and said I didn't think I could help her and it's very interesting because in fact only about two weeks ago or three weeks ago, she said to me, 'You know the first time we met you were incredibly rude to me.' And I didn't actually think that I had been. I thought that I'd just been, you know, absolutely straight and honest because I was trying to tell her that really there was no chance of her getting treatment successfully. And of course, I was wrong because actually, she'd had a child. So the difficulties of medicine are that inevitably you're taking judgements, you're making decisions and your decisions are fallible and people expect them not to be. I think the trouble with my sort of family medicine is that those decisions are incredibly responsible in a rather unusual way. You don't kill somebody but you change one of the most important aspects of their lives, don't you, in a way, in reproductive medicine.

CLARE: How did you get into reproductive medicine? You came back from Pirandello back into medicine.

WINSTON: I knew I wanted to do obstetrics and gynaecology because I'd always liked that. By that time I thought that was the one area that really was of interest to me especially and did excite me because it's such a wide area. There's a mixture of science, reproduction itself is interesting, there's the family medicine, there's sexual elements, there's a lot of different interests in obstetrics and gynecology and there's dealing primarily with healthy people and, above all, one's dealing with women and I like women. I like women as patients and I like women.

CLARE: Why do you like women as patients?

WINSTON: I don't know. I think I probably empathise with women patients. I don't say that I don't empathise with men, but I just quite like thinking in the way that I think seems to be appropriate and trying to understand. I'm sure this is also politically incorrect to say that finding women patients attractive, and I don't necessarily mean physically attractive, but you know, people that I can talk to at length and find engaging, necessarily.

CLARE: Would you relate better to women in general, leaving aside the question of patients? Tied to something you said earlier I wondered whether the irritation you had with much medicine was to do with its masculinity.

WINSTON: It's very male-dominated, yes. I feel strongly for the feminists in medicine, actually.

CLARE: Do you relate better to women?

WINSTON: I don't know that I do, terribly. I get on well with my male colleagues actually. At least the ones that I choose to be with, i.e. on my own unit, for example. I like male company. I used to play rugby, after all it's as male as you can get, and enjoy the rugby environment, which is largely the drinking afterwards. So I don't think I have a particular problem with relating with either sex but I just like women patients. I mean, that seems to be it.

CLARE: Are there aspects of masculinity you don't like?

WINSTON: I've never really thought about it. I don't think so.

CLARE: Do you find at the present time it's a difficult time to be a man in obstetrics and gynaecology?

WINSTON: I think it's becoming easier again now. I think there was a kind of doubt that men had about dealing with women, but I think now that's resolved. I think on my own unit at the moment, I would say there are probably too few women, actually. There are too many men and too few women, but basically, you don't appoint people for their sex, you appoint them because you think they're going to be the best people. Those recently, on the whole, who have applied for jobs, at least to my unit, have been male and, and consequently I think I've got too few women. But there have been other times when there have been probably more women than men so I think that varies.

CLARE: But most of the people working in reproductive medicine, *in vitro* fertilisation, for example, would be men.

WINSTON: Yes, but then that's because I think to practise IVF, *in vitro* fertilisation, you have to be extraordinarily aggressive. All the people who've done IVF have been very aggressive.

CLARE: How do you mean?

WINSTON: Starting with Patrick Steptoe. Well, because first of all nobody has any sympathy with reproductive medicine, really, outside the patients.

CLARE: You mean it's seen as a kind of luxury?

WINSTON: Yes, it's seen as a kind of luxury.

CLARE: They're not sick.

WINSTON: Yes, they're not sick, they don't need National Health Service resources, so you have to fight every stroke of the way for your resources.

CLARE: When you say aggressive, you mean, verbally, physically, the fluency that you talked about, all mobilised in terms of battling.

WINSTON: Yes, I think they are. I think if you look at most people in reproductive medicine, certainly in this country, you'll see people who are fairly trenchant characters. There are exceptions. That may be one of the reasons why they sometimes grate against each other a bit. But they've used that aggression to very good effect. It's a question of getting resources, of getting the rights of patients looked for, of demanding, for example, even of obstetrics and gynecology, that infertility is a real issue. You know, it's a major part of obstetrics and gynaecology and yet large numbers of gynaecologists refer to it as not fertility but futility, which I think is quite interesting. And when I was brought up as a young gynaecologist in training, people thought that I was mad wanting to be in a futility clinic. So that was one aspect, I think, that made me feel that that was quite wrong.

CLARE: And what is it about infertility that makes you such a battler in that sense. Why do you feel it's such a big issue, given all the other priorities in medicine?

WINSTON: Well, because it causes such enormous distress and because probably for nearly all of us, it is the only important thing we ever do. After all, it doesn't matter if you win the Nobel Prize, you're completely insignificant, you're forgotten within fifteen years. If you're a cabinet minister you're forgotten, you know. Unless you're Mozart, that's the way you're remembered and the one thing that we really do is to produce our children, so that creating the next generation is something that we're all capable of doing. I think that may be why people feel so strongly about procreation. I mean it's difficult to know quite why it causes such severe lack of self esteem when you can't have children, the desperation of the infertile couple is extraordinary sometimes. It's a very acute form of bereavement, it seems to me. I'm not a psychiatrist but the emotions that they show, the inability to communicate, the inability to walk into a room where there are pregnant women, the inability to go to the usual sorts of parties because the subject of children might come up, the corrosion of the relationship between man and woman, all that. So that's one aspect. But the other side of course to it and the reason why it attracted me was also because of the intellectual aspect. I mean there is an extraordinary interest in how we reproduce. And I came into it at the right time. As a science then, it was extremely poor and suddenly it's blossoming. It's now incredibly exciting. I was fortunate I got a Medical Research Council grant early on so I got a research track record and that made a huge difference because, suddenly from being just a clinical doctor who would end up perhaps in a peripheral hospital, I suddenly found that I actually could compete on research terms.

CLARE: Does it scare you, the fact that these people with such desperation will come and invest you often with their last great hope?

WINSTON: Yes, it does, but of course, all medical practice invests the doctor to a certain extent with a degree of imperviousness to some of those issues when he's doing the actual treatment, or taking the actual decisions. The surgeon at the operating table doesn't think with the next incision that the patient's going to die. Actually, if he did, he'd be an awfully bad surgeon. He actually has to take bold manoeuvres sometimes to do things properly. And I think there's an element of that too, even in a clinic. You take broad sweeps. You have to be careful, though, to reflect. I hope I reflect when I take those sort of decisions inside.

CLARE: I mean do you sometimes find yourself thinking, 'This couple in front of me, they've just got this whole business of having a child completely out of proportion, that it dominates their waking hours, that there is nothing else. And after all, large numbers of people live and die without ever reproducing themselves.'

WINSTON: No, I genuinely don't think I think that. No, I think I would take people at their face value and accept the fact that they're suffering. I don't want to sound like a saint because I'm certainly not a saint. But I think I try to take each individual on the ground that they want to present to me, as far as I can. I may come to the conclusion that they're a bit deranged and occasionally perhaps not even necessarily worthy of treatment in the way that they expect.

CLARE: How do you mean?

WINSTON: I'll give you one example, because it's best to think in terms of clinical models, paradigms. There's one patient who I'd been treating for a long time, several years, who struck me as being pretty desperate, and there was something about her treatment that I couldn't really quite work out, why she was really wanting treatment. She always came with her husband. They seemed to be quite a different couple in some ways and they kept on demanding IVF and I kept on resisting, thinking that they weren't right for *in vitro* fertilisation – perhaps rather an authoritarian view, but always feeling anxious about it. It seemed ridiculous in a clinic that's doing two thousand treatment cycles. Finally, because they were very, very persistent, I agreed to the idea of treatment and they went through, and this woman ended up with a termination of pregnancy at twelve weeks, at her request of course, saying that she and her husband decided they didn't want children after all. Now that's in a clinic that's got very good counselling because we have professional counsellors with psychotherapeutic training. Quite clearly, you know, I made an error, but there was a gut reaction at the back there that perhaps was right all along. I think that's what I mean. Now, of course, nobody's denying that that patient is suffering, indeed, every time I saw her, about six times between the time she got pregnant and other members of the team saw her as well, there was no doubt she suffered. She kept on saying to me, 'Well, that means you'll never treat me again doesn't it, you know, for fertility.' And do you know, I found it very difficult to answer her. I couldn't actually answer the question. I could never truthfully say whether I would or I wouldn't. I kind of avoided the question. Now, I suppose if I'd been perhaps less deficient, I would say that you know, this decision doesn't have any bearing on what we might do in the future.

CLARE: Did she give you an adequate explanation, or one that satisfied you about what had been going on.

WINSTON: No, and what's more, she lied to me, too, I know that she lied to me. She told me things about her relationship which weren't true and I knew that, actually, at the time.

CLARE: In the work that you do, I notice that you say sometimes you'll see these people over many years, though people listening will think, 'Well, look, *in vitro* fertilisation, it either happens or it doesn't,' so what's the explanation for that person? In fact, it doesn't just happen. People have two, three, several attempts at *in vitro* fertilisation spread over months, maybe even years.

WINSTON: Yes, I think the record that I've seen recently this year is somebody who's had twenty-one failures. I'm pleased to say not in my own department!

CLARE: Each of these failures being, to use analogy, a bereavement.

WINSTON: Yes, the whole process is a bereavement but it's punctuated by acute episodes which some patients brush off and others don't. It's one of the reasons why I've stood out rather against the treating of older women with donor eggs because I think they're in an acuter form of mourning and they're much more likely to miscarry and therefore any emotional disturbance they have at the age of fifty is likely to be much more heightened and I think there's an area of serious danger for them.

CLARE: This significant act of having a child, I'm interested in teasing out the elements about it. There is, as you say, the profound fact that for most people that will be their significant event in the great evolutionary cycle. They're not Mozart, they're not Shakespeare but they will leave something behind them that is part of them and yet different. But that is, of course, true in the classic Judao/Christian model of two people coming together and sperm and egg fusing and creating a new being. And as we've talked, that's been implicit so far in the model, of *in vitro* fertilisation, usually involving the eggs of the woman and the sperm of the man. But there are other techniques of course that now the technology permits, such as the use of donor eggs, eggs belonging to a completely different woman and I wondered how, given what you've said about the importance of procreation, which I would share I have to say, what do you feel about that because that is in a sense, I know you hate this phrase, in a sense it is a bit like you beginning to play God.

WINSTON: You've tested out an inconsistency in what I said first of all, haven't you, because I've implied I suppose that giving one's own genetic message . . .

CLARE: Yes.

WINSTON: Now, I think you've raised something that's terribly interesting, and I don't know the answer to it. I don't really know, and isn't this a shocking admission after all these years of practice, I don't really know how couples who give birth to children that are not genetically their own really relate to them. Now, of course I've read books, I mean there are a number of experts like Robert Snowdon's books and so on that have dealt with this issue, but I really don't know how my patients deal with that.

CLARE: Do you worry about it?

WINSTON: Well, you mentioned the Judao/Christian thing. Now, of course, the interesting thing is that under the Jewish religion, the idea of donor eggs or donor sperm, well, donor sperm certainly would be forbidden; donor eggs there's a question mark about. But also under the Jewish religion, it's quite clear that a mother who gives birth to the baby actually is the mother, so there's no doubt about that. So, if you had a donor egg you would be the mother. And the question I think might be, and maybe Judaism is raising this issue, that in fact one is bonding with that child and therefore that child is specially yours, even though it's not genetically yours.

CLARE: But take you. When I started to talk to you about you, I said to you, what of your father do you see in yourself, and what of your mother do you see in yourself. And yet, if you happened to be the offspring of Robert Winston's donor egg programme, that would be a meaningless question.

WINSTON: Yes, it would be, it would be, wouldn't it? One would presumably rationalise it by saying that one was the offspring of the environment that one was brought up in. Perhaps that would then be important. And it's interesting, we do know of course from research studies that people who have been adopted, and probably people who are the result of donor insemination, we don't know enough about donor eggs because it's not been going long enough, but people who come from those backgrounds certainly want more information about their genetic parents.

CLARE: They do . . .

WINSTON: And seek them out . . .

CLARE: That's right.

WINSTON: But other studies have tended to show that they're pretty satisfied, in the most case, for the most part with the environment that they end up in. These are issues which of course should dominate the whole practice of modern IVF because they're issues which are central. The issue is that when a fertility doctor conducts a treatment, he should bear in mind the child that's going to be produced as a result of that action and the feelings of that child should be important.

CLARE: But you've already said that you have no idea what the consequences are.

WINSTON: Yes, yes I have.

CLARE: Why I'm interested in interviewing you for example from so many other doctors in British medicine is that I, like you, do take this issue of genetic transmission, procreation, and the movement of the generations very seriously indeed. It seems to me to be really the lynchpin of all the other things as you say. You're not God in that you don't create something out of nothing, but you're becoming the nearest thing to God in the sense that you and the molecular biologists are working at where life is transmitted, at where it moves from one generation to another – the handing over of life. And you yourself said, that's what makes it so important to you because this really is what is significant about us as humans, our ability to hand on our lives to our children. Is your defensiveness about being God partly at any rate fed by an unease that you're as close to a certain kind of godlike activity as any of us is likely to get to?

WINSTON: That's a very interesting question, but I don't think so, no, I don't think I feel like that at all. In a way we're at risk of muddling two issues, if I might say so. One is the issue of the donor eggs and sperm, and the donor embryo and that seems to me to be an unresolved problem. It wouldn't be for me, I don't think. I can't imagine that I would want that kind of treatment myself but it seems to be one that people find acceptable, but I think we don't understand its full consequences. But the other issue of being close to the very beginnings of life and influencing them seems to me to be absolutely soluble. I have no doubt about that. If we believe that we're made in God's image, then this act of helping to create life, and you pointed out that it's not creation, you said yourself, 'It's not creation out of nothing' – in Jewish terms, there's a difference between creation from nothing and creation from the things which creation's already given you. God has provided. That is *imitatio dei*, it's the imitation of God which is the highest thing to which man can strive because it's the protection and maintenance of human life, which is the most sacred thing. So, in religious terms, I don't actually have any problem with the practice of IVF at all and it's one of the reasons why I found the Catholic view actually a little strange because it seems to me that the Catholic church has taken the view that to help people procreate in this sort of way is something which is potentially, morally wrong. And certainly the Jews don't feel that. Jews are very positive about fertility treatments of this sort and don't see any problem with them. They don't actually even see any problem necessarily with genetic engineering, which is very interesting. That would seem to me to be tampering with life and something which I would have great ethical difficulty with, but there isn't a religious difficulty about it, which is interesting. I don't know if I've really answered your question.

CLARE: Related to it is that one of the ironies of your work, I suppose, is that people's valuation of fertility probably has increased since the ability to treat infertility has developed. That is to say, there was a time, you and I will remember this in relation to other aspects of medicine, but there was a time when your colleagues referring to it as the futility clinic would have been referring to the fact that there was so little you could do, other than eliminate the most gross causes of infertility and then hope for the best. In that sense, of course, many, many people who were infertile resigned themselves. I suppose if they were religious they would have said God's will, and if they weren't they would have said it's just science's failure, nobody knows why we are infertile. Now the irony is there are many, many people you help but now the many, many people you don't help are left with a double disadvantage. They are not only infertile, but they've failed in a way that you mightn't have said before because there was nothing to fail. This is the question, how much of your work is about the failures as much as the successes? We think of you as the IVF man, busy helping people who are infertile to be fertile. But of course, there are large numbers who remain infertile, but they've been to you.

WINSTON: Oh, yes, I've no doubt that the most important work I do clinically, not research-wise, but clinically, is assessing people who've failed IVF and trying to help them to come to terms with no further treatment. That I think is the most important work I probably do.

CLARE: Terribly difficult, isn't it?

WINSTON: Very difficult.

CLARE: When it's all happening inside you and you're waiting over six, eight weeks to know if it's going to work, there's an arbitrary quality to it and since there's that, won't they when they fail think, 'It might work the next time?'

WINSTON: Yes, they do, of course they all do and you have to try and dissuade them of that view and there are many prognostic pointers, I believe, which aren't viewed carefully enough by clinics in general. There are, for example, a lot of hormone tests that you can do during the treatment. There are a number of ways you can assess the quality of the eggs and the number of the eggs that are produced and a whole range of other things and you can work up to a computer prediction of the likelihood. In my view you can do that even now and within five years we will be able to do that much more accurately, and I think that's something to be striven for.

CLARE: The pain of failure, when there's a method available. It is so much easier to cope with something you cannot have, if nobody knows why you cannot have it, but the more we know . . .

WINSTON: Yes, but you referred to something very interesting which intrigued me earlier, which was the idea that, you know, in the 1940s people just gave up and got on with life, and one wonders if that's really true. I wonder if there wasn't a huge amount of morbidity, of real suffering. Words like barren for example.

CLARE: Sterile.

WINSTON: Sterile, and those words do come out in literature a great deal. I mean, they've always come out and perhaps, it's just that the floodgates have been opened. In many societies still today the stigma associated with barrenness is overwhelming. In African society if a woman can't have children, she's totally dispossessed. In many societies she loses her belongings, even, her physical belongings. She's chucked out of the house. There are many societies where that happens. Now of course, it's never been that acute in Anglo Saxon society but I think the background of suffering has probably been there but we haven't realised it.

CLARE: Do you demand of a woman who comes to you that she's living with a man? In other words, do you demand the traditional family structure?

WINSTON: No, I don't. I actually have very few criteria for treatment. I've certainly seen lesbian patients who have been worried about infertility and I do get a few patients who are completely single. It would be rather unusual for us to put them through *in vitro* fertilisation. The licensing authority, the HFEA, the government authority, certainly, I think, views it rather askance. If one is absolutely truthful and candid, one probably wouldn't take absolutely what they're saying as gospel because their experience is no greater than ours. I don't want to sound arrogant, I think one has to be very careful not to be arrogant.

CLARE: But it's tempting?

WINSTON: It's tempting! But I think all I'm really saying is that I would have very few criteria for treating or not treating people. I think the one criterion I can think of would be if I suspected, or if there was a history of child abuse. I think that's almost the only one I can really think of.

CLARE: How do you cope with the disappointments? Do you talk about your work much?

WINSTON: No, I shut off completely, that's what I do and I don't talk about it at home.

CLARE: What age are your children?

WINSTON: Well, my daughter is eighteen, my middle son is sixteen and I have a child who is almost thirteen, a boy.

CLARE: Now, would they know much about it?

WINSTON: They know what I do.

CLARE: Would you have talked about it as much as you've talked now.

WINSTON: Well, they all know my team because we're quite a family group, I mean the team are. We have recreation together. For example we go skiing, some of us, together and so on and the children often come as well so there's quite a bond. So they would know quite a lot about the work but they wouldn't hear much about my disappointments or my views of these things directly from me because I actually prefer to do other things at home. I think, I actually need to do other things. Having said that, because I'm an academic a huge proportion of my writing is done in the early hours of the morning because I get home quite late sometimes and start writing at perhaps, you know, twelve, one, two in the morning.

CLARE: So what do you do if you're upset? Do you get moved by patients?

WINSTON: Yes, I do, I do get moved by patients.

CLARE: Would you ever weep?

WINSTON: Yes. My family will find that amazing because they don't believe that I am capable of crying!

CLARE: You don't show that side to them?

WINSTON: No, I don't show that side to them.

CLARE: Because?

WINSTON: I don't know.

CLARE: Would your wife know?

WINSTON: Isn't that a terrible thing to say, she probably wouldn't realise that I might be that moved by certain things.

CLARE: You have to be strong.

WINSTON: That's ridiculous isn't it? Yes, perhaps, I don't know. I don't know. I mean, it may be because . . . no, I don't know if it's because I have to . . . maybe I see her vulnerable in those areas. I don't know. I think ours is a good relationship, I don't think it's ever been under serious threat. So there isn't any particular reason why I should show either weakness or strength.

CLARE: Is she interested in what you do?

WINSTON: Yes, I think she is. She probably feels that she would like more information about what I'm doing, or what I've just done but I think also recognises, after many years, that really I want to try and cut off from those aspects of work to a large extent and don't particularly want to discuss them and have difficulty doing so. I think it's also partly because reproductive medicine has such a high profile, one's always being asked to talk about it as well and, you know, the idea of going home and perhaps, you know, putting on a Shostakovich or something, really getting away from it is actually positively helpful.

CLARE: So it isn't just that you wouldn't talk to her about it, you wouldn't talk to anyone?

WINSTON: No, I wouldn't and I actually have difficulty sometimes when people want to phone me about their fertility problems at home, friends for example. I actually probably don't feel that very easy to deal with because it's no longer in a clinical setting and I suppose part of me feels it's something of an invasion. Now, I hope I don't always feel like that because very often with some people it's the only way they can talk but I suppose if I'm honest I do have certain reservations and some resentment sometimes about having to talk to people when I actually don't choose to because it's the wrong battleground physically.

CLARE: How do you empathise with that sense of loss. The loss you had was your father. I don't know how that influences you. You've never been significantly ill yourself?

WINSTON: No, I think one of my greatest worries, which I've never verbalised to anybody, but now you mention it and I hadn't really thought about it—I haven't verbalised it because I don't think I'd actually thought about it in concrete terms but I had a desperate fear of dying in my forties, so that my children wouldn't remember me (pause) and that's no longer a fear.

CLARE: Now you've mentioned that in relation to a question about people who couldn't have children. Is that what touches you, so when you see someone across the table and they've failed, is it the notion that there won't be, in one sense, there won't be anyone who will remember them, as a father or a mother. Is that it?

WINSTON: I don't know. It may be part of it but I'm also conscious that you can channel those sadnesses and failures in other directions and I think modern fertility treatment is doing that increasingly successfully, actually. I think we're getting better at understanding. One of the things I've noticed and, and I've even written a little bit about it is that infertile couples who often may go through a very rough period together and perhaps physically with their sexual relationship, for example, often end up being very close because they've been through something like that. That actually it's a very positive aspect of their experience and often sometimes seeing couples a long time afterwards, they may still have bouts of sadness but they've quite clearly come to terms and they've got on with a new area of life, perhaps having been through the treatment thing which has actually been helpful in doing that. Patients have said that to me. I don't want to digress too much but I remember one patient saying to me, years and years ago, a Greek patient, a very well-to-do woman, saying, 'The great thing I regret you know, Dr Winston, is that you operated on me. You opened my fallopian tubes. I could have quite easily come to terms with having my tubes blocked because I knew I couldn't get pregnant but having them opened meant that I was always uncertain whether I could get pregnant or not. And it's been years before I could come to terms with it.' That actually was quite influential in my thinking. That actually changed the way I thought about infertility management quite early on.

CLARE: Well, of course in a sense that's what I meant about the treatment of infertility. Symbolically in terms of opening the tubes, it now creates for a lot of women the possibility of it happening, where once there was the certainty that it wouldn't.

WINSTON: Yes, and that's actually also the difficulty, it's also the difficulty and the strength of *in vitro* fertilisation. One of the things about *in vitro* fertilisation is you're bypassing all the bodily functions and the anatomy but you don't change the body, so when somebody has failed *in vitro* fertilisation, they're back to being sterile.

CLARE: Yes, yes.

WINSTON: Now, when you do almost any other treatment, particularly a surgical treatment, you've actually altered their body and that's one of the reasons why I'm actually very pro surgery. I think that my colleagues have greatly underrated the value in actually putting a woman's body together, because it changes her image of herself and I think sometimes that even can be useful sexually. I think that it helps women to come to terms and they don't feel an empty vessel any more.

CLARE: What I was geting at, though, in fact you took me along another interesting groove, but what I was getting at was, let me give you a parallel from my own field. Somebody will say to me across a table, 'Look, I don't think you can understand how I'm feeling because you haven't been there.' Now I have my own ways of responding to that and I'll tell you what they are in a moment if you wish. But they will say that. Now in your case, in the anger that must come out from time to time, because you've mentioned anger and I want to come back to that in a minute, presumably at times there will be a doubt, 'Look, you haven't any idea of what this is like,' and they may even refer to the fact that you've got three children. You've gone into this field, fertility, a lot of people in your profession and my profession have never rated it very highly. You empathise in some way with these people. Now, it's not just because of what you said about procreation being a crucial human moment. I just wonder what it is that you tap into. Maybe it's nothing and my theories are wrong, but I just wonder, what is it that you tap into in a person facing this loss that makes you empathic, that they feel you understand what it is they're going through? What is it in you? How have you tapped into this in the way that you have?

WINSTON: I honestly don't think I know.

CLARE: I mean you're not infertile, you're not a woman, you haven't had that kind of loss. I'm calling on your other interest, your interest in the theatre because, of course, many actors, and this is where you and I were discussing earlier the extent to which they get it right, many of them will describe, of course, calling on some equivalent experience to understand something they're asked to act. And in a way, there's a bit of that about medicine, calling on some equivalent experience to understand the predicament of the person across the table. And what is the equivalent experience for a male obstetrician with three children faced with an infertile woman?

WINSTON: I wonder if it isn't just rather wider than that? If it isn't just seeing a gap, a sadness and you feel that it's something that you understand because you've seen so much of it. Maybe just simply by experience. When I first started doing infertility medicine, I had none of these insights, if you can call them that. I mean I went into the branch of infertility medicine that I did initially, which was very research-orientated, because it was intellectually stimulating and that was for a long time. I remember my boss once saying, 'Well, you know, that guy Winston, he's doing some very interesting research work, you ought to go and watch what he's doing,' and it was a long time before I realised that, in fact, there was a huge emotional content to this work which was totally enthralling. And I get it wrong a hell of a lot of the time.

CLARE: But it is enthralling. Do you ever feel like you felt in the theatre? Do you ever feel, this is too much?

WINSTON: Yes, of course I do, and regularly. I would say that doing an infertility clinic is extremely tiring and one of the problems I have is that my clinics are far too long because there's rather a large demand. I tend to work much too long in the clinic. I probably ought to be shortening the time, but if I did that I'd have a monstrous waiting list so I compromise and I see people and keep others waiting when I think there's a problem that I might be able to deal with and I think in consequence no doubt there's patchy treatment. Some patients you probably don't treat as well as you should do and others you probably treat very well, because you spend more time or because you happen to hit it off with them. That may apply to all medicine but I think it's probably rather acute in this area.

CLARE: Do you worry yourself about disease, about illness?

WINSTON: Am I a hypochondriac?

CLARE: Well, I wasn't putting it as indelicately as that.

WINSTON: Yes, I think I probably am a hypochondriac like, probably, most doctors.

CLARE: You feel they are?

WINSTON: I think a lot of doctors are, yes. I think like all medical students one goes through the feeling that one's got cancer of the lymph glands, Hodgkin's Disease, doesn't one?

CLARE: Subarachnoid every time you get a headache?

WINSTON: Headache, yes and I suffer from migraines a bit but I don't think I have a subarachnoid any more.

CLARE: Are you a worrier?

WINSTON: I think I probably am a worrier but I don't show that either. I don't know that I think I control. At home people would be amazed to hear I'm a worrier. That would be almost unbelievable.

CLARE: How do they see you at home?

WINSTON: Well, they don't see me as a worrier, that's for certain.

CLARE: No?

WINSTON: I don't think my team do either because I think, probably, a team of people needs to feel that the person who's sort of looking after their interests is actually in control of those issues. So, for example, when, recently, my hospital was very threatened because the secretary of state was thinking of closing us down, or moving us out, I was very threatened by that actually, very threatened.

CLARE: Personally?

WINSTON: Yes, well, first of all I thought it was a kick in the teeth but also because it would have meant very great difficulties for my team. I reassured them absolutely that there would be no question that the team would break up in any way whatsoever, with total confidence, because that seemed to be the right thing to be doing. I think probably there was a hidden degree of nervousness about what might happen to us as a group. Obviously I would have fought very hard for everybody.

CLARE: Control is very important to you. That's how they see you at home?

WINSTON: Well, that's what you're saying to me and I haven't really thought of it in those terms, but perhaps you're right, yes, maybe, maybe that's right, maybe I need to show control. Maybe that's partly being an older child in a bereaved family, the need to be controlled. My mother at work, coming home quite late at night and an empty house. The youngest child perhaps not yet a teenager with two younger children. The element of fright at the dark and all that sort of thing and being in control. Maybe that does go back a long way.

CLARE: Not letting people really see how you feel?

WINSTON: Yes, because it would have been hurtful to my mother probably, too.

CLARE: Do you ever lose control?

WINSTON: Yeah, I lose my temper.

CLARE: Do you?

WINSTON: Yes, I can get very angry. I don't think I'm slow to forgive though, I think I probably am pretty forgiving. I get very annoyed with people who I haven't perhaps spoken to but as soon as I've spoken to them I lose all sense of resentment. I don't think I resent things that have happened, on the whole. (Pause.) I'm fortunate in that respect in my wife too, who's a remarkably patient individual who, I think, loses her temper with me occasionally although she doesn't show it much but rapidly comes to terms with my idiosyncracies.

CLARE: Are you the sort of person that has to be turned away from your work, at home for example or for holidays or things? Do you find it easy to turn off?

WINSTON: I do now, probably much more than I used to. I've chosen pastimes which I think help that. For example one passion is skiing and it's difficult to find a pastime which turns you off so totally. When you're on a moutain, facing a steep slope, you're facing instant death, aren't you, in the most beautiful surroundings. There's something wonderful about that. You can't think about work then.

CLARE: Do you think about death? You did, you say, during your forties.

WINSTON: Yes, I don't think I do so much now, no, I don't think I do so much now, no.

CLARE: You're fairly equable about it?

WINSTON: Yes, I think I am, really. I really do think I am. I don't see death as a terrible event. I mean suppose one of the things that does worry me now, if you're asking me of sort of death-like things that threaten one, I very much worry at not having an area in which my group is excelling. Now, that's the arrogance that comes with the research worker in me. At the moment we're doing pretty well in human genetics, but I recognise that lead is fragile so I'm thrashing around now looking for new areas all the time. I'm a competitive individual. I'm quite ambitious I think. I wish I wasn't but I am.

CLARE: But you're in a very competitive institution, isn't it, the Hammersmith?

WINSTON: Yes, yes it is a competitive institution. It's a wonderful institution though because first of all it buzzes, it's a very exciting place, and one of the things I really like about the Hammersmith and I think I can say with all truth, although it's competitive and it's very much like the American institutions, it's not arrogant, people there are not arrogant people and they're also very kind to patients. I think their clinical record on the whole is very good. You can forgive a lot I think in an institution of that kind, but it is essentially competitive.

CLARE: Did it upset you that it should at all be mooted that such an institution at the heart of London, which is known certainly throughout the world as a major postgraduate institution, that there should have been any talk about it being moved, relocated, broken up at all?

WINSTON: Yes, I thought it was outrageous. I thought it was outrageous and misguided. I think with some good reason, after all. It's an institution which has had no fewer than six government reviews in the last eighteen months, each one of which gave it full marks.

CLARE: So that would make you angry?

WINSTON: Yes, and I'm quite political too. I'm politically involved. I've become increasingly political.

CLARE: Do you like that?

WINSTON: I think what changed me was '85 particularly. That really politicised me. It was when Enoch Powell tried to introduce his Embryology Bill to ban embryo experiments. That made me very political because it wasn't the rights and wrongs in that or the morals, it was the way he was doing it and the fact that he was actually, in a pluralistic society trying to produce what seemed to me to be very right-wing legislation and it made me increasingly left-wing to the extent that I actually joined a political party, which I didn't think I would ever do. And I feel much more left now than I ever did. I feel quite concerned about those sorts of issues.

CLARE: Do you think that's representative? Do you think that there's a generation of doctors now who are beginning to realise that the political aspects of being a doctor, political with a small 'p', that these are becoming more significant again, more important again? That to fight for a unit, it isn't enough to point to its superb research and academic achievements, you've got to get out there and fight?

WINSTON: Yes.

CLARE: And lobby politically?

WINSTON: Well, I think that's true and I think actually, you know, one of the things that might politicise doctors much more now is the recognition of how the health service is changing with the internal market, and the other things. Obviously one doesn't want to get into the politics of that, but I think we, as a medical profession, were pushed over, we just actually laid back and allowed the government to ride over us. I don't understand why. It's partly because doctors on the whole are fairly conservative and I mean politically conservative, and partly because being a profession that is influential, many, dare I say, many of us perhaps expect may be some form of preferment, I don't know what it might be.

CLARE: Does that interest you?

WINSTON: Well, I mean if I'm very honest, I think to be recognised for what you've done, if you've done anything, that's open to question, gives people a warm feeling. I got a great deal of pleasure out of getting a personal chair, being made a professor and I think it would be quite wrong to pretend I didn't. I suppose now perhaps I would be most interested in trying to influence things perhaps. That's the sort of politics that I think doctors tend to get involved with, the idea of trying to influence what they see as being appropriate. I'd like to see, for example, my own branch of medicine better organised.

CLARE: Is there something that you particularly want to do?

WINSTON: I think the things I would most want to do would be to try and develop certain research areas which I see as being tremendously valuable. There's one research area at the moment that I'm sort of tentatively involved with which I see as important, the sort of genetic work we've been doing, which I think potentially might be important. I think it's quite a privilege to have done some work which actually might be influential in medicine in twenty years' time. But there is one area at the moment which I think would actually sweep the board with reproductive medicine, which would make reproductive treatments much cheaper, much more available for a whole range of people. If, for example, we could mature the human egg outside the body, from a tiny piece of ovary which had been cut away. The foetal ovary issue which has been in the press is quite irrelevant, but to do it from adult ovaries, which actually ought to be much easier, if we could do that, and then use those eggs to treat the patient at her leisure, when she was still working and not having to come for monitoring, not having any drugs, that would be a wonderful achievement. I think it would be quite important. Things like that do grab me, there's no doubt that it's partly a feeling of ambition, it's by no means selfless, but it's also because it's intriguingly interesting.

CLARE: Are you an optimist?

WINSTON: Yes I am an optimist, absolutely. I mean in my heart of hearts I never thought our institution would be closed. I think perhaps to practise medicine, and also to be quite pleased that at least one of my children might do medicine means that one has to be an optimist really.

CLARE: Robert Winston, thank you very much indeed.

ANTHONY CLARE

In The Psychiatrist's Chair

ARTHUR ASHE · JANET BAKER · KEN DODD ·
ANTHONY HOPKINS · PETER HALL · P. D. JAMES ·
DEREK JARMAN · EARTHA KITT · R. D. LAING ·
CLAIRE RAYNER · JIMMY SAVILE · TOM SHARPE

This first collection of interviews from Anthony Clare's
riveting Radio 4 series, *In The Psychiatrist's Chair* not only
offers astonishing insights into the psyches of the famous but
also turns the tables and allows the reader into the
psychiatrist's head.

'Arthur Ashe is emotionally super-controlled to the point
where he kept his AIDS condition secret even as he talked of
his fascination with death. Sir Peter Hall, no less death-
fixated, was thus spurred on to cram his days full of diverse
activity to over-achieve. Ken Dodd acknowledged just weeks
before Inland Revenue dropped in that well, yes, of course he
liked money, but he didn't hoard it. A riveting read which
allows us a more leisurely appreciation of what was actually
revealed'   *Publishing News*

'The element of dispassion gives Clare's own conversations
their best moments. He is admirably quick to see when
someone is trying to put him off the scent and is not afraid to
keep probing at a tender area . . . In these exchanges . . .
there is the raw stuff – the fears, the doubts, above all the
bloody perseverance – of actual human life, and this makes
gripping radio'   *Independent on Sunday*

A Selected List of Non-Fiction Titles Available from Mandarin

While every effort is made to keep prices low, it is sometimes necessary to increase prices at short notice. Mandarin Paperbacks reserves the right to show new retail prices on covers which may differ from those previously advertised in the text or elsewhere.

The prices shown below were correct at the time of going to press.

All these books are available at your bookshop or newsagent, or can be ordered direct from the address below. Just tick the titles you want and fill in the form below.

Cash Sales Department, PO Box 5, Rushden, Northants NN10 6YX.
Fax: 01933 414047 : Phone: 01933 414000.

Please send cheque, payable to 'Reed Book Services Ltd.', or postal order for purchase price quoted and allow the following for postage and packing:

£1.00 for the first book, 50p for the second; FREE POSTAGE AND PACKING FOR THREE BOOKS OR MORE PER ORDER.

NAME (Block letters)..

ADDRESS..

....

☐ I enclose my remittance for ....

☐ I wish to pay by Access/Visa Card Number ☐☐☐☐☐☐☐☐☐☐☐☐☐☐

Expiry Date ☐☐☐☐

Signature ....

Please quote our reference: MAND